Marijuana Rx

THE PATIENTS' FIGHT FOR MEDICINAL POT

Marijuana

Rx

THE PATIENTS' FIGHT FOR MEDICINAL POT

Robert C. Randall and Alice M. O'Leary

THUNDER'S MOUTH PRESS • NEW YORK

Published by
Thunder's Mouth Press
841 Broadway, Fourth Floor
New York, NY 10003

First edition

Library of Congress Cataloging-in-Publication Data
Randall, R. C. (Robert C.)
    Marijuana Rx : the patients' fight for medicinal pot / by Robert
Randall & Alice O'Leary.
        p.   cm.
    ISBN 1-56025-166-2
    1. Marijuana—Therapeutic use—United States.   2. Marijuana—
Therapeutic use—Law and legislation—United States.   I. O'Leary,
Alice.
RM666.C266R36   1998
615'.7827—dc21   98-27499
                                                               CIP

Manufactured in the United States of America

To our mothers
Thelma Jones Randall and Martha Whitaker O'Leary

Contents

Part III Synthetic Solutions

Part IV New Allies

Part V Coming of Age

Foreword
By Lyn Nofziger

STRANGE AS IT may seem, here is one right-wing Republican who supports carefully controlled, medical access to marijuana.

When our grown daughter was undergoing chemotherapy for lymph cancer, she was sick and vomiting constantly as a result of her treatments. No legal drugs, including the synthetic "marijuana" pill Marinol, helped her situation.

As a result we finally turned to marijuana which, of course, we were forced to obtain illegally. With it, she kept her food down, was comfortable, and even gained weight.

Despite advances that have been made in controlling the side effects of cancer chemotherapy treatments, the simple fact remains: each of us is an individual with similar but unique biological chemistries which react differently to the medical drugs we are given. Those who say Marinol and other drugs are satisfactory substitutes for marijuana may be right in some cases, but certainly are not right all of the time.

Lyn Nofziger served as press secretary to Ronald Reagan during the presidential campaign of 1980. Following the election of President Reagan, Mr. Nofziger served as the White House director of communication and chief speech writer for the President. He continues to work for Republican candidates throughout the country.

A doctor should have every possible medication—including marijuana—in his armamentarium. If doctors can prescribe morphine and other addictive medicines, it makes no sense to deny marijuana to sick and dying patients when it can be provided on a carefully controlled, prescription basis.

Marijuana clearly has medicinal value. Thousands of seriously ill Americans have been able to determine that for themselves, albeit illegally. Like my own family, these individuals did not wish to break the law but they had no other choice. The numerous attempts to legitimately resolve the issue—via state legislation and federal administrative hearings—have often been ignored or thwarted by misguided federal agencies. Between 1978–1981 more than thirty states enacted legislation recognizing marijuana's medical potential. Several states conducted extensive, and expensive, research programs which demonstrated marijuana's medical utility—particularly in the treatment of chemotherapy side effects. Frances L. Young, the chief administrative law judge of the United States Drug Enforcement Administration, ruled marijuana has legitimate medical applications and should be available to doctors.

In the early 1990s, many hundreds of doctors applied to use marijuana through the government's investigative research program at the FDA. Our government's reaction was to close the program in 1992.

Ironically, by allowing this issue to fester for so long and handling it so badly, the federal government is responsible for the growing number of ballot initiatives, such as California's Proposition 215, which attempt to resolve the problem by allowing individuals to "grow their own" or by establishing unregulated "clubs" where marijuana can be procured.

This is no way to treat serious illnesses or to deal with a serious issue but it is difficult to condemn the American people for voting affirmatively for such measures when all of their previous, lawful efforts have gone unheeded.

The medical marijuana issue calls out for responsible, honest leadership at the federal level. Until that time seriously ill individuals who can benefit from this substance will continue to rally around any possible solution. We owe it to them to provide safe and controlled access to this drug.

Acknowledgments

THIS BOOK is a personal reflection. It was not our intent to create the definitive history of medical marijuana in America but rather to record the efforts of some remarkable people who tried to right a wrong, often at great personal expense or peril. The medical marijuana issue has been a part of our lives for more than twenty years and it is impossible to acknowledge everyone who has contributed to our efforts. Through the years we have been in contact with thousands of patients. To each of them we say thanks. To anyone who ever took the time to write a letter, make a call, or take some action on behalf of medical marijuana we say thanks.

There are some who deserve additional thanks. The law firm of Steptoe & Johnson has made an invaluable contribution both personally and to the nation as a whole by providing countless hours of pro bono representation, first to Robert and then to our group, the Alliance for Cannabis Therapeutics (ACT). Richard J. Dennis provided financial support that allowed us to expand the issue immeasurably and gave us security at a dark hour of our lives. Dr. Richard North has been a brave and ethical physician. Kevin Zeese was a steady and much appreciated friend. Daryl Reinke and Craig Hosmer have been the finest friends and their help throughout the years was much appreciated. Mark Heutlinger's advice was always useful. Thanks to Dr. Jeff Stall, Dr. Vilma Vega, Nurse Maureen Murray, and Nurse Pat Kelly for helping Robert survive a difficult illness so that we could write this book.

To our families we express our deep love and sincerest thanks for their understanding and support over the years.

To our agent, Alan Kellock, we say thanks for believing in this book. And to our editor, Maura Feeney, we say thanks for her hard work and invaluable contribution.

Finally, thanks to Boni P. and Richard T., whose gift on a cool autumn night in 1968 truly began this entire adventure.

September 1998

I

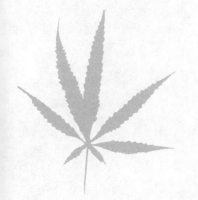

Beginnings

I

Beginnings

1   Machine of the Gods

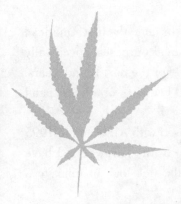

I HAVE NEVER been reborn before.

It is as daunting as dying.

The Death Wave, which swamped me in late '94, swallowed me whole in '95, and ever so slowly receded in '96, has—at long last—landed me on the unexplored shores of an unexpected Future.

Instead of dead, I'm tan as a red man and fat as a Buddha of Happiness. Living in a condo on Florida's intracoastal waterway. Dazzling days. Hot sun. Sapphire sky. Perfumed nights, heavily scented with citrus and lunar light. It is good to be alive.

Still, it is too soon to tell if Fate is affording me a brief reprieve or granting a full pardon. Clearly, my rendezvous with reincarnation has been rescheduled; my Odyssey to Oblivion interrupted by the magic of modern potions.

It is not the first time Fate has flown me, deus ex machina, beyond the reach of a despairing plot to make my life a more interesting play. We are storytellers to the gods. And the gods like a good story, particularly one of great struggles, battles, blindness, death, and love.

The safari of my soul has had all those elements. In my half century of life I have engaged a giant foe, the U.S. government, and wrestled from it a forbidden elixir, marijuana, to stave off blindness. I have plotted grand strategies to help others procure this medication and have engaged in great and small battles to that end. I have watched good friends fall on the battlefield, many of whom would never rise again.

Personally I have faced the two greatest fears of man: blindness and death. For the moment, at least, each of these adversaries is held at bay.

My name is Robert Randall. In 1976 I became the first American to gain legal access to marijuana for medical purposes, specifically to treat glaucoma, a blinding eye disease. For the next twenty years, together with my partner and mate Alice O'Leary, I worked to expand this unique privilege to others.

Then, in November 1994, I was diagnosed with AIDS and in 1995 nearly died. But, having survived my dip in the River Styx, I have been reawakened to phantasm Life; to the tick-tock of time, to a cautious reacquisition of the future.

As my future is unresolved, my past is clear as crystal. And, while fate holds me in this delicate balance between beginnings and endings it seems prudent to reflect upon those people and events which conspired to grant me a box seat at the play.

This is our story of medical marijuana in America. The gods have granted me a reprieve to bring you this story but I am not so prideful as to think this is a one-man show. The medical marijuana story encompasses many people in many places. You will learn about a White House aide and a British Lord, a ten-year-old with cancer and an 80-year-old with glaucoma, an Arizona cowboy and a Pennsylvania doll shop owner, and more. This story is about the kindness of strangers and betrayal by friends. It is about the brutality of the system and banality of bureaucrats who are charged with managing it. Medical marijuana reveals the failure of elites and the success of common citizens intent on righting a wrong.

And, in the final analysis, it is about much more than marijuana.

It is a story of a remarkable public consensus which was ignored, denigrated, and trampled on in order to maintain a deeply entrenched policy. It is about the failure of government to trust its citizens and the casualties of that failure.

I am cast in the dual role of central player and chief storyteller, a position of some precariousness. My style is part drama, part narrative. There are scenes and vignettes from memory, which I present as faithfully as possible in dramatic style. But there are thoughts great and small, there is fact and speculation, and, most of all, there is more than twenty years of time to cover.

Indulge me, as the gods have, and you will find a fascinating tale.

2 Busted, Broke, and Going Blind

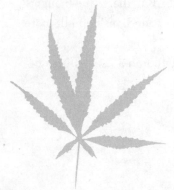

August 24, 1975
8th St. S.E.
Washington, D.C.

"I was going out to buy a bra when I noticed this commotion up at your end of the block." Susan was pouring a glass of sherry for each of us in her small living room, "As I got closer I saw these men, these policemen, and they were all carrying those little silver evidence cases, and . . ." she paused to cork the sherry, "and I wondered what in the hell was going on!"

She continued, "I was walking down the opposite side of the street, towards the bus stop?" Still vibrating from eight hours in a cramped Volkswagen, Alice and I nodded in recognition. "When I got directly across from your building I realized they were running in and out of your apartment! Well, I thought there must have been a burglary or a fire. I rushed across the street," she paused to swallow, "and asked the cop at the door what was wrong. He said, 'What's it to ya, lady?' real unpleasant. When I explained I was taking care of your plants and things, that's when he told me to go upstairs."

Between liberal doses of sherry, Susan provided the details of the previous day's events. She had had the misfortune to stumble on the scene early and was present during nearly the entire search. Finding herself in the midst of a drug bust she employed her considerable feminine wiles and managed not to implicate herself in the scene. When the agent-in-charge asked Susan if she had ever seen marijuana she replied, with more coyness than candor, she was not certain.

Susan watched as at least eight members of the vice squad tore apart our apartment and gleefully seized various items of "contraband": 1) four (4) "suspect" marijuana plants; 2) five (5) pipes; 3) four (4) tabs "suspect" LSD; 4) four (4) ounces "suspect" marijuana; 5) one (1) flour sifter; 6) one (1) postal scale.

These items were carefully listed on the "Seized List" which was left with the search warrant. Other items, including a bottle of prescribed Librium (a sedative) and a month's supply of birth control pills, were missing but not listed. The cops also took pictures of the apartment and pieces of mail.

It had, in fact, been a very busy Saturday for the vice squad. They had first tried to bust the next-door neighbor. His plants had drawn the attention of police during a routine patrol of the alleyway just two days before. The plants, ten of them, had been placed on the fire escape the day we left for vacation.

The patrolman summoned the vice squad who climbed onto the fire escape to investigate. From there it was easy to look down onto our deck where four marijuana plants were discreetly hidden behind coleus, morning glories, and tomato plants.

The neighbor saw the Friday afternoon visit from the vice squad and immediately disposed of his contraband plants. He tried to reach Alice and me, but we were blissfully enjoying the American wonders of U.S. Route 50. When the police returned on Saturday with formal search warrants the neighbor would escape arrest.

• • •

Of course the roots of this adventure predate the "bust" of August 1975. As with any good story, the seeds are sown early and allowed to grow. In my case the story began at my conception, when heredity determined my vision would be marred by a condition called glaucoma.

There are two kinds of glaucoma: narrow-angle and open-angle. Narrow-angle glaucoma often comes on quickly, in an acute situation which sends most people scurrying to an ophthalmologist.

In open-angle glaucoma, the process is more sinister. The inner pressure of the eye is elevated, pinching the optic nerve and starving the eye for nourishment. As a result, sections of the eye begin to die leading to progressive blindness. But the progress of the disease is slow and there is rarely any pain so the afflicted individual has time to compensate for the growing blindness without realizing that he or she is going blind. Over time the individual develops more and more blind spots until the brain can no longer compensate.

Further complicating the situation is our limited knowledge of open-angle glaucoma. For decades it was thought only the elderly developed the disease. Now we know glaucoma can strike at any age. Juvenile glaucoma is uncommon but not unusual. Often the disease is hereditary, manifesting itself younger in each generation.

So it was with me. Throughout my family there are cases of visual problems and some blindness but as I was growing up in the 1950s and '60s there was little understanding of how these problems may have been passed on to my generation. Thus my early complaints of eyestrain in high school and college were never taken seriously.

I can recall waiting for an eye exam when I was about 19 years old and reading a pamphlet called *Glaucoma: The Sneak Thief of Sight*. The symptoms seemed so familiar I asked the doctor if I might have glaucoma but he seemed amused. "You're studying too hard, young man," said the friendly optometrist. "You need to give those eyes a rest. That will clear up the eyestrain in no time."

But it didn't.

September 6, 1972
Dr. Ben Fine's Office
Washington, D.C.

"How long?"

"Two to five years," the doctor relpied. "Perhaps a bit longer if the medications work well. And they are always working on new drugs. You may get lucky."

I was 24 years old and had just been told I would be blind before my thirtieth birthday. I looked across the desk at the kindly physician who had finally discovered the reason behind my "eyestrain": advanced open-angle glaucoma.

Dr. Ben Fine gave me a handful of prescriptions and I emerged onto the busy streets of Washington, D.C. nearly blind from the eyedrops he had instilled. I had come to D.C. in 1971, intent on becoming a political speechwriter. Instead I was driving a cab to make ends meet. As I climbed behind the wheel of my Red Top cab, I suddenly realized this means of livelihood had come to an end. I quietly sat in the cab, contemplating my future and waiting for my eyes to clear enough so that I could drive home.

Dr. Fine was a competent doctor, one of Washington's most respected ophthalmologists. In the following months he tried varying combinations of eyedrops and other medications in an effort to stabilize my disease, which was stubborn and aggressive. Fine had to resort to the maximum strengths of available medications to bring my eye pressures to near normal levels but the medications didn't always work. At the time of my diagnosis, I had already lost a significant amount of eyesight and I soon learned the telltale signs of elevated pressure: milky vision, tricolored haloes around lights, or complete "white-outs" which were virtually blinding.

For more than a year the doctor struggled to control my disease and then, remarkably, things began to stabilize. My intraocular eye pressure (IOP) was regularly in the "safe range" and my loss of vision had stopped. Fine couldn't understand what had happened but he was disinclined to look a gift horse in the mouth. He was pleased that the medications had finally begun to work. He didn't know I had added another medication to the regimen, albeit an illegal one—marijuana.

I had first smoked marijuana in 1968 while a student at the University of South Florida (USF) but I had had little contact with the illegal substance after moving to Washington in 1971.

In late 1973, after a new friend gave me a marijuana cigarette, I discovered, quite by accident, that marijuana helped my glaucoma. It was evening and looking out the window of my Virginia apartment I saw the now-familiar tricolored haloes around a nearby streetlight. My pressures were elevated despite the eyedrops and other medications from Dr. Fine. This had become "something to live with" and I didn't think much of it. I turned on the stereo, lit the joint, and settled back to listen to the music.

A few minutes later I rose from the chair and headed to the kitchen. On the way I glanced out the window again. What I saw stopped me in my tracks. Actually it was what I didn't see that stopped me. The haloes around the nearby streetlight were gone.

It was a singular moment. I immediately drew the connection between the use of marijuana and the now-absent haloes. Indeed, parts of my brain absorbed the connection so quickly and so assuredly that I was certain I must be stoned, which of course I was. I tried to follow the exploding synaptic spasm but was quickly left behind. The thought was too fast, too large and complex to pursue and understand, to place into words. Stuporific, I could do little more than smile at the building delusion. Marijuana beneficial? A delicious thought perhaps, but nothing to hang your sight on.

But the thought would not go away and over a period of months, through nothing more than cause and effect, the prospect became more believable. My observations were confirmed by Fine's regular ocular readings. My eye pressures were well controlled for the first time since his diagnosis.

Whatever confusion and reluctance I might have had in accepting marijuana's therapeutic promise ended when the droughts began. Droughts: long, barren periods when marijuana could not be bought for blood or money. My lack of faith in marijuana's medicinal value was finally overcome during the Spring drought of 1974.

Days would pass without so much as a twig of the substance and each of those days would be followed by an evening filled with brittle dancing lights. On random evenings I would visit friends lucky enough to have found some of the weed. On those nights the rings would not appear. Or, more impressively, they would dissolve, vanishing before my eyes. For two months, until the drought broke, day in and day out my understanding deepened. By the summer of 1974 there were no more doubts. I began a program of self-medication. Marijuana had suddenly become more than a recreational drug. The goofy relaxant had become a critical medication.

I considered telling the doctor about this discovery but worried about the impact of such a revelation. Would Fine dismiss me as a "druggie" and stop treating me? If I told Fine and he continued to treat me, knowing that I was using an illegal substance, would that make Fine part of a criminal conspiracy?

It was too risky. Best to keep the information to myself and let Fine believe the prescribed medications or some quirky element was the reason why my eye pressures were doing so well.

Actually in 1974 many things were "doing" well. The immediate aftermath of my glaucoma diagnosis had been difficult. I could no longer drive a cab and had no means of support. I was forced into temporary disability—a kind term for welfare. But in 1974 I was writing drama reviews for a weekly newspaper chain and would soon find work as a part-time college professor.

In that year I asked Alice to live with me in a two-storey apartment on Capitol Hill. Alice and I had known one another since college where we associated rather than dated. But in my final year of school I thought it was too soon to be entrapped by stability, to decide the future. First I wished to find out what was beyond college, so Alice and I separated for two years. She went off to graduate school to study theatrical design; I ventured to Washington, to my cab and diagnosis.

By the time Alice arrived in Washington she knew herself and had worked in various theaters as a lighting designer and technical director. Rounding the age of 25, we found the hormonal surges of youth were giving way to fuller emotions. We had played through an elaborate dance and finally we mated but did not wed. We had long been friends and settled slowly into lovers. The arrangement worked well.

Alice came to live with me accepting the likelihood I would go blind. I told her of my marijuana discovery soon after she moved in. At first she thought it was a convenient way for me to rationalize an ever-increasing marijuana habit. But soon she became convinced of my increasingly critical need for the drug and she often helped in locating my illegal and expensive medication.

Procuring marijuana became a regular part of our life and trying to cover the dry spells became particularly important. In the Spring of 1975, in an abandoned flower pot on the sundeck, a lone marijuana seed sprouted and began to grow, literally, like a weed. This uninvited, "volunteer" plant was the obvious solution to my problem—grow enough marijuana to cover the dry spells. We planted three more seeds and soon there were four healthy marijuana plants growing in the lengthening days of Washington's springtime.

Marijuana was illegal and it was a risk to grow the plants outdoors but we felt safe. The deck was on the second story, well concealed from public view and terrific for gardening. As the marijuana plants grew we took pains to conceal them among vines, coleus, tomato plants and more. Alice frequently checked from the back alley to see if the marijuana plants were visible from below. They were not.

We felt safe and content. Things were going well enough to think about a vacation. So, in August 1975, we entrusted the cats and plants to Susan's care and prepared to head out of town. As we loaded the car Alice asked, "Should the plants come in?" I argued the sun was good for them, they were well obscured. And so they stayed, sunning in seclusion until the vice squad arrived and took them away.

August 27, 1975
D.C. Superior Court
Washington, D.C.

"Just tell me when this whole thing has gone over $500, Paul."

"It already has."

It was Wednesday, less than 72 hours since we had returned from vacation to find our apartment ransacked and a search warrant on our kitchen table. Now, in the hot August sun, we stood on the steps of the D.C. Superior Court with our attorney, Paul Smollar. We had been arraigned, booked, and released on our own recognizance. We were criminals.

On Monday morning Alice had called the only lawyer she knew, John Karr. He had done some legal work for the American Theater where Alice worked as technical director and lighting designer. She did not know if Karr handled criminal cases but it was a place to start. Karr was on vacation in Spain but his junior partner, Paul Smollar, listened to the story of our bust and agreed to represent us.

Paul had patiently accompanied us through the mechanics of our arrest and arraignment. Shuffling from room to room, we faced a sea of poor, maimed, hostile, or inept individuals waiting for the wheels of justice to process their future. We drew little comfort in realizing we were completely out of place, with the possible exception of the inept part.

The next day we returned for the formalities. Paul was professional and assuring. He seemed certain the entire situation could be resolved easily. There would, however, be numerous legal procedures to endure. He advised us to relax and enjoy the upcoming Labor Day holiday. He was flying off to Maine for a week. Karr would be back after Labor Day. "Relax," he told us, "It's a simple enough case. Some of these drug cases can be tough but this one shouldn't change your life too much."

Making our way back to our car, I thought about the first meeting with Paul on Monday afternoon. "Paul, there's one thing you need to know." I spoke hesitantly, unsure of how the young lawyer would react to what I was about to say.

"What's that, Bobby?"

I was startled at the familiarity, unsure if the nickname conveyed affection or an impression of immaturity. I plunged forward.

"I smoke marijuana for medical reasons."

Paul's lips unconsciously moved into a friendly smirk. "I have glaucoma and" . . . I could see the lawyer was trying hard not to chuckle, "and marijuana has helped control it. Marijuana is helping me save my eyesight."

The final words came out strong and sure, startling the lawyer just as much as the entire premise had. Paul collected himself and said the only logical thing.

"Prove it, Bobby. Just prove it."

3 An Interesting
Intellectual Exercise

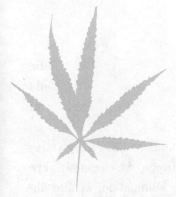

WHAT WOULD BE the consequence of proving marijuana had medicinal value? I had no burning desire to find out. In the abstract it was a compelling curiosity and on quiet days made for playful diversion. It was an attractive toy because one could easily sense it encompassed powerful energies.

Powerful enough to challenge The System?

In the abstract perhaps, but life was too precious to spend with such questions. In 1975 I was gnawing through my third year of glaucoma treatment, worried about the possibility of surgery. Even playing the outside of Dr. Fine's prognosis I was rushing through my allotted time rapidly. There was no need to spend my last years of remaining sight pursuing the question of marijuana's medical utility.

But needs change. Life can turn on a dime and ours had been forever altered by the bust. Now the question was no longer abstract. How could I possibly prove marijuana's medical utility?

There were certain advantages to getting busted in Washington, D.C. There was a wealth of information available and all at the cost of a local phone call or a short car ride. On the Tuesday following Labor Day I contacted the National Organization for the Reform of

Marijuana Laws (NORML) and quickly received a fat packet of information by mail which included a brief mention of a NORML lawsuit brought against the federal drug agency, the Bureau of Narcotics and Dangerous Drugs (BNDD).

The suit was challenging marijuana's classification as a prohibited drug and it was doing so specifically on the basis of marijuana's medical utility. I was intrigued at this little glimmer of hope and decided to visit NORML's office.

September 5, 1975
M St. NW
Washington. D.C.

In the fall of 1975, NORML was well-established in a three-storey office building on M St. N.W., just on the fringe of Georgetown. The group received funding from The *Playboy* Foundation, wealthy individuals with liberal leanings, membership fees, and the sales of T-shirts and buttons. I made my way up the handsome slate stairs that led to the receptionist's desk, explained that I had been arrested for marijuana possession, and asked if there was anyone I could talk to about the situation. Much to my surprise, I was ushered into an office where the founder of NORML sat behind a huge desk piled high with manila folders and other papers.

R. Keith Stroup was a young, activist lawyer who had cut his teeth working on the National Commission on Product Safety. He had founded NORML in 1970, fashioning the group as a public-interest lobby which would use all legal means available to reform the nation's harsh and unjust marijuana laws and protect the marijuana "consumer."

Stroup listened to my story of marijuana's beneficial effects in treating glaucoma and I waited for the smirk and chuckle, But, unlike Paul Smollar, Stroup did not look bemused. He merely nodded and began thumbing through the stack of files, finally pulling out a bulky folder labeled "Medical Use" which he opened and quickly glanced through before handing it to me.

"Yeah, there are some reports," he said, "and there are some people you can contact." He quickly jotted down some names and phone numbers from a bulging rolodex on the corner of his desk.

I gratefully accepted the information, thanking Stroup as I prepared to leave. But Stroup felt compelled to add one further thought.

"I think what you're considering, this marijuana/glaucoma thing, might make for an interesting intellectual exercise. But we've been at it for years without any luck. Just don't count on anything working out. Don't," he searched for the right words, "don't end up hurting yourself trying to prove something."

Alice and I greeted the folder from Stroup like beggars at a banquet. It contained numerous old newspaper clippings. Marijuana was variously described as a general, all-purpose tonic, a wonder drug, an elixir of youth, a painkiller, even as a tooth decay preventative. It seemed the drug could do a hundred helpful things.

Amidst these glowing articles, some plain silly, others approaching serious comment, was one from the *Medical World News* dated September 1973. The article reported the story of Dr. Fred Blanton, a south Florida ophthalmologist who had conducted "unauthorized" experiments on several willing glaucoma patients using marijuana brownies. Blanton reported his findings, which were impressive, in 1972. His fellow physicians, however, were not impressed. They promptly convened a medical ethics investigation and Blanton's license to practice medicine was suspended for several months. Strict limitations were imposed on him for several years after that.

The article went on to note that marijuana's ability to reduce inner eye pressure had first been discovered by researchers at UCLA in 1970.

• • •

That article from *Medical World News* had a curious effect on me. Initially I felt a stab of sorrow when I realized I was not the first to discover marijuana's unique property as a glaucoma control agent. But it was a micromoment followed by a rapidly expanding sense of elation. A trail existed, a trail worth investigating. A trail that could lead to challenging The System.

Before I acquired that manila folder from Keith Stroup I was in a very shallow orbit of personal experience. I knew marijuana helped me and Alice knew. That was it. As sure as I was about marijuana's medical benefits I was disinclined to challenge The System even though I knew that others were similarly afflicted and facing blindness. Why make waves? There was no need, no inclination. My only goal was to save my sight.

But the arrest had infuriated both of us. We had done nothing more than grow some plants to help prolong my sight. We had not harmed anyone. Yet our home was violated, our property seized, and our reputations impugned. We were facing considerable legal expense. All of this made us very angry. But it was nothing compared to the anger that was about to settle upon us.

September 8, 1975
National Institute on Drug Abuse
Washington, D.C.

"Phyllis Lessin speaking."

Keith had appended a short, written biography to each name. Phyllis was listed as a member of the President's Commission on Biomedical Research. I had finally tracked her down in her new post at the National Institute on Drug Abuse (NIDA).

"Glaucoma? Oh yes, NIDA has done lots of research on that. In fact, I was working at UCLA when the discovery was made. Marijuana affects glaucoma positively, you know?"

I was surprised at her frankness and amazed she could answer my questions so quickly.

"Would you like a copy of the *Marijuana and Health Report for 1974*? The 1975 book won't be out until 1976, but the current book has some information on marijuana/glaucoma research that might help you."

The book arrived a few days later with Phyllis' business card attached to the cover. The table of contents led me to a small section in the back entitled "Therapeutic Aspects."

After providing the reader with a brief historical account the report went on to list areas of medical treatment which might be benefited by the use of marijuana. The first entry was "Intraocular Pressure."

In 1971, Hepler (*et al.*) reported that normal subjects sustained a drop in intraocular pressure following the smoking of marijuana. . . . This finding has been confirmed by other investigators. Hepler has started a program for treating patients with ocular hypertension or glaucoma, particularly those whose intraocular pressure is not reduced with conventional medication for this purpose.

I was stunned. There it was, in hard, unyielding black and white, printed under the stamp of the Department of Health, Education and Welfare. Delivered, by law, to Congress!

The report went on to list the other research work which supported the UCLA Hepler studies. All of the conclusions had been the same—promising. The report to Congress went on to suggest an aggressive program was under way to develop an eyedrop based on one of marijuana's ingredients, something called THC. It had already been made into a eyedrop by a University of Georgia researcher named Keith Greene. The report noted research rabbits in Athens,

Georgia were being tested with these eyedrops. It also noted, rather sadly, that the bunnies still got high.

I wondered how the researchers knew the bunnies were "high."

It was the *Marijuana and Health Report for 1974* that set my course. It was one thing for me to know marijuana worked as a glaucoma control drug. It was understandable that a pro-pot lobby would make whatever claims possible. But to find that federal agencies knew, had known for five years, was staggering. For the next couple of weeks I continued to dial myself through the bureaucracies. Everyone I called who knew anything at all about marijuana knew that it had a favorable impact on glaucoma.

"It works," they all said. . . . "No question, really."

I wondered, being afflicted with the disease, why this relationship—so obvious to those inside the government—was being concealed from me and my doctor? Some of the voices said not enough research had been done to release the drug to the public. After all, the bunnies still got high. I was endlessly reminded that most people with glaucoma were elderly. The rationale was hard to fathom. The concept that older Americans were somehow less able to endure euphoria struck me as suspect. Euphoria did not seem such a dreadful side effect for a drug which might prolong or secure an individual's sight. Would euphoria complicate an ailing soul's life as much as blindness? As for releasing the drug to the public, the report repeatedly noted marijuana was regularly used by more than ten million Americans for pleasure. It seemed marijuana was already "released."

Other federal officials appreciated my situation, but thought it best to plead guilty and quietly continue my own program of self-therapy. One author of the NIDA Report, Dr. Robert Peterson, counseled that working through the bureaucratic structure could be "sheer hell."

Both sides of the marijuana control argument—pro-pot and federal government—were saying the same thing. "Don't count on anything working out," Keith had said. "You'll never make it," added Bob Peterson. Neither understood that there was little choice. Without marijuana I would go blind. I knew that and Alice knew that. Hell, the entire drug control bureaucracy knew that. But everyone counseled me to quietly accept my punishment and continue on as I had before, paying exorbitant prices for a weed while looking furtively over my shoulder for narcs and vice cops trying to make a second arrest.

It was wrong. Dead solid wrong. No one, save Alice, could seem to appreciate that. When I moved in my own orbit of personal knowledge of marijuana's medical use the prospect of quietly going my own way was fine and dandy. But things had changed. No one in the federal government denied or even appeared to doubt marijuana's beneficial impact on glaucoma. Many of the bureaucratic scientists working at NIDA, the agency charged with marijuana research, would confess, without prodding, over the phone, what they would not venture to say in public: that after a decade of research devoted to finding marijuana's harm, none had been found. Years of research, millions of dollars and not one demonstrable harm. Indeed, it seemed, just the opposite was true. The most demonstrable effects of marijuana were beneficial, such as its ability to reduce intraocular pressures.

All of this made me very angry and I began to chart my course through the maze of The System.

September 20, 1975
8th St. SE
Washington, D.C.

After several weeks of reading research papers and talking with bureaucrats it was time to contact the principal researchers—the individuals who might actually help me prove my case.

Dr. Robert Hepler was the UCLA ophthalmologist who first reported marijuana's ability to lower intraocular eye pressure. He had serendipitously discovered this while investigating the long held belief smoking marijuana caused the pupils to dilate. It was reasoned such a physical phenomenon could be useful to police officers in identifying suspected marijuana users. Hepler disproved the myth.

Phyllis Lessin was the first to mention Dr. Hepler and she had repeatedly encouraged me to call the UCLA physician. But I was nervous about calling him. If I struck out with Hepler there was no where to go.

I decided to begin with Keith Greene, the Athens, Georgia researcher whose marijuana eyedrop was getting the bunnies "high." Greene was unavailable but I spoke with his colleague, John Bigger. Like everyone else, Bigger was sympathetic but there was little he could do. The Georgia researchers were restricted to rabbit research. No human testing was allowed. He did provide enlightened information about the efforts to create marijuana eyedrops but made it clear such medications were a long way from possible human use.

With Athens out of the running, I placed a call to Dr. Mario Perez-Reyes at the University of North Carolina-Chapel Hill. Mario Perez-Reyes had a thick accent and a quick interest. After listening to my story, Perez-Reyes explained he had never experimented on a person with glaucoma, "only normals." He wasn't sure his license allowed for experiments on glaucomics.

"Besides, I only work with pure THC, not with smoked marijuana. If you were to come here to Chapel Hill I would only be able to give you an injection." This qualification did little to diminish my interest. The doctor stressed he would need a complete medical history before making any final decision. I promised to comply and Perez-Reyes promised a prompt response. The line clicked dead.

Perez-Reyes made it seem so simple. I was buoyed with the ease of it all. I mustered my courage and placed a call to Robert Hepler

"Hello, Dr. Hepler's office. Can I help you?"

I assumed blurting out my life story to a secretary would get me nowhere so I tried a more direct approach. I gave my name, where I was calling from and then said, "I'm calling about the glaucoma experiments?"

There was a brief pause. "Just a moment please, I'll connect you."

Assuming I would speak with an assistant or a nurse, I was startled when the line clicked and a voice said, "Hello, this is Dr. Hepler speaking."

My experience with lawyers, bureaucrats, and Perez-Reyes had taught me there was no easy way to enter this conversation. I plunged headlong into the reason for my call.

"Dr. Hepler, I was recently arrested for possession of marijuana and I have glaucoma . . ." Static rumbled through the line and I faltered. Hepler was distant in more than miles. Coolly, without any tone of intent, he responded, "How exactly did you use this marijuana, Mr. Randall?"

"Yes, well I was using about five joints a day when I could get it. The effect seems to last four, maybe five hours. I noticed it a couple of years ago because if I don't smoke I get these rings, these tricolored haloes. Smoking causes the rings, the haloes to go away, and . . ." I began to grab for words.

"What kind of glaucoma do you have?" Hepler asked, still cool but with a bit more interest.

"Open-angle. The pressure has been recorded as high as 35. Normal pressure is 20 or less, isn't that right?" I knew that was right but I was desperately trying to engage the physician in conversation. The curt "yes" from Hepler did nothing to dispel my growing nervousness.

"If I stop smoking the pressure builds up fairly fast. Within a day or so, after I run out, the rings are usually back. It seems, at least to me, I think . . ." The words finally ran out. I had the sinking feeling I had made a mistake in calling.

"What medications are you on, Mr. Randall?" I listed the medications I was taking, drugs that had failed, and whatever else I could recall about my medical history. "It sounds like a very serious case of glaucoma. And you sound young. How old are you, Mr. Randall?"

"Twenty-seven, sir." There was that silence again but somehow it seemed warmer.

"Hmm . . . Well, Mr. Randall, I'm not certain we can do anything for you here. Why don't you give me your address, though, and I'll send you some of our research findings. It will interest you." Hepler's tone had clearly changed and he had slipped into a practiced bedside manner with fatherly tones. He asked for my medical history and we exchanged mailing addresses. Upon saying good-bye Hepler added, "Keep those pressures under control."

September 24, 1975
Dr. Ben Fine's Office
Washington, D.C.

Both researchers had requested a medical history which could only be obtained from Dr. Fine, my treating ophthalmologist. Four weeks after the bust, I found myself in Fine's office for a routine ocular check. I was not surprised the readings were elevated. Marijuana was hard to come by and it had been a stressful time.

As Fine turned to jot down the figures, I let go with my news. "Dr. Fine, I was arrested last month for marijuana."

The doctor "tsked" once or twice under his breath. I couldn't be sure if it was at me or the law. I had been coming to Fine's office every few weeks for three years but I rarely saw the man for more than five minutes. If a medication needed changing the visit might be fifteen minutes. Fine was probably in his late fifties. I had no idea about the man's politics or interests but he was a good doctor.

Fine's back was still turned when I unloaded the second barrel. "I was using marijuana to treat my glaucoma." He stopped writing and turned to face me. "Young fella. I don't care what you do or how you live your life, and I don't know one way or another about this law. But you shouldn't be using marijuana to treat your glaucoma."

"But there is evidence," I protested, "evidence that marijuana helps lower eye pressures. I've talked with officials at NIH and . . ."

"Look, I don't know one way or another about marijuana being good for glaucoma. But I don't think you should be using it as a glaucoma drug." Fine managed to say this without being stern, but there was no questioning his definitiveness.

I plunged forward. "I've already contacted a couple of researchers, one in North Carolina and another at UCLA's Jules Stein Eye Institute." Fine's brow arched and he took the sheet of paper from me that had the addresses for both Perez-Reyes and Hepler.

"This place is very well-considered in the field," he noted, pointing to Hepler's UCLA address. "I take it you want me to write up something for these doctors?" I nodded. "Okay, I'll do that, but I'm just not sure you should get wrapped up in something like this. You don't have a lot of eyesight to waste chasing after . . ."

"Would you be willing to testify in court if these researchers demonstrate that marijuana helps me?" I knew I was pressing.

"Ah, well . . . sure. Sure! If you can prove to me that this stuff really works. Facts are facts. Show me facts and I'll testify, be glad to help you. But you've got to show me the facts."

Fine, true to his word, prepared a letter outlining my medical history, noting the broad fluctuations in eye pressure and aggressive use of medication. The same letter was sent to both Perez-Reyes and Hepler. Hepler's went out first, a deference no doubt to the California doctor's prestigious address. The Perez-Reyes letter followed a few days later. Both concluded, "If with your medications you can hold his pressure at a lower level and more uniformly over a longer period of time, we feel that this would be most helpful."

4 Memory Hole

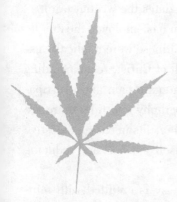

WHILE I DIALED my way through bureaucracies in Washington and researchers throughout the country, Alice was collecting historical information and contemporary news articles from the nearby Library of Congress. Clearly there was scientific evidence, both historic and current, to support claims of marijuana's medical utility. Moreover, there was ample scientific data to show that marijuana was no more harmful than currently approved medications. Indeed, there was evidence to show it was a great deal less harmful than some of the drugs I was using at Dr. Fine's direction.

In a sane society the discovery of such a medication would be cause for celebration. Yet federal officials who spoke to me about marijuana's medical utility were not happy I had found a means of preserving my sight. They were very sympathetic to my plight but none gave me a snowball's chance in hell of succeeding in my quest for legal acquittal from criminal charges. "Pay the fine," they said. "Don't rock the boat," they advised.

In retrospect it was reminiscent of the memory hole in George Orwell's chilling view of a totalitarian future, *1984*. In Orwell's clas-

sic book the memory hole was used to destroy all evidence of the
past not in step with government policies. In many respects this was
the status of marijuana's medical utility in 1975, a trend that sadly
continues today.

"There was a time in the United States when extracts of cannabis
were almost as commonly used for medicinal purposes as is aspirin
today." So began a 1971 book entitled *Uses of Marijuana*.* In fact,
the history of marijuana's medical use predates the written word.

Every civilization since the dawn of man has employed the unique
therapeutic properties of this plant. The Chinese were medically using cannabis 28 centuries before the birth of Christ, recommending
it for a variety of disorders including rheumatic pain and constipa-
tion. In cultures widely separated by geography and time there are
consistent reports of marijuana's medical benefits in easing digestive
upsets, enhancing appetites, relieving muscle spasms, and reducing
melancholia.

British physician William O'Shaughnessy is credited with rein-
troducing cannabis to Western medicine in 1839 with a forty-page
article entitled "On the Preparation of the Indian Hemp or Gunja."
O'Shaughnessy, a man of wide interests and varied occupations, was
traveling in India and noted the use of cannabis there for treatment
of convulsive disorders, as an analgesic, and as a muscle relaxant.
It was this latter quality that led to one of the most famous therapeutic
applications of cannabis: the use by Queen Victoria to treat men-
strual cramps.

O'Shaughnessy's reports, and later articles by Victoria's physician
J. R. Reynolds, promoted considerable interest in cannabis by European and American physicians. But the cannabis tinctures of the
late 1800s and early 1900s were unstable and quirky. As the Industrial Age began to place its imprint on every aspect of the culture
there was a demand for uniformity and repeatable expectations even

---

Uses of Marijuana, Solomon Snyder, M.D., New York, Oxford University Press, 1971.

in the medicines of the time. Powders, tinctures and elixirs gave way to pills and injectable solutions. Many of our most common medications were synthesized during this time from natural products— morphine from poppies, digitalis from foxglove, and aspirin from birch bark. But, try as they might, doctors, scientists, and pharmacists could not synthesize cannabis.

It was during the turbulent 1920s and 1930s that the low hiss of the memory hole began. The Great Depression was ravaging the country and the broad cultural effects of alcohol prohibition were manifesting themselves in crime sprees and violence. As the "Noble Experiment" of alcohol prohibition began to collapse, threatening the layoff of enforcement personnel, one enterprising agent, Harry Anslinger, noted with considerable alarm the growing menace of marijuana—a "drug" particularly favored by Negroes, Mexicans, and purveyors of the hideously subversive new music, jazz.

Mr. Anslinger must be given credit for creating opportunity where none existed before. Cannabis, a plant with a 5,000-year history of benign medical use, was suddenly characterized as an evil and addictive menace. In an effort to foment social hysteria, lurid press stories were published and propaganda films like *Reefer Madness* flickered across America's movie screens. It was a fearful time and Anslinger played upon that fear with terrific success. In such a climate it was easy for a young Orson Welles to create a believable Martian invasion. It was even easier to create a "Devil's Weed."

Anslinger and the Federal Bureau of Narcotics (FBN) convinced the U.S. Congress that marijuana needed tight controls. It was claimed the use of marijuana led to violent behavior and appealed to only the lowest echelon of society. It had to be outlawed.

The Marijuana Tax Act of 1937 was proposed and during congressional hearings there were only two dissenting voices. One was from the birdseed industry, which, in fact, won some concessions. The other was from the American Medical Association (AMA). The

AMA lobbyist, Dr. William Woodward, made two points. First, that marijuana was not dangerous enough to warrant a legal prohibition and criminal sanctions. Second, and more specific to his professional interests, Woodward told Congress that marijuana had important medical properties and expressed concern that the proposed prohibition would restrict marijuana's therapeutic use while inhibiting research with the plant. "There is a possibility," he said, "that a restudy of the drug by modern means may show other advantages to be derived from its medicinal use."

Woodward's efforts succeeded in preventing an absolute prohibition of the drug. In theory, the Tax Act, which became law in October 1937, did allow the continuing medical use of cannabis. Anslinger and the FBN, however, quickly used their newly granted authority to promulgate sixty pages of regulations that severely hampered legal access to the drug. Doctors, therefore, turned their attention to other, more easily obtained medications. Pharmaceutical companies quickly lost interest in attempting to synthesize cannabis. By 1941, with the helpful prodding of Mr. Anslinger, cannabis was removed from the *United States Pharmacopeia and National Formulary*. The memory hole had opened.

The nation, understandably, was considerably distracted during the 1940s by wars, both hot and cold. In the 1950s the communist menace became the Number 1 public fixation and marijuana remained in the background. As the country struggled its way through the 1960s the need for reorganization of drug laws and, particularly, drug agencies became obvious. Legislation was drafted during the presidency of Lyndon Johnson and, with some minor modifications, was sent to the Hill by newly elected President Richard Nixon in 1969.

The Comprehensive Drug Abuse Prevention and Control Act of 1970 (CDAPCA), as originally drafted, divided drugs into four schedules of legal control based on a scientific assessment of each substance's "potential for abuse." The proposed scheduling scheme alarmed several well-heeled Washington attorneys, including Joseph Califano, who worked for pharmaceutical interests. They strongly objected to the CDAPCA's classification scheme because—based on a purely scientific assessment—legal drugs like Valium might end up in the same schedule as an illegal drug like marijuana. And that, they said, would confuse the public.

To remedy this problem they proposed segregating legal medicines from illegal drugs by creating a fifth control level to be known as Schedule I. By law, Schedule I drugs had "no accepted medical use," and were "unsafe for use under medical supervision." The purpose, quite clearly, was to create a regulatory fire wall between officially prohibited "street drugs" and legally prescribed, highly profitable medicines. Drug warriors insisted this approach eliminated any possible public confusion, and would politically be viewed as a hard line on drug abuse.

Nixon, who was planning the 1970 midterm Congressional elections as a national referendum on the liberal politics of "pot, pornography and permissiveness," jumped on the idea of a rigid scheduling scheme based not on scientific assessment, but on law enforcement perceptions of "abuseability."

The deal was all but done when Ted Kennedy and other Senators objected to the seemingly arbitrary conclusion that marijuana was as dangerous as LSD or addictive as heroin. Echoing the concerns of Dr. Woodward more than three decades before, they simply asked, "Where is the scientific proof?"

The Senators were able to access 5,000 years of history, from the first medical writings through 1937, literature of vastly divergent cultures containing a detailed and consistent appraisal of cannabis. In nearly every mention, cannabis was described in benign terms; its multiple medicinal properties enumerated; its mildly intoxicating and possible adverse affects carefully indicated. Significantly, there was nothing in this immense historical record which would warrant marijuana's classification as a Schedule I drug.

"Folk medicine," responded the Prohibitionists. Whoosh goes the memory hole.

After 1937?—A black hole. At least, that's what Senator Kennedy and Congress were told. It was an almost credible lie. After the 1937 Tax Act there was no opportunity for private sector marijuana-related research. So, Senator Kennedy and the liberals responded, maybe we should do some research and find out just how dangerous marijuana really is.

Eventually, a compromise was reached. Marijuana would be temporarily placed on Schedule I as a drug with "no accepted medical use," and "unsafe for use under medical supervision." But a presidential commission would investigate marijuana's proper classification and make appropriate recommendations after a consideration of the facts. To make this compromise workable Nixon agreed to authorize a government-financed research effort designed to scientifically evaluate marijuana. This would, it was guaranteed, fill in any gaps in our knowledge.

Behind this boring public dance over marijuana's proper classification lurked a far darker reality: a CIA project with the code name MKULTRA.

It is not possible to know much about MKULTRA. It was approved in April 1953 but even at that point it was already operational under the name MKDELTA. Beyond the reach of official CIA controls, MKULTRA had free rein and big budgets. The Army was looking at the big picture of large scale chemical and biological warfare. MKULTRA was the CIA's attempt to individualize chemical conflict and to explore the possibility of pharmacologically altering minds— individually or collectively—to alter political outcomes. It was a matter of national security.

Marijuana—sliced, diced, pulverized, brewed, tinctured, suspended, irradiated, atomized and otherwise—was clearly part of the earlier MKDELTA effort. Like the pharmaceutical companies in the mid-1930s, the spies discovered that marijuana's unique chemistry defied easy synthesis. Eventually they concluded that the best way to administer the drug was via inhalation. Tobacco cigarettes were laced with liquid marijuana and given to unsuspecting subjects. The primary goal was a "truth drug." Ultimately, marijuana failed in this particular role.

MKDELTA, and its bastard son MKULTRA, provided the U.S. government with ample information on marijuana. But in 1970, when Congress asked for information on marijuana nobody mentioned MKDELTA. Whoosh went the memory hole. By denying the existence of virtually any information on marijuana, however, the intelligence complex opened the door to a congressional insistence for research to explore the very information MKDELTA was designed to obscure.

After much debate Congress enacted the CDAPCA, a massive piece of legislation. Within it, Title II to be exact, is the Controlled Substances Act of 1970, establishing the five schedules of drugs. A Presidential Commission was appointed to review marijuana's classification as a Schedule I drug. Chaired by former Pennsylvania Governor Raymond P. Shafer, the Commission reported its findings in March of 1972, recommending that marijuana be rescheduled and decriminalized. "Of particular significance . . ." the report noted, "would be investigations into the treatment of glaucoma, migraine, alcoholism and terminal cancer."

Nixon, in the midst of a reelection bid, dismissed the Commission's recommendations. Whoosh goes the memory hole.

In 1973, as the Watergate crisis triggered congressional interest in less than savory CIA operations, Nixon's CIA Director, Richard Helms, saw the writing on the wall and ordered all MKDELTA/ULTRA files destroyed. By the time the Senate began investigating CIA behavior in 1975, nearly all traces of MKULTRA had—officially at least—been systematically erased. Whoosh goes the memory hole.

At the time of our arrest in August 1975, we knew none of this. We were certainly aware of the use of marijuana laws as a societal control mechanism although now the focus had shifted a bit to encompass not only blacks and musicians but also a new emerging facet, the counterculture, a broad collection of individuals which included white, middle-class college students who called themselves "hippies"—a term which accurately described Alice and me during our college days in Florida. But cannabis had been long absent from the medical scene. The Shafer Commission recommendation on therapeutic use, brief and buried in the report, was barely known to the public. The NIDA report to Congress, provided to me by Phyllis Lessin, had cursorily dismissed the plant's vast history of medical use with a single line. "In many parts of the world," the section began, "marijuana has been, and still is, used as a folk medicine." Five thousand years reduced to "folklore." Whoosh.

It was, I could tell from the vocal tones of federal officials, rather inconvenient of me to think federal policy should be modified just because *I* had glaucoma. Authorities became particularly vexed when reminded that *I* wasn't the only one who had glaucoma. Two to four million Americans were afflicted with the ailment. More than 10,000 people a year were blinded as a result of it. Shouldn't they have a chance? Well, yes, we're working on eyedrops now but the bunnies still get high and. . . . Whoosh goes the memory hole.

I wasn't a bunny and I didn't have the time to wait for some researcher to make an eyedrop. Inconvenient or not, I had little choice but to follow my lawyers' advice.

Prove it Bobby, just prove it.

5 Getting Started

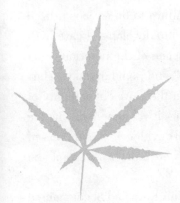

October 16, 1975
D.C. Superior Court House
Washington, D.C.

On a mild Indian Summer morning, Alice and I once again found ourselves in the judicial complex of the District of Columbia. It had been seven weeks since our arrest, booking, and arraignment.

Our attorneys had discovered two critical flaws in the search warrant and prepared a motion arguing that all evidence seized inside our home had been illegally obtained. Their request to the court asked that all such evidence be suppressed—removed from the case. It is a routine legal procedure, an attempt by defense attorneys to quash evidence and provide their clients with the least possible legal jeopardy when the case finally comes to trial. For us it was a pivotal moment. Success would mean dismissal of all evidence seized inside our home: one or two ounces of marijuana and several "tabs" of the psychedelic drug lysergic acid diethylamide—LSD.

The presence of the LSD had been worrisome from the first. It complicated matters on any number of levels. Alice and I did not deny our experience with the drug, another part of youthful drug experimentation during college. But those days were gone. I had discovered such "trips" were extremely stressful for my eyes. Alice disliked the duration and unpredictability of the drug. The tabs seized by D.C. police had been a gift from a college acquaintance of questionable stability. They had been stashed away and forgotten until the vice squad uncovered them in August 1975.

We had cursed ourselves many times over for our foolishness in not destroying the unwanted drug. Our failure to do so jeopardized the legal case which I was working so hard to develop—a case built on medical need for marijuana. The presence of the notorious psychedelic drug, commonly known as "acid" and popularized by Harvard professor Timothy Leary, would give the prosecutor plenty of opportunity to undermine the medical necessity argument during the criminal trial. It was essential that the LSD evidence be suppressed and as we arrived in the courtroom we were all too aware of the importance of this "routine" hearing.

We were pleasantly surprised to see John Karr had accompanied Paul Smollar. We had assumed our case didn't really warrant the attention of Karr & Graves' senior partner, and though we liked Paul well enough we found John's presence reassuring. John Karr had the friendly, rumpled look of a well-seasoned lawyer. He was engaging and confident.

When our case was finally called Alice and I followed the attorneys to the defendant's table and sat quietly as John presented the major points of the Suppression Motion.

The first witness was called, one of the arresting vice squad agents. All went well for about ten minutes as the agent answered questions from both John and the District Attorney. Then, without realizing what he was saying, the agent stumbled into one of the major arguments in the Suppression Motion—whether the police had permission to enter the premises or simply search the sun deck.

He had been going on about how the agents had gotten into the house (still a mystery) when he contradicted himself. John leapt to his feet, objecting forcefully. The judge ordered the witness from the room and counsel to the bench.

For the next forty-five minutes, as Alice and I sat quietly just beyond easy listening distance, John, Paul, the prosecutor, and the court clerk huddled around the bench. An occasional hand would gesture wildly from the packed group of bodies. Every so often a break in the enclosing circle would appear and the judge would peer through to size up the defendants.

Then it was over. No more witnesses. No explanation. John and Paul packed their folders and papers into their briefcases. John told us to "expect a decision in a few weeks." Making our way out of the courtroom, Alice quietly remarked that the judicial procedure was "not exactly a Perry Mason moment."

As we emerged into the warm sun on the courthouse steps, John turned to me and asked a question Alice and I had been dreading. "How do you intend to pay for the case?" I explained about my glaucoma, the federal reports, my success with finding researchers, and my feelings about challenging The System. The stern look which had accompanied the initial question began to fade as the senior partner listened carefully to my story. John Karr was intrigued.

"Well, let's see where this goes. We won't worry about the money just yet." Then he and Paul turned to leave, hustling down the steps to hail a cab.

The departure was abrupt and left me wanting guidance, feedback, and reassurance I was doing the right thing. I had a million questions about procedures and possibilities. But the lawyers were scurrying along the sidewalk, intent on seizing possession of a just-emptied cab at curbside.

"John," I looked around quickly as I raised my voice to make myself heard, "What should I do about this marijuana/glaucoma thing?"

"Prove it!"

While we sat in the D.C. courthouse, wheels were grinding on the other side of the continent as Robert Hepler wrote the following letter.

Dear Mr. Randall:

As I considered your particular problem, I was struck again with the fact that you would be an ideal subject for our glaucoma research project. Please let me know if there is any chance that you might be coming to the West Coast in the near future. If we could have you in the vicinity with us for two weeks or so I think we could obtain a great deal of valuable data. I am wondering whether it would be possible to utilize research grant funds to provide transportation and housing out here for a brief period of time. Perhaps I might give you a call later this next week to discuss this possibility with you.

Sincerely,
Robert S. Hepler

P.S. Please let me know if you could possibly participate. If so, I'll explain the project in greater detail if it looks like we could get travel funds for you.

RSH

The letter arrived just a few days after the Suppression Hearing and greatly cheered us. The prospect of two weeks of study, paid for by a government grant, was more than I had hoped for. The postscript in Hepler's letter was handwritten, demonstrating, at least to my thinking, an eagerness on the part of the researcher.

A week later another letter arrived from Hepler.

Dear Mr. Randall:

I have thought about the matter of your arrest on marijuana charges, and I hope that the court will grant every possible interpretation in your favor. It appears probable the use of marijuana in the past has significantly aided the management of glaucoma in your only remaining eye. Our research so far strongly suggests that marijuana is effective in lowering eye pressure, and it may very well provide a means of help which will make the difference between sight and blindness in at least some cases like yours.

I have heard of some other individuals who, like yourself, have been afflicted with severe glaucoma and, like yourself, have in desperation used marijuana to help control their eye pressures. Certainly in some instances this has been successful. Furthermore, I think that it should be noted that such individuals appear to use marijuana without any harmful side effects upon themselves or upon society. It certainly does seem unfortunate, under these special circumstances, to penalize an individual like yourself and to deprive you of future access to an agent, use of which might very well prolong your sight.

Please do not hesitate to get in touch with me if I can help at any time in the future.

Sincerely,
Robert S. Hepler

Both researchers, Hepler in California and Perez-Reyes in North Carolina, were willing to conduct the experiments that I knew would demonstrate my medical need for marijuana, evidence which could be submitted in Court. The lawyers had told me to "Prove it." Just six weeks before I had wondered how I could possibly do that. Now

I could see the path. Come hell or high water, I was about to challenge the nation's marijuana laws.

November 28, 1975
Raleigh-Durham Airport
Raleigh, North Carolina

It was the day after Thanksgiving. I stood in the chilly morning sunlight at the Raleigh airport looking for Dr. Mario Perez-Reyes. The doctor had described his car as a red Pontiac Ventura and soon it appeared at the curb. As I walked toward the auto, Reyes reached across the seat, popped the door lock, and thrust out a hand of greeting.

Of Mexican birth, Reyes had a coppery complexion and strong facial features that suggested Aztec heritage. His focus was clinical pharmacology, but his educational background was impressive, with medical certification ranging from Internal Medicine to Psychiatry.

For a number of years Dr. Perez-Reyes had been among an elite circle of researchers in America permitted to employ the derivatives of marijuana on human test subjects via injection or oral transmission. He was linked to The Triangle Research Center, a large conglomerate of government offices and laboratories where, among other things, various components of marijuana were synthesized and made available to researchers throughout the world.

Perez-Reyes had already published a number of articles concerning the general effects of intravenous (IV) infusion of marijuana derivatives. In the fall of 1975, he was concluding a study on the effects of IV cannabinoids on intraocular pressure, attempting to confirm early studies conducted at UCLA which demonstrated a direct pressure reduction in the normal eye following use of marijuana or several different marijuana derivatives.

Perez-Reyes had extensive experience with many marijuana derivatives but his current experiments focused on delta-9 tetrahydro-cannabinol (THC), delta-8 THC, cannabinol, and cannabidiol. Delta-9 THC is commonly referred to as marijuana's "psychoactive" ingredient, the part that makes people high. In fact, other ingredients in marijuana also have psychoactive effects but on a much milder scale. Perez-Reyes had observed that marijuana, or a collection of its active ingredients, could indeed aid in the reduction of intraocular pressure (IOP), confirming the UCLA results. But Perez-Reyes went on to demonstrate that delta-8 THC could provide the same measure of IOP reduction with less psychoactive impact. He had observed this in approximately twelve paid volunteers, all "normals"—healthy with no glaucoma.

I would be Perez-Reyes' first glaucoma patient.

As Perez-Reyes drove through the quiet, post-holiday streets toward his laboratory he spoke of varying problems he had encountered with the bureaucracies which control marijuana experimentation. In passing he mentioned his part in the current investigation of THC's ability to reduce the negative, often deadly, side effects of cancer chemotherapy treatments.

"Yes," I said, "I read about that in NIDA's report. It seems to be an important discovery."

A small chuckle escaped from Perez-Reyes. "It was an accident. Did you know?" I shook my head as Perez-Reyes continued to explain. From the researcher's account, the whole evolution of this chemotherapy link was pure serendipity. A young cancer patient in Boston, undergoing treatment, mentioned to his doctor that smoking a joint allowed him to eat and rest. Without marijuana he suffered the same fate as most chemotherapy patients: horrendous nausea and vomiting, sometimes for hours at a time. Unable to eat, patients quickly lost weight and would often abandon the potentially life-saving treatments because of the brutal bouts with nausea and vomiting.

The boy's oncologists, to their credit, immediately began investigating ways to legally provide the relief offered by an illegal drug. The federal government, unwilling to acknowledge marijuana's medical value, offered the doctors a substitute—delta-9 THC, synthesized for drug abuse experiments and conveniently available in pill or IV form. The Boston physicians had turned to Perez-Reyes for help in establishing a proper dose. He was clearly proud of his work in this area.

We arrived at the Triangle Research Institute and entered a nondescript building where Perez-Reyes led me to a cluttered work area and introduced me to his assistant. She asked me to remove my shirt and "hop up" on the examining table

While the assistant attached an elastic band around my arm and various electrodes to my upper body to measure metabolic rates, Perez-Reyes explained the procedures he would follow during the experiment. "Once every five minutes I will come in and ask you to describe your feelings. You will get very high," he was speaking carefully and looking at me intently. "Take as much of the drug as you feel comfortable with. If you feel you are losing control, call out and we will stop at once. As soon as we stop you will begin to come down again very quickly. Do you understand? This is very important." I nodded. "THC can hit you like a train. Do not be embarrassed to call out. Okay?"

After a last check of serum and delta-8 THC containers, Perez-Reyes wiped my arm with a cool alcohol swab, and a long thin needle sliced perfectly into a vein.

The final step before beginning the experiment was measuring my eye pressure, which Perez-Reyes recorded in the 20s, not as high as they could have been but well above the normal range.

After once again reminding me to call out should the experience become too threatening, Perez-Reyes joined his assistant in a corner of the room, out of my sight. I waited, staring at the offensive florescent light overhead, trying to feel the beginnings of promised euphoria. Perez-Reyes came and went like Carroll's rabbit. Every five minutes, as promised, he would pop into my field of vision and ask how I felt. Each time, I responded there was nothing to report, no distinctive feelings of euphoria, no marked changes in the psyche. Nothing.

On Perez-Reyes' fourth entry, he reminded me with a gentle smile that he could quickly stop the experiment and eliminate any adverse reactions. In a flash I comprehended the game. All this time, some twenty minutes or so, Perez-Reyes had simply run serum into my vein. There had been no THC. This was the investigator's control. But the repeated warning gave it away. With new anticipation, I awaited the introduction of some unknown glory.

Perez-Reyes' assistant appeared on the next five-minute check. This seemed to confirm my assumption that the real test had finally begun. I replied that I felt nothing but asked for a glass of water which was quickly produced.

The assistant disappeared and I continued to wait. I was not prepared for the event that followed.

Perez-Reyes returned to the table followed by his assistant. Once again he asked me if I felt anything unusual. I considered the question carefully. "No, nothing distinctive." Perez-Reyes reached over and carefully pulled the needle from my arm.

"Mr. Randall, I do not know what is wrong. You say you do not feel high, yet I have given you 10 milligrams of THC. You do not feel odd or strange, nothing is abnormal to you?"

"Nothing distinctive or overpowering," I replied, confused by the doctor's frustrated excitement.

Perez-Reyes pulled a chart from a nearby bookcase and held it before me. "Let me explain what has happened. This is my chart for experiments dealing with eye pressures. I gave these people 6 mg. of delta-8 THC and every one of them noted profound alterations in their thought processes. Some could not tolerate a full dose, some had a negative response. But you tell me you feel nothing after 10 mg. What am I to think?"

I gazed at the chart. I had the sinking feeling that I had somehow sabotaged the experiment. Worse yet, my hoped-for court evidence was teetering in the balance.

Perez-Reyes once again inquired about my mental state. "You say you are not stoned?" "No, I'm not stoned," I replied. Perez-Reyes had me lay back on the table and once again measured my eye pressure, fumbling a bit as before but when he finally recorded the IOP my hopes soared. From the dangerously high 20s, my eye pressure had plummeted to a normal range. The hoped-for court evidence once again loomed in my inner vision.

In fact, the North Carolina evidence was never presented in court. Despite the reduction in eye pressure, the lawyers were concerned about the researcher's lack of federal approval to conduct experiments with glaucoma subjects. Legally, it was felt, Perez-Reyes was on shaky ground and evidence from his experiments could 1) muck up the case, and 2) get Perez-Reyes into considerable trouble.

Nevertheless, the North Carolina experiment was important. It was the first official demonstration that marijuana lowered my eye pressure and bolstered the early efforts to build our defense. Two weeks later I would be on my way to California to visit Robert Hepler, a noted ophthalmologist with all the necessary permissions from government agencies.

November 28, 1975
8th St. SE
Washington, D.C.

At 6:30 P.M., I finally arrived home and climbed the stairs to the second floor apartment. Alice greeted me warmly with good news.

"We won the suppression motion!"

Paul had called earlier that afternoon. The judge had reached his decision and would rule in favor of Randall and O'Leary. The written decision would be forthcoming in the next few days.

This was good news indeed. The worrisome tabs of acid and ounces of bagged marijuana were gone, vanquished from the legal case. Suddenly it was a much cleaner situation: four marijuana plants on the deck.

I poured myself a glass of cola and moved into the living room. There on the table was a fat, neatly rolled joint, a welcome home gift, Alice explained. I lit the joint and began to tell Alice about my experiences. Several minutes later, for the first time that day, I felt high.

6

Are You an Agent of God?

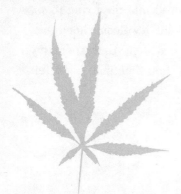

December 8, 1975
UCLA Neuropsychiatric Institute
Los Angeles, California

"Are you an agent of God?"

With a thick No. 2 pencil I blackened the NO box. I was halfway through the 500-question Minnesota Multiphasic Personality Inventory (MMPI) test, administered to determine if I was sane enough to "get high" on Uncle Sam's pot. It was my first morning on the Marijuana Ward. Soon I would meet Doctor Robert Hepler.

UCLA's Marijuana Research Project was among the first elements of MKDELTA to move beyond the "black world" of CIA-funded secret studies into the almost "white world" of publicly acknowledged drug research.

Designed as a "longitudinal" evaluation, the UCLA Marijuana Research Project's mission was to explore marijuana's effects on basic human physiology. How, for example, did marijuana affect heart rate, blood pressure, body temperature, basic motor and cognitive skills?

Put another way, UCLA and similar programs were to publicly discover what the CIA already secretly knew. The emphasis for these bureaucratically directed explorations was, of course, on scientifically proving marijuana's widely reported harms.

Among the questions posed to the UCLA Marijuana Research Project was the matter of marijuana's effect on pupillary dilation. Folklore suggested marijuana, like belladonna and some hallucinogens, might enlarge the pupil of the eyes. If true, perhaps pupil size could be translated into "probable cause" or used to identify people intoxicated on marijuana.

Dr. Tom Ungerleider, a UCLA psychiatrist working on the Marijuana Research Project, mentioned the proposed pupil study to his next-door neighbor, Dr. Robert Hepler. A neuro-ophthalmologist, Hepler was intrigued by Ungerleider's comments. And, as Fate would have it, the Jules Stein Eye Institute—located directly across from the UCLA Neuropsychiatric Institute—was one of the few eye centers in America able to accurately measure and precisely record alterations in pupil size on film. Hepler agreed to help out.

For nearly five years teams of six to twelve research subjects, all males between the ages of 25–45, flowed through the Marijuana Research Project's doors. Dr. Hepler and his staff dutifully recorded alterations in pupil size before and after marijuana use. They quickly discovered marijuana did not enlarge the pupils. In fact, it did just the opposite, causing a barely perceptible, but clinically significant pupillary contraction, a common side effect of several glaucoma control medicines used to reduce ocular tensions.

Hepler made the critical connection and began taking the eye pressures of subjects admitted to the Marijuana Research Project. The results were striking. After smoking marijuana there was a sudden, often very significant decline in ocular tensions. Very unusual. While many drugs increase intraocular pressure only a handful are known to effectively lower it. As early as September 1971, Hepler communicated his findings in a letter to the *Journal of the American*

Medical Association (JAMA). He wrote, "The purpose of this letter is to present preliminary data concerning the most impressive change observed so far, namely, a substantial decrease in intraocular pressure observed in a large percentage of subjects. . . . The possible implications, including the mechanism of action, and even possible therapeutic action in the treatment of glaucoma, are obvious."

In 1973 Dr. Hepler received government permission to expand his study to include a small sampling of glaucoma patients. But finding glaucoma patients—generally in their sixties and seventies—willing to smoke marijuana was difficult. Attempts to advertize for patients even got Hepler in trouble with the professional ethics board of the California Medical Association. The handful of glaucoma patients willing to participate in the study were all marijuana-naive, first-time smokers. To further complicate matters, glaucoma patients—unlike the young male subjects held captive in the Neuropsychiatric Institute—could not be incarcerated and closely monitored over extended periods. Despite these difficulties, Hepler found marijuana, when smoked, was highly effective in lowering the elevated ocular tensions of glaucoma patients.

After five years of study involving hundreds of normal subjects, and brief, confirmatory tests on ten glaucoma patients, Hepler felt he had a fair understanding of marijuana's IOP lowering properties. But, what Hepler really needed to confirm his conclusions was a glaucoma patient who was not marijuana-naive and whose IOP could be carefully tracked over a period of days. He was despairing of ever finding such a candidate when my call arrived in October 1975.

December 8

"Hello, Robert. I'm Dr. Hepler. Welcome to UCLA."

I looked up to see a tall, middle-aged man with glasses and a small moustache standing in front of me. Hepler was dressed in a starched white coat and gray slacks. He spoke with an easy, midwestern plainness.

"I've reviewed Dr. Fine's records," he said, as he finished washing his hands, "Let's see if things are as grim as they seem."

The resulting exam—conducted with the most modern equipment—was thorough. It began with a measurement of my IOP, which was already elevated above normal. Hepler then began to explore the inner surfaces of my eyes using a combination of narrowly focused light and powerful lenses. While surveying the damage, Hepler, without realizing it, let out an audible groan.

"Not so good?" I asked.

"It's a wonder you see anything at all," Hepler replied. "There's a great deal of injury, and almost no healthy tissue left."

I found Hepler's candor bracing. It was the first time an ophthalmologist other than Dr. Fine had looked into my eyes. As the examination proceeded I began asking questions. To my delight Hepler provided concise, understandable answers.

For the next hour Hepler continued examining my shattered vision, and I continued to explore my disease through Hepler's eyes. I found the examination exhilarating. Dr. Fine was an excellent practitioner. But Dr. Hepler was something more.

After considerable discussion Hepler made minor alterations in my medical routine adding a diuretic, Diamox, and a different eyedrop, epinephrine. The doctor promised me I would not get into any difficulty. He then led me to the end of the corridor and introduced me to Bob Petrus, Hepler's associate and ocular technician. Hepler returned to his own office and the waiting room filled with patients.

"Dr. Hepler and I have discussed this." Petrus explained. "We want to get as many IOP checks as we can, and for as much of the day as we can. So, beginning now you'll come back here every two hours from 8 a.m. until at least 10 p.m. Under the best of circumstances we'd like to do it every two hours for 24 hours each day. But interrupting your sleep so often could disrupt your natural cycle. So, we'll be checking your pressures every two hours over 14 hours each day. That should give us enough baseline data to work with. Obviously, Dr. Hepler or I won't be available early in the morning or after 5 or 6 o'clock in the evening. But I'll leave instructions with the resident on call. He'll take your pressures and leave the information for me each morning. Any more questions?"

For the rest of that first day I was checked every two hours and a chart was made of my diurnal (daily) IOP curve. The results were not promising.

Intraocular pressure is measured by a process called Tonometry and calibrated in terms of millimeters (mm) of mercury (Hg). Normal IOP for most individuals is between 10 and 20 mm Hg and can vary slightly in each eye. Upon waking, my 8 a.m. pressures were around 17–18 mm Hg—high normal but acceptable. By 10 a.m., however, they had already risen over 20 mm Hg—above the accepted limits of "normal" pressure. By noon my IOP was around 25 mm Hg, and during the afternoon it remained elevated in a range of 24 to 33 mm Hg. Then, around 6 p.m. the IOP began to rapidly increase. By the 8 p.m. pressure check it exceeded 30 mm Hg, and by 10 p.m. it was nearly 40.

Despite the best glaucoma control drugs known to modern medicine, my IOP was dangerously elevated for 12 of the 14 hours tested. Hepler had promised he wouldn't let me get "into any difficulty" but left on these medications I would quickly go blind.

December 9

It was shortly after breakfast. I had already seen Bob Petrus for a pressure check and had been led by two graduate students to a room where white plastic chairs were arranged in a semicircle. They were just sitting down when there was a knock at the door.

"So, is this our newest research subject," said an aging man whose leathery skin was brown as a mummy. "Hello, Mr. Randall. I'm Dr. Cohen. Dr. Sidney Cohen."

A famous man, at least in drug research circles, Dr. Cohen's name littered the literature. For decades Sidney Cohen, M.D. had gotten government grants to conduct all kinds of research. The Marijuana Research Project was his fiefdom. I felt the room chill. "I'm just stopping by to say hi, and drop something off. Dr. Hepler was very keen on your coming. I hope it's worth the trip." He spoke like a man concerned over budgets and implications.

Having said hello, Dr. Sidney Cohen drew one of the graduate students aside, mumbled a few words, palmed something off, then vanished. I would not see him again.

"Shall we begin?" the grad student said returning to his chair. We sat in a tight triangle. I thought them an odd pair. Both were only slightly younger than me. One was heavyset and bearded; the other was blond, tanned and muscled.

"Let me have your wrist, please," the blond said. Puzzled, I extended my paw. The blond took my pulse. The beard took notes and said, "You have smoked marijuana before?" I nodded.

"Ready to light up?" the blond pulled out a fat, perfectly rolled machine-made joint and offered it to me. His bearded friend struck a match. Both men watched intently as I took my first drag from Uncle Sam's stash. The smoke was harsh and I started to cough.

"That's not unusual," the blond said reassuringly. "It's not the best grass. If you want I'll get you some water."

"No," the beard interrupted. "No water. Not until his next pressure check. Just smoke naturally, ok?"

I took another drag. Then another. And then, without thinking, I reflexively held out my hand and tried to pass the joint to the bearded man on my right. The bearded graduate student, without thinking, reflexively reached for the joint. The blond nervously shifted in his chair. As the bearded fellow's eyes met mine both of us suddenly realized the significance of our gestures.

"Thanks, but I'll pass," the beard said trying to extract himself from an awkward moment. "I smoked earlier." The weak comment only amplified his unintended action. These were not agents of an all-powerful State, but grad students at UCLA.

The 10 a.m. pressure check by Bob Petrus was unremarkable. My IOP was 22/22; elevated. "Just about where it was yesterday," Petrus said with seeming satisfaction. "How do you feel?"

"Fine. To be honest I don't feel anything." I paused. "Does the government make placebo joints?"

Petrus wavered. "Why do you ask?"

"Because I think the joint I just smoked wasn't really marijuana," I said. "It smells like pot and tastes like pot, but I don't think it was pot, just a placebo. I don't feel anything."

"Well, let's just see where this takes us," Petrus replied. "I'll see you back here at noon."

At noon the pressures were 30/23, in line with the previous day's readings.

"So, what I smoked was a placebo?" I said, guessing.

Petrus was elusive. Obviously, he'd not had time to consult Hepler. "I'll see you back here at 2:00."

After lunch—an institutional sandwich and small carton of milk—the two graduate students appeared, collected me and took me back to the room of many white plastic chairs.

Without prompting, I extended my wrist. The blond took my pulse. The beard took notes. "Ready to try this again?" the blond asked.

"That first joint was a placebo, right?" I wanted answers.

"Yes," the beard said without the slightest hesitation. The blond shifted nervously in his chair. Without reading the warning the beard continued. "You can tell because the real marijuana cigarettes have a small "M" printed on them. See?"

He held out another perfectly rolled machine-made government joint and pointed. I strained to focus, and finally saw a discreet, nearly invisible "M" in exactly the same place tobacco cigarettes were imprinted with a brand logo. The beard struck a match and I smoked my first real government joint. This time I consciously avoided the impulse to pass the cigarette to the two grad students.

"Let me take your pulse." The blond held my wrist. The beard took notes. Seemingly puzzled, the blond asked, "Feeling anything?"

"Not really. Maybe a slight buzz. But, no, not really."

The grad students glanced at each other. "Well, whatever," the blond said. "It's nearly time for your next pressure check."

My 2 p.m. pressure was 30/23 (30 mm Hg in the right eye, 23 mm Hg in the left), right about where it had been the previous day. "You feel anything at all, Robert?" Petrus asked.

"Nothing."

Petrus excused himself to confer with the blond grad student. They spoke in muffled tones. Petrus shrugged, then returned. "I think we'll keep you here until your next pressure check at 4 p.m. Is that ok?"

The blond led me to an empty room reserved for the resident on call. "They'll phone me when you need to come back," the blond said.

The 4 p.m. pressure was still tracking the previous day: 30/22. Elevated. No alterations. "You feel anything at all, Robert?" Petrus asked.

"Well, my mouth's dry. But, no, I don't feel 'high' or anything. And I'm getting a headache."

"Ok," Petrus said with a hint of exasperation. "That will be it for today. I'll discuss this with Dr. Hepler. Like last night the resident will take your evening pressures and we'll review those results to-morrow."

It was clear that my situation was confusing to the researchers. It was confusing to me, too.

The first joint had been a placebo so the lack of response was understandable. The second joint, however, the joint with the discrete red "M," must have been the real thing. But there had been no effect on my pressure. None. And how could that be?

The third day of testing, December 10, was a repeat of the first, a day of continuous pressure readings with no placebos, no pot. My ocular pressures were steady, predictable, and high, dangerously high, especially in the evening.

Thursday, December 11

My 8 a.m. pressures were 20/20. I returned to the ward, smoked a placebo joint and returned for my next pressure check. At 10 a.m. my pressure was already elevated. By noon it was 26/26; dangerously elevated. Clearly, the placebo had no effect.

"Ok. It's time to try something different," Petrus said. He handed me a small, round gelatin pill. "Take this."

The pill was almost black with a sinister cast. I wanted to protest, but took the pill.

"I think you should stay over here this afternoon," Petrus said. He guided me to a waiting room. After an hour's wait, I went to the bathroom. I was washing my hands when I noticed my eyes were profoundly bloodshot. I returned to the waiting room, my mouth bone dry, as the first uneven vibrations broke.

Two elderly women, one white, one black, had entered the room. I acknowledged, but did not engage them. Instead, I pretended to read a magazine while eavesdropping on their conversation. Before long I felt myself trapped in a Flannery O'Connor short story, sensing the subtle, elaborately polite tensions between the women of different colors. I became very absorbed in their dramas, nearly missing my 2 p.m. reading. As I raced to Petrus' small office for my reading, I realized my heart was pounding. I felt anxious. Terribly anxious.

"26/26," Petrus said with a trace of annoyance, "Let me check your pulse."

I extended my wrist. Petrus timed out the rhythm. "120." Petrus seemed content. "Your eyes are red. How do you feel, Robert?"

"Anxious."

My answer made Petrus smile. "Do you feel 'high'? Let me put that differently. On a scale of 1 to 10, how 'high' do you feel?"

"What do you mean by 'high'?" I was suddenly confused. What did "high" mean?

"Self-defined. You know what being 'high' is like. So, on a scale of 1 to 10 how 'high' do you feel?"

It seemed a simple question. And, clearly, something impressive was happening. Time was slowing; extending. My heart was racing; my mouth desert dry. I had entered an unevenly vibrating universe and the resulting anxiety was nearly overwhelming. After some reflection I suddenly realized being "high" was fun. What I was experiencing, while powerful and oddly appealing, was not fun. Indeed, it was just the opposite of fun. I was working desperately hard to maintain an outward shell of tranquility.

"One. Very definitely, a one."

Petrus seemed perplexed. "I'll see you in two hours," he flatly said.

I returned to an empty waiting room. With no distractions I moved inward to the small center of myself. From this safe place at the core of my being I monitored the raging psychic storm. My brain randomly jumped from anxiety to anxiety. Disassociated, I watched the show. From experience I knew it would be folly to engage such drug-induced demons.

At 4 p.m. my pressures were 27/27. Perfectly in sync with my diurnal curve. Perfectly out of sync for someone given a massive oral dose of synthetic delta-9 THC. All of Hepler's data suggested a large dose of THC would cause an abrupt collapse in ocular tension. There was no collapse. No discernible IOP affect whatsoever.

"This only gets more interesting," Petrus said. "Quite unusual. Do you feel anything at all, Robert?"

"Anxious. Very anxious."

"I think we're all beginning to feel a bit anxious," Petrus mumbled. For the first time I sensed I had entered an utterly virgin territory beyond Petrus' experience. Petrus, seeming to read my thoughts, said, "I think Dr. Hepler and I need to confer."

THC, the black sinister-looking pill, was a complete and utter failure. By 10 p.m. my pressure readings remained on the well-tracked pattern of 35/36, dangerously high.

The next day I was given another, stronger THC pill, this one with 30 mg of the synthesized hallucinogenic substance, 10 mg more than the previous day's dose. Once again the regular routine of pressure readings dominated the day. Once again there was failure. My eye pressures remained locked into the steady diurnal curve which was plotted four days ago upon my arrival at UCLA.

My lack of "high" was confounding to the researchers. The 30 mg of THC produced even less psychic anxiety than the previous dose of 20 mg. It was North Carolina all over again. Just as with Perez-Reyes, I began to have the feeling I was somehow savaging the experiment.

The weekend loomed ahead of me. Hepler and Petrus would not be around. Pressure checks would be suspended. No tests whatsoever. The weekend gave all involved time to consider the previous week's results. There was little encouragement in the data. Neither smoked marijuana nor massive doses of oral THC had significantly altered my ocular baseline.

For Hepler and Petrus this result was jarringly out of sync with all their previous research. For nearly five years they had consistently found that marijuana when smoked, or oral THC, when ingested, significantly lowered the ocular tensions of normal research subjects and glaucoma patients. Why was I different?

If Hepler and Petrus were perplexed, I was alarmed. It seemed no useful data would come from this trip to UCLA. No data. No case.

December 15

Monday's 8 a.m. pressure readings were right on target: 17/18. At 9 a.m., I was handed a fat, perfectly rolled machine-made marijuana cigarette imprinted with a discreet red "M". I deeply inhaled the harsh smoke and felt a slight buzz.

At 10 a.m. my IOP was 17/23. Below baseline. "On a scale of 1 to 10 how 'high' do you feel, Robert?" Petrus asked.

"Maybe a 2–1.5 to 2."

Hepler appeared, concern evident. "Robert, we don't understand what's happening. What are your thoughts?"

"I don't think I'm getting enough marijuana."

"But we've given you two large doses of oral THC, and there was no effect." Hepler was leading the witness, looking for clues.

"Dr. Perez-Reyes had the same problem."

"You've seen Mario," Hepler seemed stunned. "Perez-Reyes in North Carolina? But he doesn't have government approval to do research on glaucoma patients. Why isn't this information in your chart?"

"Look," I said, "this is in confidence. I visited North Carolina just after Thanksgiving."

"And Perez-Reyes gave you THC by infusion?" Hepler was annoyed but he was also intrigued. "What did he find?"

"That I didn't get 'high' on THC."

"You didn't get 'high' on infused THC?!" Hepler was disbelieving. "Do you know how much THC you received in North Carolina?"

"Between 10 and 12 mgs. over 40 minutes. Dr. Reyes said it was twice as much as he'd ever given anyone else."

"And you didn't feel 'high'?!"

"No. No 'high.' Perez-Reyes was so concerned by my lack of re-action he stopped the test. I think that was a mistake."

"At that dose, by infusion, I can see why he stopped the test. Did someone check your pressures?" Hepler was intent.

"Yes. Dr. Reyes took my pressures . . ."

"Perez-Reyes took your pressures? He's not an ophthalmologist, and he doesn't have government approval." Hepler suddenly sensed he was being territorial. "Ok, so what did he find?"

"Well, Dr. Reyes said my pressures had declined about 30 %. But, to be honest, he wasn't very good at taking eye pressure. So I'm not sure the data can be used."

"Ok. We're getting a bit off track. Let's review. You didn't get 'high' on infused THC. And you didn't get 'high' on oral THC. Is that right?" Hepler was systematically eliminating possibilities.

"That's right. And I haven't gotten 'high,' not really 'high' on the couple of marijuana cigarettes I've smoked since I've been here."

"You smoked a joint with 2 % THC an hour ago. Do you feel 'high' now?" Hepler was struggling to put it together. Why was I different?

"Not 'high.' Maybe I'm THC-tolerant. Is that possible?" I was also searching to explain why marijuana, which worked so well for so long at home in Washington, would suddenly stop working at UCLA.

Hepler paused. "Maybe you're not hitting your therapeutic load."

"What's a 'therapeutic load'?" I had never heard the term.

"It's the amount of a drug required to trigger a therapeutic affect. If you are under your 'therapeutic load' you don't get an effect—at least not an effect we can measure. The fact you're not getting 'high' suggests . . ."

"We haven't hit my 'therapeutic load'?" I grasped the import of what Hepler was saying.

"You've smoked marijuana daily for nearly two years, right?" I nodded. "So your liver is saturated with THC." Hepler was trying to solve the puzzle. "Maybe we are simply having a 'therapeutic load' problem. Wait here while I talk this over with Petrus. And I'll need to make a few phone calls." Hepler vanished.

Twenty minutes passed. Hepler reappeared with Petrus in tow. "Ok, Robert. We're going to test this 'therapeutic load' theory. We need to resolve this problem." Hepler seemed determined.

Petrus led me to an empty room. "This should do," he said, gesturing me into the room. Like a magician, Petrus began removing a large number of small manila envelopes from his lab coat pockets. Then he handed me a stopwatch and a printed form. "You know how to work a stopwatch?" I nodded. "Fine. Here's what we're going to do."

Petrus opened one of the small manila envelopes and pulled out a fat, perfectly rolled machine-made government joint imprinted with the discreet red "M." "See this serial number on the envelope?" I nodded. "Ok. You write down the serial number here. Then you take your pulse." He quickly showed me how to time my pulse. "You record your pulse here. Then, start the stopwatch and smoke the joint. When you've finished the joint record the elapsed time here—how long it took to smoke the joint."

Coping with the rush of clerical instructions, I looked up from the preprinted form, "Ok, then what?"

"Then you smoke another joint. And another. You can smoke as many joints as you want. And you're not to stop smoking until you either feel 'high' or think your eye pressure has fallen. You understand the procedure?"

I repeated the instructions. "Fine. I'll check on you in an hour or so. If you have any questions or just need a break I'll be in my office. This is an ad lib experiment. Let's hope it works." Petrus closed the door and I found myself alone in a pleasant room, in a comfortable chair surrounded by ten manila envelopes. I started the stopwatch, struck a match and lit the first joint.

For the next hour I dutifully opened manila envelopes, recorded serial numbers, took my pulse and timed how long it took to smoke each new joint emblazoned with the "M." I was half way through my third joint when I paused just long enough to realize I was 'high.' But, I reckoned, why stop at three? By the time I finished the sixth joint I was absolutely, unmistakably stoned. Utterly blitzed. Still, in keeping with the spirit of the experiment, I pressed on. I was finishing my seventh joint when Petrus reappeared.

"How are you doing, Robert?"

"I'm quite fine," I replied with an irrepressible smile. "Is it time for a pressure reading?"

"Yep. Let me look at you. Your eyes are certainly red," Petrus said as he reviewed my carefully completed form. "Seven joints?! You've smoked seven joints in just over an hour? Impressive. Now, on a scale of 1 to 10 how 'high' do you feel?"

"Oh," I said, distracted. "How 'high' am I?" I giggled at the rhyme. After an awkward pause I looked around the room, out the window towards the far away Pacific, back at Petrus. "Really 'high.' Maybe 7 or even 8." I couldn't stop grinning.

"Have you ever been 'higher'?" Petrus seemed delighted.

"Oh, yes. But, this is about as 'high' as you can get on pot."

"Excellent. Now, are you ready for your pressure check?" Petrus led me to his small office, splashed topical anaesthetic and dye into my eyes, carefully positioned my head on the chin rest of the tonometer and took a pressure.

"Your IOP is 17/17!" Petrus was gleeful. "Let's see. That's nearly 10 mm below your baseline; about a 35 % reduction!"

At 2 p.m. my IOP had barely budged: 20/20. My 4 p.m. IOP was 14/14, by far the lowest IOP reading Petrus had recorded; a full 50% below my pre-pot baseline.

"So, it was a therapeutic load problem," Hepler said triumphantly. "We just weren't getting enough marijuana into you. And, clearly, something other than THC or in addition to THC is helping to lower your pressures. Seven joints of 2 % THC," he calculated, "means the most THC you could have gotten was around 14 to 16 mgs., and half that was lost in the process of smoking."

"Marijuana works?" I ventured.

"It seems marijuana works very, very well," Hepler, now also smiling, replied. "And we've still got two more days to refine the data."

For the next two days Hepler and Petrus devised a series of procedures that confirmed the theory and refined the process. Having resolved the problem of therapeutic load Dr. Hepler was able to quickly establish a proper dose schedule for me—three joints every four hours to control the dangerously elevated intraocular pressures.

I spent thirteen days at UCLA but it was the last two days that were the most critical. Consistently hitting the therapeutic load had pushed my eye pressures far below the 'non-pot' baseline. It was precisely the kind of data needed to prove that marijuana worked.

Precisely the kind of data to submit in court.

December 18

It was my final morning and I entered Hepler's office with some sadness.

Hepler, reviewing the data, looked up with a smile. "We've learned a great deal over the past ten days," he said. "Clearly, marijuana plays an important role in helping to control your eye pressures. I think, based on what we've found, it's safe to say that without marijuana you'd either be blind or forced into risky surgery."

I listened to the words in awe. They were precisely what I had hoped for, exactly what was needed for the court trial.

"Beyond that," Hepler continued, "I think we've learned something important. It appears oral THC has some real limitations.

Clearly, THC isn't the only thing helping to lower your eye pressure. To be honest, that was a surprise. We've never seen that before. Until you came along we basically assumed oral THC and smoked marijuana were about the same. Clearly, they're not. You agree with that?"

"Absolutely," I said. "Oral THC didn't help at all. And, while it didn't make me 'high,' it certainly created a lot of anxiety. Marijuana works better with a lot less psychic distress. I like marijuana. I didn't like THC. That's what I learned."

"Well, I just wish my medical students picked up this stuff as fast as you did," Hepler said. "I hope we've helped answer some of your questions, Robert. And I hope you can put our data to some good use."

"In court," I replied.

Hepler hedged. "Whatever. I'm sure we'll be talking after New Year's. By the way, Robert, Merry Christmas. And good luck."

I returned to my tiny room to finish packing. "We've arranged for one of the graduate students to drive you to the airport, Robert," the nurse said.

My flight was at 3 p.m., but the grad student said he'd like to stop by his apartment on the way to the airport. We drove out of Westwood, down Santa Monica Boulevard, and turned into a small apartment complex. "We have some time. Why don't you come in for a few minutes."

The small studio apartment was surprisingly neat. Outside UCLA the grad student seemed more human. "We kinda talked among ourselves," he said, "and we informally decided you shouldn't go home without some help." The grad student reached into a drawer and pulled out a baggie stuffed with pot. He loaded up a small pipe and handed it to me. "Enjoy."

Unlike the fat, perfectly rolled, machine-made government joints, the grad student's fresh California pot was smooth—sweet and tasty. After a few tokes, I passed the pipe to the grad student who took several hits before handing it back. "It's a long flight," he explained, "so smoke as much as you think you need. I can always get more."

By the time we arrived at LAX, I was very mellow. My eye pressures, I felt certain, were well-controlled. It was, all in all, a friendly end to what had been a fascinating experience. Now, it was time to go home, put the pieces together and make legal and medical history.

The gods had been exceedingly kind.

7 Building the Case

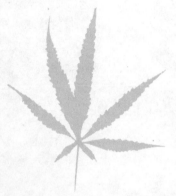

IT WAS A short trip from UCLA to the New Year. I arrived home on December 19, 1975, the holidays descended, and before we knew it the American Bicentennial Year had begun. It was a curious portend and would provide an interesting backdrop for the coming events.

During the first week of the New Year Alice and I compiled the raw data from my UCLA tests into a presentable format. There was no denying the failure of conventional medications nor the near-miraculous results when legal quantities of Uncle Sam's weed were added to my medical regimen.

January 16, 1976
Paul Smollar's Office
Washington, D.C.

The lawyer and an associate were reading through the charts and summations of the UCLA data. After five months of repeatedly explaining marijuana's beneficial effect on my glaucoma there was, at last, some specific data on which a case could be built. "Bobby" had proved it. Alice and I waited expectantly.

It was a dismal day and the dreary view from Paul's window provided a bleak backdrop to the expectant air in the small office. On mid-winter days Washington can be especially gray. The incessant brightness of the overhead fluorescents did little to lift the somber mood or improve visual acuity. The five or ten minutes it took for the lawyers to absorb the report seemed an eternity.

Paul finished the last page and looked across the desk at me. "Bob," he said quietly, "this is history!"

It was an instant of glorious communication. Bobby was gone, replaced by a newly respected Bob who wasted little time in stating his demands.

"It's not enough to win the case. We want to sue someone. Without a guarantee of legal access to marijuana nothing is gained. I need a noncriminal supply, at a reasonable price."

Paul looked delighted. All the implications, each facet of the thesis asserted a fascination and within seconds the lawyer and associate were engaged in a flurry of rapid incantations. Like patients in a hospital bed surrounded by doctors and interns, Alice and I listened to our future discussed in Latin terms and judicial procedures with familiar words such as "publicity," "history," and "great case" punctuating the discussion.

I edged my way into the conversation and was soon engaged in a free-for-all brainstorming session. Fantasy gives flight. Quash the Superior Court with a federal injunction or ask Congress for special action?

"Sue the bastards!" It was Alice who had spoken, softly and directly. We men turned in her direction. "The government has mindlessly set out to destroy Robert's sight. Sue them! The historical evidence is there, the current research is there, and now we have the UCLA data. Let's get their attention and sue for $17.76 million."

Paul was uncertain the government could be sued for acting to prevent an illegal act. Alice looked crestfallen as the conversation expanded into my UCLA experiences with different doses of marijuana cigarettes. The lawyers were intrigued and conversation flowed back to the question of what to do about marijuana supplies. Paul observed that a "not guilty" decision will do nothing to resolve the problem. Perhaps a judge would go so far as to allow cultivation but it seemed doubtful and if I ever left Washington, D.C. how would that affect my situation?

"Why not ask the government for their marijuana?" It was Alice again, a bit more tentative following the $17.76 million dismissal. Once again we stopped in mid-conversation. For a moment there was silence. Paul spoke first, struggling to reject the idea on legal grounds. I tried to support him. But the harder we tried the more rational, obvious, and suitable the question became. As Paul walked to the elevator with us he continued to talk excitedly about the prospect of making Uncle Sam provide the pot, "straight from the farm in Mississippi." As the elevator car arrived he briefly congratulated Alice for her suggestion. It was a nice gesture on the lawyer's part, but as the elevator descended Alice wished aloud that the lawyers would spend more time considering her suggested suit for $17.76 million.

We were cocky and confident following that meeting. Without a clue as to what lay ahead we naïvely felt the curtain had come down on Act 1 and we greeted the lawyers' enthusiasm as resounding applause for a job well done. But there was plenty of work ahead—the play was far from over and the act had barely begun.

Throughout the first five months of our adventure there were endless fears about money. I was making $68 a week as a part-time professor. Alice had secured temporary employment at the Smithsonian Institution, part of the extra work force needed to prepare for the Bicentennial. But her job would end soon. The legal case was becoming more complicated and I couldn't help but wonder how we would manage to afford it. So, in that first meeting of the momentous 1975 year I decided to stage a frontal attack and asked Paul how much this might cost us. The uncontrollable laughter with which he responded did nothing to ease my fears. "There's no way you could ever afford what has to be done."

He was more than right about that. Over the next few weeks I would begin making inquires about possible funding. Keith Stroup would direct me to The Playboy Foundation and Stewart Mott, an heir to the GM fortune and well-known Washington philanthropist. Keith also offered a tax-deductible fund via an arm of NORML called The Center for the Study of Non-Medical Drug Use. It seemed an oddly named group to fund a fight for medical marijuana but I wasn't about to quibble.

Alice, meanwhile, identified celebrities who might be sympathetic. Musicians and rock stars seemed an obvious place to start. Alice is a great believer in "cosmic circles," events or encounters that continually circle back on one another to form the links in the chain of our lives. In June 1972, Alice and I attended an anti-Vietnam War demonstration on Capitol Hill, just eight blocks from what would be our home three years later. We arrived as the festivities were winding down. The crowd had generally dispersed but a small group was still clustered on the stage, sitting Indian style in a huge circle, surrounding a radiant and resplendent Joan Baez. She was dressed in a brilliant white shirt and blue denim overalls. Her smile was dazzling and the aura about her was captivating.

As we approached the group the folks sitting nearest to Baez suddenly got on their feet and left. Alice and I quickly slid into their spot. Alice had her camera and began clicking away. One resulting picture captured Joan Baez and me, side by side.

Alice believed this was a cosmic circle. She had a copy made of the photograph, wrote a letter, and sent it on its way. It was a start, she noted. I appreciated the gesture but thought little of it. I was far more focused on the court date which loomed in the very near future. The money, I reasoned, would sort itself out and a successful trial would insure contributions.

Our trial was scheduled for March 15, 1976, a date which gave me some pause. It was, after all, the Ides of March, the day on which Caesar had been brutally slain so many years before. It is also the day when, by tradition, the buzzards return to Healy, Ohio. Neither occasion promised much hope and as we moved through January and February we would often make jokes about the cataclysmic date that loomed in our future. We were trying hard not to believe in omens.

Never mind, Fate was orchestrating a curve ball that would save us from the buzzards. The daggers, unfortunately, were not quite sheathed.

Dr. Hepler had provided a strong, positive letter summarizing the UCLA findings and supporting my medical use of marijuana, which he called my "special substance." It was helpful but the lawyers wanted more. I explained this to Hepler and discussed ways in which his letter could be made stronger. I then drafted a formal statement for him and asked that he have it notarized. Several weeks went by before the sworn statement was returned but it was worth the wait. Hepler had taken my draft and made it even stronger. It was a powerful, ringing endorsement.

Attention then turned to my personal ophthalmologist Dr. Fine. Would he agree with the conclusions that Hepler had reached? In September 1975, just after our arrest, Dr. Fine had boldly committed himself to supporting the facts and, after looking over Hepler's sworn conclusions, he had the look of a man burdened by the receipt of what he had asked for. I offered to prepare a similar document for Fine, eliminating the sections on research and drawing a conclusion, based on Hepler's authorized research, in which Fine would agree to prescribe marijuana, if it were legal. Fine stalled and stalled and stalled. February was slipping away; our court date was fast approaching.

After considerable delay Paul offered to intervene. The result was unexpected and traitorous. It was suggested another round of medical tests be conducted, this time with the highest possible doses of conventional medications. The site? Johns Hopkins University in nearby Baltimore.

I felt betrayed, stabbed in the back by both Paul and Fine. Who would pay, I asked? Fine said he would arrange for Hopkins to carry the cost and made it quite clear that without the Hopkins tests we would not have his support. How would we be able to conduct the tests and analyze the results before the trial date? Not to worry, said Paul. A request for continuance had already been filed.

It was the fatal blow. I was going to Baltimore. On the Ides of March, instead of Superior Court in Washington, D.C., I would be at Johns Hopkins University's Wilmer Eye Institute.

March 15, 1976
Wilmer Eye Institute
Johns Hopkins University
Baltimore, Maryland

I had just enough time to assess my surroundings when Dr. Gary Diamond entered the hospital room and introduced himself. I provided the young resident with a thick folder of medical records including the UCLA data and supportive letters from Dr. Hepler. Diamond looked confused. It was clear he had been given very little preparation for this new patient. He read aloud from a memo prepared by his superior, Dr. Irvin Pollock. It was Pollock who Fine had spoken with and the last line of Pollock's memo gave an ominous impression that the goal of my stay at Hopkins would be to secure a means of treatment with conventional medications so that Fine would not have to testify in court.

I reflected on the folly of such an approach as Diamond went through the initial evaluation procedures. Surely Fine realized that the discovery of such a conventional treatment left the doctor open to malpractice. Fine was a competent physician. After 3½ years of treatment I could not understand why the man would suddenly doubt his own talents so severely.

My pressures were extremely high, reading 40+ in each eye. I mentioned my "special substance" to Diamond who asserted that marijuana's effectiveness, if any, must be caused by a psychological release of anxiety.

"Actually, according to years of study at UCLA, all the evidence suggests a consistent physiologic effect." I tried to keep an edge from my voice.

In the early afternoon I was led to an examining room and a short while later Dr. Pollock arrived with Diamond and another resident. The three examined my eyes and performed some additional tests. Pollock then proceeded to address the room with his conclusions and amidst the scientific jargon was a basic assault on marijuana.

"Tetrahydrocannabinol," he began, "only has a reduction power of around 25%. Now, in Mr. Randall's case this would seem inadequate."

I was impressed with the authority that the voice conveyed but I could not allow the statement to go unchallenged. "Well, the actual level of reduction, at least in my case, was between 35 and 50%. And this can be added to the reduction available from conventional medications. Add them up and marijuana makes the critical difference."

The mood shift was sudden and perceptible. I was asked to return to my room while the doctors "conferred about the treatment protocol." Things were not off to a good start.

At around 5 p.m. the room suddenly filled with eight to twelve residents, all clad in white coats, all ogling for a look at the new patient. From the mass of white a hand suddenly extended towards me and a voice announced, "I'm Dr. Miller. I'll be in charge of your case." I never saw him again.

Dr. Diamond emerged from another part of the mass and moved to measure the pressure in my eyes. Still high. Time to begin testing.

"We're going to change your medication now, Mr. Randall."

"To what?" Dr. Diamond stared at me for a number of seconds. He seemed surprised at the question.

"The nurse will bring it as soon as we've finished rounds."

"What will the nurse bring?" The room became remarkably still. I felt as though I had asked for the Holy Grail. Diamond shifted once or twice.

"We're shifting you to Pilocarpine 4%, four times a day and Glaucon 2 %, two times a day."

I couldn't restrain myself. "Isn't that basically what UCLA tried? All you've done is replace the Pilo Ocusert with straight Pilo."

Having asked for the Holy Grail, I was now defiling it. That was clear from the hushed silence, the absolute sense of inappropriateness. As if one, the doctors turned and left the room. Through the small sliver of a window, I looked out at the fading light of the day. Beware the Ides of March indeed.

For five days I was "tested." Neither my eye pressures nor my relationship with the doctors improved. Johns Hopkins was not about me—it was, in fact, about lawyers and doctors, ophthalmologists in particular. I was at Johns Hopkins strictly for Dr. Fine. He desperately wanted something else to lower my eye pressures so that he would not have to testify on my behalf. He could not bring himself to believe that with all modern medicine had to offer it was a weed, a smoked weed, that was the key to my medical treatment. This simple fact went against everything Fine had been taught.

There were only two differences between Dr. Fine and the Hopkins residents: age and familiarity. Fine was probably twice the age of the Baltimore residents. More importantly he knew me, had treated me for more than three years. Our dealings were tempered by this fact. In the Hopkins residents I saw ophthalmologists in training and what I saw was a conspiracy of conservatism, a willingness to accept only what they were taught and nothing more. It was only in Hepler that I had seen the curiosity and drive for knowledge that separates practicing physicians from true caregivers and even in Hepler there was some waffling. In the course of my twenty-year adventure these observations would remain as steady and predictable as marijuana's ability to lower my eye pressure. Many ophthalmologists, unlike physicians who treat cancer, AIDS, pain or paralysis, have little if any interest in the unknown.

But Hopkins did have its rewards. It was at Johns Hopkins that I met my first glaucoma patient. In all the years with Fine I had never spoken with the other patients in the waiting room. Nor did I meet any patients at UCLA. At Chapel Hill I didn't stay long enough to even see another patient. At Johns Hopkins things were different.

March 15, 1976
Wilmer Eye Institute
Johns Hopkins University

Vincent Mustachio, 53, walked into my hospital room and threw his suitcase on the bed next to mine. After introductions and a change to more suitable hospital garb, Vince Mustachio found himself at the mercy of my endless questions. He didn't seem to mind.

The West Virginia resident had come to Hopkins for glaucoma surgery, his third. Mustachio had glaucoma in just one eye and it had responded to conventional treatment for nine years. Then things went haywire and his pressure became severely elevated. His doctor sent him to Wilmer Eye Institute for filtering, a surgical procedure in which a hole is poked in the eye to allow the aqueous fluid to escape and, hopefully, lower the pressure. In Vince, like many others, it had failed.

Now they would try, for the second time, a procedure called a freeze. Using an agent chilled to $-60°$ the chamber above the eye is frozen and, it is hoped, the ducts regulating the input of aqueous humor are numbed into inefficiency. If successful the resulting scar tissue will help curb the ability of the pressure to increase.

The first "freeze" was a failure and Vince's pressure elevated to 70 mm before they sent him back to Wilmer. This time they would use an agent chilled to $-80°$. Vince was not looking forward to it.

I peppered the man with questions about the procedures, genuinely fearful they would be a part of my own future. Vince was friendly and accommodating.

In the midst of this general conversation, Vince Mustachio began to tell me about the night at the factory when "a couple younger fellows asked me if I wanted to smoke some marijuana." Off they went to the parking lot.

"It was kinda interesting, that marijuana." Vince explained. "But, believe it or not, it reduced the pressure. Usually the pressure gets so bad at night that I wake up with a headache. The night I smoked marijuana I woke up feeling just fine."

I stared at the man on the bed across from me. I couldn't believe my ears. Not only was Vince the first person with glaucoma I had ever met but now he was explaining to me how helpful marijuana was.

"It was good for my glands too," Vince rubbed his crotch area. "Took away the swelling and pain. The pressure in my eyes only went away for maybe four, five hours. My glands, they felt better for a month!" Vince chuckled. "Prostate. You know," waving again at his crotch.

I gave a nod of understanding and leaned back on my bed in thought. I wasn't sure what to say. Vince indicated he had used marijuana even before the filtering procedure. He knew it lowered the pressure but he had surgery anyway.

"Vince, why didn't you keep on using the pot? Maybe you wouldn't have needed the surgery." It was a gentle probe.

There was a pause. "Don't like the high," Vince responded.

Twenty-four hours later I looked over at my roommate, recently returned from surgery. Vince was clearly in pain and nothing the nurses brought him seemed to abate it. Vince's toes curled in pain and his moans in the night were low and sorrowful. His eye was swollen and black with bruises. It was my future if things didn't go well at trial and it was a scary sight indeed.

As I watched Vince in agony following the surgery I knew his explanation of disliking the "high" was not a complete answer. The euphoria that can accompany marijuana use could not be worse than the suffering this man endured. In the days following Vince's surgery I probed for a deeper reason and, with time, it emerged. Vince feared arrest and, most of all, he feared losing his job.

When the management at Vince's glass factory found out about his glaucoma Vince's job had been changed. After 27 years with the company, and five additional years at Pittsburgh Plate Glass, Vince Mustachio was told he "lacked experience and education" for advancement. Indeed, the company suddenly discovered Vince was unqualified for the job he had held for several years. His wage was reduced and his hours cut. Vince was hanging on for dear life. At home were two preteen children and a wife. The last thing Vince needed was a narcotics arrest or even a hint of wrongdoing.

So, Vince Mustachio was trapped in a world of ever-increasing medical problems brought on by the failure of prescribed medications and modern surgery. I wondered then and still wonder today how differently Vince might have felt about marijuana's "high" if the doctor could have prescribed it for him. I have little doubt that his feelings would have been very different.

I remained at Hopkins for nearly six days. It was a dismal, depressing, sometimes brutal exercise in denial. It wasn't me that was in denial. It was the medical community. They brought out the big guns, leveled them straight at me, and missed every time. None of conventional medications managed to lower my eye pressures to an acceptable range but they did manage to irritate my eye causing it to spasm and twitch. The drugs increased my urinary output, caused diarrhea, altered my concentration, induced nausea, caused sleeplessness, and blurred my vision. Despite all that, I can truly say Hopkins opened my eyes. I did not want to be like Vince but more importantly I did not want there to be other Vinces.

March 20, 1976
Wilmer Eye Institute

The last pressure check was a mere formality. A morning check, as UCLA proved, recorded only normal readings unless I woke up several hours before it was taken. Dr. Diamond seemed pleased and I refused to explain how ill-placed that pleasure was.

"Well, what will the Hopkins conclusion be?"

"That is something I cannot tell you. I'll report to Dr. Fine and he can, if he wishes, share the recommendation with you."

I tried to be jovial. "Look, I have these lawyers and they'll want to know right away . . ."

"Mr. Randall!" The cutoff was sharp and angry. "You are a patient. Dr. Fine asked us to check you. He'll be the first to get the results. This is a matter between physicians."

The pomposity was too much. I snapped and the words spilled out. "Alright, Dr. Diamond, I'll draw the conclusion. You've failed.

There are no conventional medications that can produce decent results. Thank you for your trouble." I turned and walked away. In my mind I could hear Paul advising me to be gentle with the Hopkins' doctors. Be bright. Be cheerful. Cooperate for the sake of "the case."

To hell with Paul! Like Brutus and Cassius, Paul and Fine had conspired to send me into this den of assassins. These "doctors" would sooner watch me go blind then to acknowledge one iota of interest in marijuana's ability to lower intraocular eye pressure. It was a stunning observation in professional elitism and institutional jealousy. Johns Hopkins v. UCLA—cross-continental competition. Not once in five days of tests had any of the "doctors" inquired about the UCLA tests. Not one word of interest had emanated from these learned mouths. Like a great white gaggle of educated geese they would gather around the bed of Vince and other hapless souls, congratulating themselves on a well-done surgery and blaming the patient for having such uncooperative and weak eyes. It had been an appalling week and it made me more determined than ever to succeed.

Standing in the cool March air at the front entrance I saw the familiar shape of Alice's yellow VW entering the Wilmer driveway. As we headed south on the Baltimore-Washington Parkway Alice handed me a joint. For the first time in a week I began to feel my pressures subside but the medication could do little to soothe my anger.

It was a dreadful week but I learned a great deal. Most important was my exposure to Vince and other patients in the hospital. They expanded my horizons, helped me understand how intelligent and rapidly cognitive people can be. I began to understand that my allies would not be found in the halls of justice or medicine. The strength and support would come from the people. To understand such a concept in the Bicentennial Year was not without some considerable awe.

I also learned to never, never, never allow doctors and lawyers to "confer" on your behalf. Neither trusts the other but they trust the client/patient even less. Given half an opportunity they will conspire against you—all in the name of justice and science, of course.

In that long, barbarous week there was one ray of hope. It, too, came on the Ides of March as Alice rattled about our apartment, trying to adjust to my absence. The phone rang and she fully expected to hear my voice. Instead it was a woman asking if this was Alice O'Leary. When identity was confirmed the caller identified herself. "This is Joan Baez."

It can be safely said that Alice never expected this call. Dumbfounded she could only muster, "Far out!" It is a moment of inarticulateness that will haunt Alice forever. No doubt it was a reaction Joan Baez had encountered before.

After recovering from an inartful beginning, Alice thanked the singer for her call, explaining she never anticipated such a personal response to her letter. Joan Baez responded that Alice's letter was "beautifully written" and how was Robert? She seemed concerned to hear I was hospitalized and promised a monetary contribution.

The conversation was brief. Alice explained we needed considerable financial and organizational assistance and Joan Baez suggested we try the Quakers or perhaps Amnesty International. Alice realized there was little more the woman could say. What could she possibly know about medical marijuana? Her call, with its explicit conveyance of support, was more help than any organization could do for us, at least at that point in time. After more pleasantries, she was gone.

A few days later we received a check for $100, which was immediately delivered to the lawyers, and a gracious handwritten letter that Alice still cherishes. The money was a very small part of what we owed the attorneys but the source was impressive. In fact, it would be the only contribution we ever received from the music industry until fifteen years later when David Geffen would support our work with AIDS patients.

On that cold March day, however, the world seemed brighter and warmer for just an instant because someone of stature had been touched by our story. For Alice it was an affirmation, a closing of a cosmic circle that signaled she was on the right path. Each of us, in our own way, received an affirmation that week. Come hell, high water, or even the Ides of March, we were committed to our course. Neither of us has ever looked back.

8 Full Court Press

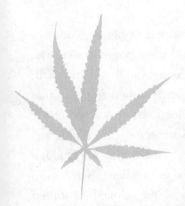

IN THE EARLY Spring warmth of the Bicentennial Year, with Hopkins behind me and the trial rescheduled for May 7, we settled down to the task of tying up loose ends.

The criminal case seemed well controlled. The successful suppression motion had dispelled all the contraband seized inside the house, greatly simplifying the overall defense. With Chapel Hill, UCLA, and Hopkins we had secured the scientific evidence that supported the claim of medical need. One remaining question was the troubling aspect of the charges against Alice. The lawyers clearly could build a case on my behalf but what defense could Alice claim? It was agreed I could fall on the sword and swear the four plants were mine and mine alone but it was a perilous course and involved outright perjury. Alice did smoke. Without the benefit of a marriage certificate she and I could be compelled to testify against one another. It was a messy aspect of the case that would not be resolved until the trial itself.

Following the January meeting with Paul the case had become two separate actions. There was the criminal case, and then the matter of ongoing, legal supplies of marijuana. Paul had run with Alice's suggestion of asking the government for their marijuana and had chased down the various petitions, forms, codification, regulations, protocol demands, policy assessments, and procedural and administrative requirements needed for permission to use the government's marijuana. The early enthusiasm for demanding "Uncle Sam's pot" was quickly diminished by a growing mountain of legal work necessary to satisfy government demands.

While I languished at Hopkins, Paul made a call to the National Institute on Drug Abuse (NIDA) and found a sympathetic soul who led him to believe that all would be simple and quickly dispatched. Paul was assured NIDA would happily provide Robert Randall, that poor soul, with the marijuana he needed. Paul was elated and easily convinced. I wondered how anyone could be so naïve. If NIDA was so willing to help, where had they been since December? Through my continuing talks with Phyllis Lessin, the good folks at NIDA were well aware of the undeniable UCLA findings. Yet no one had offered assistance until the lawyer called with a vague, no doubt artlessly articulated insinuation of "legal petition." When a lawyer calls, offer to cooperate—Bureaucracy 101.

There is only one way the government will be moved to compassion. It involves public exposure and it is accomplished via The Media. As early as September 1975, I had realized media attention would offer personal protection, the modern day equivalent of seeking sanctuary in the church. But the timing was critical. Too much exposure prior to the trial would burn out the circuits and reveal strategies too soon. So I waited for the proper moment, continually rethought the options, and trusted the Fates.

Fate, it seemed, was an accommodating partner to the tale. In late February, just two weeks before the soon-to-be-postponed court date on the Ides of March, I received a call from Karen Spadacene, an old college friend then working at the Washington office of the Australian Broadcasting Commission (ABC). Karen wondered if I would have any interest in meeting with Jeffrey McMullen, a rising young star of the government-financed television network. McMullen was doing a story on the release of the *5th Annual Report on Marihuana and Health*, the report Phyllis Lessin had promised to send me some months before.

The report was released in early February with some fanfare. The director of NIDA, Robert DuPont, held a press conference to announce marijuana didn't seem as bad as everyone thought and it seemed to have some interesting medicinal properties. This bombshell was big news in a town still reeling from the candid comments of First Lady Betty Ford who acknowledged that all of her children had probably smoked pot and she would have tried it herself if it had been widely used when she was a teenager.

McMullen came to Washington from his New York office to tape a segment called "The American Way" for the Australian version of "60 Minutes," a show called "Weekend Magazine." He had already decided to focus the story on the health and medical aspects of marijuana and had arranged for an interview with Dupont. After listening to Karen's retelling of our story, he realized that he had serendipitously found the "human" angle to the story—someone battling the government to get a medically needed but legally prohibited drug. It was a perfect match.

On March 4, 1976, the day after Paul informed me of the mandatory Johns Hopkins hospitalization, I met Jeff McMullen at a nearby gift shop where we filmed Robert-buys-rolling-papers and Robert-walks-in-his-neighborhood shots. Then we settled down in a nearby park, across the street from Washington Police Precinct #1, to film a few questions. It was all over very quickly and my first filmed interview was "in the can."

The ABC interview was perfect. It gave me an initial taste for the power of my story. I could see the effect it had on the film crew, I could sense the power in Jeffrey's questions. The fact that it would be telecast halfway around the world was okay too. I knew it wasn't

time for local or national coverage of my story. There were still those
loose ends to tie.

April 3, 1976
Ben Fine's Office
Washington, D.C.

Dr. Fine waited patiently while I read the first draft of his legal
statement that would be submitted to the government and the Court.

"Well, Dr. Fine, it seems okay except for this last line. You say
surgery is the last alternative available which can control my intraocular pressures. I don't really like the impression that leaves. After
all, the UCLA tests show there is another alternative."

The doctor squirmed a bit. "Well, young man, you *have* declined
surgery."

My exasperated glance made Ben Fine squirm even more. From
our first meeting, long before the ophthalmologist heard of my use of
marijuana, Fine had emphasized his dislike of surgery as long as
medications could control the pressures.

Seeking some retort, Fine snatched a piece of paper from the desk
"And, of course, the conclusion at Johns Hopkins is the same." The
physician handed me the letter from Gary Diamond, pointing specifically to the last page, "it is our conclusion that maximal medical
therapy . . . was not successful in controlling Mr. Randall's pressures."

This time my glance was withering. I was annoyed with Fine's
efforts to split hairs. "But there *is* another medicine."

"Oh, well, yes there is your 'special substance.' "

I sincerely wished that ophthalmologists could learn to say marijuana.

"Dr. Fine, if marijuana was legally prescriptible would you write
a prescription for me?"

"Oh, well, that would be different and, yes . . . perhaps I would."

"Well, couldn't you just say that at the end of your statement? 'If marijuana were legal I would prescribe the drug for Mr. Randall.' " It seemed exasperatingly simple to me and I tried to keep the edge from my voice. I genuinely liked the man and appreciated the difficulties he was facing. I wanted to help the doctor find a comfortable posture in an uncomfortable situation.

The words lingered in the air and there was an awkward silence. It seemed the appointment had run its course. I realized it would take some further effort to nudge Fine along. But time was running out. The trial was now scheduled for May 7, just four weeks away. Paul was planning a simultaneous filing of a petition with the federal government for legal supplies of marijuana. Without the cooperation of my attending physician both legal actions were in serious jeopardy. Fine's involvement was critical and I was becoming frustrated with the man's reluctance to accept the obvious. Hell, it wasn't Fine's sight at stake. What was the problem?

I left Fine's office with a promise that the doctor "would work on" the affidavit. Fine did work very hard but not very fast. He would drag his feet and delay until well past any reasonable point of expectation. Our trial date would be postponed for a second time because of Fine's inability to state the obvious and sign on the bottom line. He would occupy innumerable hours of time in those few weeks between the first of April and the first of May all over a simple statement of facts: yes, I treated Robert Randall, nothing worked until he went to UCLA, based on those findings marijuana might be worth looking into. Simple. So simple it made my head spin.

My relationship with Fine was a microcosm of countless patient/physician relationships which would unfold across the nation in the coming years. The medical prohibition of marijuana enfolds those with medical needs into the complicated and moral issue of "drug use." Those who use marijuana are "druggies" and should be avoided. This was at the heart of Ben Fine's inability to say the word, "marijuana." By using the term "special substance" he managed to keep himself, and me, removed from the "drug culture." But the rhetorical ruse was not always successful. As the months wore on I could see Dr. Fine had no taste for this ethical dilemma. I was a troublesome spot in his smooth-running life.

Finally, on May 10th, Dr. Fine signed the much-needed affidavit. After weeks of wrangling with Fine and footdragging by Paul, I drafted a three-page statement for Fine that incorporated the fundamental points. How innocuous that document seems today. Ironically he would agree to sign the document after returning from an ophthalmology conference held in Sarasota, Florida, my birthplace. When he announced his intention to travel to the conference I was torn between feelings of fear that he would be swayed by other doctors to drop his controversial patient and a mystical sense of tranquility that somehow the good forces which led to my conception and birth in that lovely Gulf Coast town would enter Ben Fine's heart and make him see the path of justice and the American Way. Fanciful, Mrs. Minniver stuff. Alice's cosmic circles perhaps. Call it what you will, Ben Fine returned from Sarasota and signed.

Ben Fine had agreed to provide an affidavit for my trial but he was still reluctant to handle marijuana if I managed to break through the bureaucracies and secure legal access to the drug. Throughout April and May I was scouring Washington for an ophthalmologist willing to take my case. It seemed hopeless.

Numerous individuals suggested I call the National Eye Institute (NEI), part of the NIH complex. I had resisted the call, primarily because I did not want to be classified as a research subject. But time was running out. The NEI contact name which kept surfacing was Carl Kupfer, head of Intramural Research.

The best I can say about NEI is that they took my call. It was not the negative reply Kupfer supplied to my questions that rankled me. That was becoming routine, almost expected. It was his incredibly rude manner, his abrupt disingenuousness that was so distasteful. The man was probably an excellent administrator and certainly proved himself a competent bureaucrat when he referred me to the National Institute of Mental Health eye care program.

It required several calls to determine that there is no eye care program at the National Institute of Mental Health.

While I scouted doctors Paul was busy finalizing the petition. He was dismayed by the discovery of some rather large holes of authority within the regulatory agencies. Gone was the oft-stated belief that somehow I could be exempt from the laws of the land based on the democratically appealing action of "petitioning the government." Not surprisingly there was a Catch-22: No one within the DEA or FDA has the power to override an Act of Law legislated by Congress, and Congress had legislated marijuana a Schedule I drug, available only for research purposes. Schedule I drugs, by Congressional fiat, "have no accepted medical use in treatment" and the petition was requesting just that—marijuana for use in medical treatment. It was a perplexing problem.

Having confronted this legalistic hurdle Paul did the lawyerly thing—he went on vacation. He assured us the senior partners at the firm were "looking into" the problem and that nothing would happen while he lounged the beaches of some forgotten Caribbean island. Generous to a fault, we gave the senior partners a week of silence and then called just to inquire how things were going.

On Friday May 21, 1976, at 6:45p.m., just fifteen minutes before friends arrived for dinner, John Karr finally returned my call. Pleasantries were exchanged, I inquired about the status of the case, and John dropped the bomb: the petition had been filed midweek.

We had formally embarked on our historic mission and no one had even bothered to call.

9 Trials and Negotiations

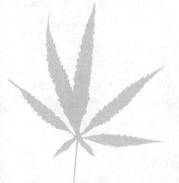

WITH THE PETITION filed and the court case scheduled for July 16, I turned my attention to the media.

When I tried to engage the lawyers in a discussion of media involvement there was little interest and some resistance. Just as Dr. Fine seemed to regard my use of my illness as a challenge to authority, the lawyers seemed to feel I was using the media to exploit my case. One video segment in Australia was followed by a press account in a Melbourne, Australia newspaper, and I was frequently warned not to be a "press hog." It infuriated me as I felt increasingly isolated and, worse yet, often forgotten.

Alice had argued for months to "go public." She had trouble understanding the delicate dance of timing I was trying to master. From her perspective the case was not going to get any stronger. The evidence had been collected and there was no denying the validity of the data. Now working as a research associate to the Washington editor of the Australian paper *The Age*, Alice had often discussed the case with her boss, Creighton Burns, who also had trouble understanding my reluctance to release the story. He had even put us in touch with a reporter at *The Washington Post*. Yielding to the older man's experience, I agreed to talk with the reporter, Janice Johnson. In late April she prepared a story and was about to release it when I asked her to hold off because of Fine's waffling. After the unexpected filing of the petition, I phoned the reporter to give an okay for release, but two weeks went by and still no story appeared.

We had agreed that Keith Stroup at NORML could probably move the story fairly fast. Well-connected, empowered with a bulging rolodex of impressive bulk, Keith was in touch with the Washington media. I had no doubt Keith could put me in touch with someone. On June 4 I picked up the phone and dialed NORML's office.

"I think I'd like to let the story out, Keith."

"Yea, well great. I was talking with Dave Anderson of UPI last night. Told him a little bit about it. He thought it was dynamite. He could get it into 500 papers by tomorrow morning. I'll give him a call. Can he reach you at home today?"

Ironically, *The Post* would call later that day to send over a photographer. Janice Johnson's article, with photo, would appear on June 8, just four days later. It would be another five days, June 13, before the UPI story was actually released. The dam had begun to crack and break. Things were finally moving.

The June 8 article in *The Post* was seriously flawed. It overlooked my December 1975 visit to UCLA and gave the impression I was refusing to be tested because, "I have no desire to become a permanent research subject." Ms. Johnson seemed to have missed the part about the UCLA program being closed in early 1976. I was the last glaucoma patient tested.

Nevertheless the story triggered a sequence of media interest that was intense. Throughout the day on June 9th I was interviewed by every major TV station in Washington. The crews came and went from John Karr's office, filming the lawyer and his client. The TV assault was followed by radio. In the cab on the way home I listened to myself on the radio as the cabby asked what I did for a living. It was starting to get weird.

The UPI story fueled the fire. Radio stations called from throughout the country. Journalists phoned for interviews.

As anticipated, the media focus began to work wonders on the federal agencies. The petition had languished for three weeks without so much as a peep of interest from the DEA or FDA. Suddenly, however, we were Number One on the runway. In true bureaucratic form, DEA lobbed the ball to FDA's court. Not our jurisdiction, said DEA. FDA began a litany of regulatory incantations and then pointedly noted that before we could even begin to approach the regulatory gates there must be a doctor in charge of my care who was willing to administer the marijuana. The ball had returned to our court.

Interlaced through all of this was the constant need to find marijuana and control my intraocular pressure. This was increasingly difficult. Our dealer had been busted in April. Amazingly enough he continued to deal but his prices rose to accommodate the added overhead of his lawyer. Friends, accustomed to simply smoking for fun and perhaps not quite believing my tale of medical need, seemed oddly uncaring. One night at dinner, I watched as one friend passed two ounces to another. When I asked if I could buy a small amount there was no reply. As they departed one left a small bottle of twigs, the other a single joint. It was a moment of despair shaded with deep anger. If they will not understand, who will?

The lawyers, worried about the bureaucratic hurdles ahead of us, had begun to talk about obtaining a "special exemption from Congress" which would allow me to use marijuana medically. Oddly enough this struck them as easier than meeting the demands of the agencies. In true lawyerly fashion they turned to their client and advised him to "find a Congressman to help, Bobby."

I fumbled my way through several calls to the Hill and got nowhere fast. Some had read the news articles and seemed fascinated with the case but couldn't help. Others thought I was plain loco. Finally Keith Stroup referred me to Brian Convoy, an assistant to Senator Jacob Javits, ranking minority member of the Health Committee, a

senior Republican in the U.S. Senate, and widely respected states-
man. Brian *was* interested in my case. He had labored for several
years on the Shafer Commission, the presidential commission that
had recommended decriminalizing marijuana, and was keenly aware
of the politics that accompanied any action involving marijuana. He
was intrigued with the possibilities my case offered. But before pursuing the exemption idea he thought he would just make some inquiries into the status of my case at the DEA, FDA, and NIDA—all
in the name of Senator Javits, of course.

As we slid into July 1976 the whirl of activity surrounding our
case was reaching cyclonic proportions. On a day in early June, as
we waited for the photographer from *The Washington Post*, I turned
to Alice and said, "These are the last quiet moments of our lives."
The building cacophony was certainly proving that to be true.

July 16, 1976
Calendar Court
Washington, D.C.

Jim McManus of CBS News was getting nervous. It was 4 p.m. and
the deadline for feeding transmission to New York was close at hand.
From across the hall I watched as McManus sent a sound technician
off to make a phone call. It had been a long, long day of going
nowhere.

The technician returned shortly and advised McManus, quite
loudly, that New York was intrigued. "Stay as late as necessary and
feed whatever possible." I heaved a sigh of relief.

All day we had waited for the District of Columbia court system
to find a courtroom and a judge. The case had been given priority
status because of the presence of an out-of-state expert witness, Dr.
Robert Hepler of UCLA. But "priority" seemed to mean nothing to
the slow-moving wheels of the D.C. judicial system.

At the start of the day I thought everything had come together beautifully. The court date, July 16, was sandwiched in between the closing of the Democratic Convention in New York and the opening of the Summer Olympics in Montreal. Hepler had agreed to testify and, with Keith Stroup's help, funds had been procured from The Playboy Foundation to cover the cost of the airline ticket, hotel room, and expert witness fees. As we arrived at the court building in the early morning hour we were greeted by Jim McManus, complete with film crew, sound crew, and courtroom artist. Metromedia News arrived slightly later. Yes, it was going beautifully, I thought.

Now it was nearly eight hours later. The first half of the day had been pleasant. McManus regaled the small group with talk about his years at the Nixon White House. The artist, Aggie Whelan, told some fascinating tales about the trial of Nixon's Attorney General, John Mitchell. Everyone wanted to know about my experiences with the federal government's marijuana at UCLA.

But as the hours dragged on everyone grew weary. There had been endless hours, it seemed, of frustrated silence.

At 4:15 John Karr emerged from the clerk's office, beaming from ear to ear. The time and place had been set: Monday morning, July 19, at 10 a.m.

CBS and Metromedia gathered their gear and headed down the hall. Alice, John, Paul, and I piled into Alice's aging VW and set off to the offices of Karr and Graves, where Hepler had patiently waited all day. John had planned to summon the doctor as soon as a court had been assigned rather than force the ophthalmologist to wait around in the corridors. Now it would be Monday before Hepler testified.

"We'll head over to the Lawyer's Club for drinks and dinner," John announced "Paul, make sure Hepler's reservation can be extended at the Hotel."

"He won't be able to stay, John." I uttered the words not as a warning but simply as a statement of fact. Paul agreed. Hepler had

mentioned a tight schedule, an ailing wife, and four small children.
John lapsed into a sulky silence.

When Hepler confirmed the inability to stay John swung into action, picked up the phone and called the judge who was scheduled
to hear the case on Monday. Pleasantries, explanations, and then the
Big News. "Well, Judge Washington, the only solution I can see is
a deposition. Uh-huh, yes sir. All right. Thank you."

It was 4:45 p.m. on a Friday afternoon in mid-July. I looked at my
lawyer and became convinced the man was mad. The prosecution
would never allow this to go forward. My eyes gazed out the window,
across the Treasury Building to the White House lawn. The case
would be postponed to mid-September, I thought, maybe longer. For
a silly moment I wondered if Jimmy Carter would be President before
I went to trial.

The lawyers were engaged in a flurry of activity as Alice, Hepler
and I sat quietly in the maelstrom. Hepler stood up and moved into
the hallway to stretch his legs. I followed, making idle chitchat about
the insanity of legal procedure. We agreed it was a wonder good law
was ever made in this type of environment.

It was just before 5 p.m. when John flew out of his office, Alice
following close on his heels. Stopping at Paul's office he issued instructions. "Paul, you'll have take the subway, there's no room in the
car." Turning quickly he descended on Hepler and me. "Let's go,
it's all arranged."

Fighting rush hour traffic and Washington, D.C. potholes, the VW
once again made its way across town. John gave directions to The
Old Pension Building, a monstrous brick structure on the edge of
Washington's newly opened Judiciary Square subway stop. Built in
the 1870s to service Civil War veterans, the Pension Building is a
cavernous arena where the maimed and mangled had once collected
their country's tribute. Taken over by the District of Columbia, it had
been configured into smallish courtrooms and other administrative
offices.

The VW pulled up to the curb. No cameras, no sketch artists, no reporters greeted us. Hustling along the sidewalk, we worked hard to keep up with John Karr who, unhesitatingly, made his way to Courtroom 38, presided over by Judge James A. Washington. We were the first to arrive.

The courtroom came to life in fits and starts. Courtroom reporters, delighted with overtime, arrived quickly and would pack slowly when the procedure was done. A bailiff sulked in and looked at the defendants with disdain. Overtime was not enough to pay for the inconvenience of this session.

The prosecutor and assistant arrived. A surprisingly young and angular man in a plaid suit, the prosecutor placed his briefcase on the communal table and extended a hand to Alice and me. "Richard Stolker," he said with a smile. I took his hand. Alice recoiled from it. She would not cozy up to the man who wanted to send her to jail.

It is 5:30 p.m. when the judge arrived. "What purpose has brought us together at this late hour, Mr. Karr?" John explained the need for a deposition and Stolker objected. Depositions are taken only for the convenience of someone at a distance from the court. Dr. Hepler was here. If he was not willing to stay then the judge should issue a court order compelling the physician to remain in town until Monday.

I sunk under the weight of it. I didn't dare turn around to look at Hepler.

For ninety minutes the attorneys argued back and forth. Judge Washington seemed determined to let the prosecutor run through his full range of arguments. Finally, at 7 p.m. the judge had heard enough. The doctor was here. The defendants had requested priority several days before the trial date and it had not been heeded. The State was at fault. Hepler should not be further burdened by the State. The deposition would proceed.

Shortly thereafter, Hepler took the stand. John began with the foundation questions. How long at UCLA? Nine years as a full professor. And what awards and citations? The question completely stymied the doctor. I could almost see Hepler trying to recall a citation from the Lion's Club or perhaps an award from the Eagle Scouts. Hepler replied that he had none. My stomach gave way. I wanted to throw up.

John then proceeded to mismatch the date of Hepler's research by five years, placing its beginning in 1975. Hepler, tired and tense after a long day, could not find a way to set it right. Paul began to scribble in large block letters on a legal pad. I was doing the same. Alice reached across the table for the *1975 Marihuana and Health Report*, opened it to the page describing Hepler's research and held it out to John.

The flurry of activity at the defense table prompted a sense in John that something wasn't quite right but he remained as smooth as silk and proved quick on his feet.

"Dr. Hepler, is the report mentioned in this government publication a report you published?"

The assistant to Richard Stolker caught her breath and leaned into the prosecutor. "He *is* the one," she whispered loudly, "He's the same H-E-P-L-E-R!!"

I almost laughed aloud. Hepler's name had been a matter of public record in the case papers for some weeks and the prosecution had to wait for this moment to figure out if he was *the* H-E-P-L-E-R. There could be hope after all.

For the next hour things went smoothly. John led Hepler through the definition of glaucoma, an explanation of IOP, a brief review of Hepler's research, how I had first contacted the doctor, and what my tests at UCLA revealed. The testimony was compelling and well presented.

At 8:00, the judge called a short recess. Hepler and I wandered into the cavernous center hall. The day's fading light was still visible outside. A gentle rain was falling. It was a quiet moment after a long day, a day not yet over.

"The prosecutor is young," Hepler observed, "I fear he is green and I shall feel his lash." I laughed and agreed.

"I can't thank you enough for this, Dr. Hepler."

I could barely see the man. My IOP, so intimately discussed before Judge Washington and the small collection of people in Room 38, was soaring. The rings were giving way to a milky vision, a white-out, just as Hepler described.

"When did you last medicate?" the doctor inquired.

"Twelve hours ago," I replied. "I never anticipated the day would be this long. I don't even have my drops with me."

The ophthalmologist let go a "tsk-tsk" and automatically patted his pockets. But he was in his civvies. No white coat with extraneous bottles of medication. There's nothing to be done except persevere.

The prosecutor *was* green and began the cross-examination with a curve ball. "Are you a forensic chemist, Dr. Hepler?"

Clearly confused, Hepler acknowledged that he was not.

"If you are not a forensic chemist, how can you tell us about marijuana?" The silence in the courtroom went well beyond the normal silence one would expect during a trial. There was a stunned quality among all that watched. Even Stolker's assistant seemed a bit green about the gills. Hepler could find no answer.

Feeling his oats and mistakenly thinking he somehow had the good doctor on the ropes, the prosecutor moved on.

"Where do you get your marijuana from, Dr. Hepler?" The voice was shaded in suspicion.

"The government."

"Which government?!" It was more a demand than a question. "Are you authorized to conduct this research, Dr. Hepler?"

"Mr. Stolker!" It is Judge Washington. "This line of questioning seems a bit extreme. We have already seen that Dr. Hepler's research has been published in the official reports of the Department of

Health, Education and Welfare. It strikes me as highly improbable that such an agency of the government would accept and publish the findings of a scientist who was not fully authorized to proceed with such research. Unless you have clear evidence to the contrary I suggest you accept Dr. Hepler as an expert witness and proceed with a line of questioning more germane to the case."

Humbled but not bowed the prosecutor bumbled his way through an embarrassing display of cross-examination for almost two hours. The clock was nearing 10 when he finished lamely, "Do you know marijuana can cause chromosomal damage, Dr. Hepler?"

"No. I know there is some evidence to suggest that but it has certainly not been proven."

The state, thankfully, rested.

John Karr rose with two final questions. Playing off the tenor of Stolker's last question John asked, "Do you know marijuana lowers intraocular pressure, Dr. Hepler?"

Hepler understood and took the bait well. "Yes, absolutely. The evidence proves incontrovertibly that marijuana consistently lowers the intraocular eye pressure in humans."

"Would you prescribe marijuana for Mr. Randall if it were legal?"

"Yes."

It was over. With one final bit of formality Judge Washington looked squarely at Alice and me. "Be in court at 10 a.m. on Monday morning or forfeit your constitutional rights, face issuance of a bench warrant, and loss of bail."

As we recovered during the weekend the first "feature" article on my case was released in *The National Observer*, a newsweekly now defunct. *The National Observer* was a combination of breaking news stories and analysis. My story was the lead, prominently featured above the fold and headlined "Pot Could Save His Sight." A large photo accompanied the article. Just below was an article entitled

"Carter: Part Lion, Part Fox." I hoped Mr. Carter would take note of which story the editors felt was the stronger of the two.

The article was written by Daniel St. Alban Greene, a reporter who, by his own admission, had first come to get a cheap story: pot-smoking radical professor gone bonkers and attacking the establishment. Unfettered by daily deadlines and seasoned enough to work with the editor rather than for him, Greene could take the time to check out some of the other angles to my story, i.e. the government agencies.

The question was simple. "What's the story on this Randall case? Does marijuana really work like he says?" The result was akin to walking into an anthill. Greene was immediately attracted by the mixed emotions and organized chaos he aroused. The more he stirred the mound the greater the confusion. The answer was always different.

In the end *The National Observer* piece was terrifically sympathetic. Not a single government official would be quoted by name but Greene succinctly summarized the prevailing attitude of the moment: the government *might* allow Randall to use marijuana but only in his doctor's office. My response to that proposed solution was to threaten a lawsuit.

He also neatly captured the real problem with my request:

Yet there is a broader issue involved here, as Randall well knows: his initiative—if successful—could be a long step toward legalizing marijuana—first for therapy, eventually for unrestricted use.

"Obviously I have a very high stake in getting access to marijuana," he reflects, in his verdant, second-floor living room. "At the same time, I'm totally cognizant of the broader implications. I'd be happy if other people with glaucoma would petition the government, too, or at least make their views known. It's time for marijuana to be discussed rationally."

The die was cast. Dan Greene's article was the first to link the question of legalization with medical use but it would not be the last as this continuing tale will show. The link was anticipated but in that summer of 1976 it was not the foremost thought in my mind.

The big problem is getting people to understand without my becoming either a pathetic figure or a hero. I'm neither. I'm simply a human being placed in this odd situation because of a convoluted law.

That was the essence of my situation. I was amazed I'd had the presence of mind to insert it into the flow of conversation and even more amazed that Greene could pluck it out of weeks of talk and wrap up the article with it. Appearing at the end of the piece, the quote seemed to round the story into a proper emotive context. If Dan Greene were the judge the case would be over.

July 19, 1976
Courtroom 38, Pension Building
Washington, D.C.

The morning was droning on as prosecutor Richard Stolker presented the case of *U.S. v. Randall/O'Leary*. The arresting officer, Patrick Mooney, was first on the stand. He managed to "mis-state" numerous "facts" about the location of the plants and the layout of the apartment. Among the items he admitted into evidence were several over-exposed photographs of mail arranged on a table in the living room. These constituted "evidence" of who lived at the apartment. No one seemed to care that the overexposure rendered them unreadable.

Mooney was followed by another detective and then a Forensic

Chemist from the DEA, David C. Noll. Next up was Lesley Ray Brett, a narcotics detective for the D.C. police. Incredibly it seemed that Stolker was going to use Brett to counter Hepler's testimony. He moved through a series of questions designed to have Brett declared an expert witness. He then turned the detective over to John Karr for cross-examination.

Under cross-examination it seemed Detective Brett had not read any scientific books or articles, relying instead on the popular press and the DEA for "that kind of information."

In a masterstroke of judicial interpretation, Judge Washington allowed Brett as an expert but not a medical expert. Hepler's testimony, for the moment, was unchallenged.

Next on the stand was Margot Kelly, our landlady. Margot was not pleased to be called as a witness. Born in Germany she emigrated after the war and was happily building a real estate empire in Washington, D.C. Margot had no desire to deal with authorities any higher in the government than the appraisal office.

Margot Kelly looked nervous as Stolker approached her like a snake oil salesman. Oozing pseudo-charm he first established that she owned the property and then asked Margot who lived at 709-A 8th St. SE on August 23, 1975?

"Mr. Randall and Ms. O'Brien."

Stolker automatically moved to correct the woman, "You mean Ms. O'Leary?"

"Objection!" John said the word so forcefully that it startled Alice and me, who were giggling at Margot's frequent error. The woman had never bothered to properly learn Alice's name and, after more than two years, we had given up trying to correct her.

"The prosecutor is leading the witness, your honor."

"Sustained."

Stolker was flustered. Margot was clearly confused. At the defense table John momentarily beamed at Paul. Alice and I were befuddled.

Alice leaned into John and whispered, "John, she always gets my name wrong." John dismissed her with a wave of the hand that was sharp and clearly said, "Shut up."

Stolker backtracked and asked Margot if the occupants of 709-A 8th St. SE were in the courtroom. When she acknowledged they were, he had the woman point them out and verbally instructed the record to show that Mrs. Kelly had pointed to Alice and me.

He then asked Margot if there was a lease for the apartment. "Of course," Margot responded, a bit indignantly. "Do you have a copy of that lease?"

Margot nodded and opened her purse. Large and white, it was a constant feature of Margot's appearance. Alice and I had often wondered what it contained and now we would learn. We watched in fascination as papers and keys emerged from the seemingly endless depths of that purse.

At last she produced the lease. Stolker asked her to read the names on the lease. "Robert Randall and Richard Talcott."

Richard and I had leased the apartment in 1973 but Richard had moved to New York six months later and I had asked Alice to share my life and apartment. It never occurred to me to change the lease.

Stolker blanched. "Talcott? Who is Mr. Talcott?"

"Objection."

"Sustained."

Stolker looked done in. "Your witness."

"I have no questions, your honor."

"You may step down, Mrs. Kelly."

Margot was barely off the stand when John leapt to his feet. "Your honor, I move that the case against my client, Alice M. O'Leary, be dismissed. The government has failed to prove she resided on the premises in question."

Alice and I were stunned but no more so than Richard Stolker. A brief argument ensued. Stolker pointed to the pictures of mail. Unreadable, noted John. Furthermore, Ms. O'Leary's name was not on the lease and the landlady stated a Ms. O'Brien lived there.

"Your honor," John concluded seriously but with a wicked glint in his eye, "For all we know, Mr. Randall may have a fetish for Irish women. That is certainly no crime."

Stolker was not amused. "Your Honor, Mrs. Kelly," he seemed to gulp at the Irish name, "Mrs. Kelly visually identified Ms. O'Leary as living with Mr. Randall."

John quickly countered, "Your honor, that is not adequate proof of a crime." His Honor agreed. With a few words and a quiet tap of the gavel Alice was free to go. "We will take a ten-minute recess."

It happened so fast we could barely react. We had worried for months about Alice's defense and now, in an instant, she was free. John was ecstatic and looked like a ballplayer who had put one out of the park. Even the judge seemed pleased as he gave his gavel a genteel tap and smiled in our direction.

Alice was removed from harm's way. Now it was full steam ahead with my defense—not guilty of possession of marijuana by reason of medical necessity. That was the goal, pure and simple.

The dismissal of charges against Alice *was* a Perry Mason moment. John was masterful. Fate gave an opportunity and John seized it. All through the Spring we had discussed "Alice." It was as though she was a thing, an offending appendage the lawyers would prefer to lob off in one quick surgical strike. I had seen her wince in conferences when she was discussed by the lawyers as if she weren't there, a piece of chattel, a bother. Now she was "free to go." But go where? Ironically her dismissal from the case led to her dismissal from the room. There was a slim possibility she could testify about my need for marijuana, she could describe how the marijuana helped me and how my vision clearly suffered when it wasn't available. This would be especially needed if Hepler's deposition was not allowed, a point still under contention. As a potential witness she could not view the testimony of other witnesses. So Alice was relegated to the cavernous hall of the Old Pension Building. It was a frustrating and difficult time for her.

Inside Courtroom 38 things droned on. Prosecutor Stolker seemed chastened after the dismissal of charges against Alice but he moved along valiantly. During the remainder of that first day he would question our friend Susan—the woman who had been on her way to buy a bra when she happened onto the bust—and recall the forensic chemist from the DEA to clarify some now-forgotten point about marijuana.

The trial was then delayed for two days while attorneys prepared written arguments about the admissibility of Hepler's deposition.

The trial resumed on July 22 when testimony was taken from Dr. Fine, Judge Washington ruled that Hepler's deposition could be used, I testified, and the closing arguments were given. Stolker's ability to stun the assembled spectators continued well into his closing argument when he railed against the "smokescreen of medical testimony," rhetorically asked if "the known risks of surgery are worst than the unknown," and concluded that "treason is a victimless crime."

John focused on the facts. Robert Randall incontrovertibly has glaucoma, which was not controlled by available medications. Two doctors indicated they would prescribe marijuana if it were legally available. Government-sanctioned tests had shown that marijuana did indeed lower the intraocular pressure of Mr. Randall to within the safe range. If Mr. Randall did not use marijuana, did not break the law, he would go blind. It was an act of necessity, John said. He reached deep into the legal foundations of our system, to the English Common Law and the Magna Carta. He spoke of the legal tenet of "necessity," those rare instances in which one *must* break the law because to do otherwise would bring greater harm upon the individual than the law itself was striving to prevent.

Judge Washington listened intently. We would later learn he had been the former Dean of Law at Howard University. This was not an average case and, through some twist of fate, we had not drawn an average judge. The argument intrigued him but his questions gave little clue as to his leanings. He was a careful, measured man, who gave great weight to each side.

Finally all the words had been spoken and the trial was over. Judge Washington said he would consider the case over the weekend. Court dismissed. Now we waited.

The case got wide media coverage. Jim McManus had reappeared on Monday. Film was fed to New York and Alice and I appeared on the *CBS Evening News* with Walter Cronkite. From that moment forward I gained new credibility in many eyes, most notably Alice's father who, after being told about the arrest, was prepared to fly to Washington and rescue his youngest from the heinous drug den into which she had unwittingly fallen. McManus' report was straightforward, well done, and handsomely embellished with sketches by Aggie Whelan. Cronkite, of course, made no comment on the case but the sheer fact that he had selected it gave the situation some weight. The mantle of credibility which Walter Cronkite could bestow was a testament to a medium—television—that was still young in 1976.

"Good Morning America" extended an invitation on Friday, July 23rd, and a segment was scheduled for July 29th but Judge Washington's delay in issuing a verdict forced postponement of the show. "Company policy," explained the producer. "We won't interview when a court decision is pending." She promised a rescheduling "as soon as the judge decides."

The "weekend" would stretch on for weeks and we could only wait for Judge Washington to render the decision. There was more press coverage as Dan Greene's article was reprinted in several major newspapers, most notably on the front page of *The Chicago Tribune* on August 1, 1976, just under the banner with huge letters "He Smokes Pot—to Save Eyesight."

It was getting very interesting.

August 11, 1976
National Institute on Drug Abuse
Rockville, Maryland

The Parklawn Building loomed before me. Somewhere in that monument to 1960s office architecture was Phyllis Lessin of NIDA. It had been slightly less than a year ago that I had first connected with Phyllis by telephone. She had been helpful then and was proving to be equally helpful now as I worked my way through the petition process, still seeking legal supplies of government marijuana.

Dan Greene and other reporters had made it clear to me that my petition was occupying many working hours at NIDA, the DEA, and the FDA. Also housed in the Parklawn Building was Dr. Ed Tocus, the FDA's point man for my request, who had told Dan Greene in early July that I would never be allowed to remove marijuana from a government research project to the sanctity of my very own home. "We have, in the past, allowed heroin addicts to take a small amount of heroin home while they detoxed but that was an exceptional situation," Tocus told Greene.

I had not appreciated the analogy of my own situation with that of a drug addict. It was a clear attempt to poison the well. Nor did I understand how the government could look kindly upon the "exceptional" situation of withdrawing from heroin but seemed utterly unable to muster compassion for someone going blind.

But Tocus and the FDA were not my destination today. I located the elevators and proceeded to Phyllis' office.

It is always a curious process to finally see someone who has only been a voice at the other end of a telephone line. I had pictured Phyllis as a matronly woman with a pillbox hat. Instead of a pillbox hat I found a pillbox office with a Phyllis Lessin who was much younger than I expected. She looked less serious and more humane than I anticipated. We were probably very close in age.

I had traveled to NIDA to discuss my options. They were not good. There was not a single ophthalmologist in Washington, D.C. who had the slightest bit of interest in pursuing research on marijuana. The feelers had gone out from all directions. Ben Fine looked. My lawyers looked. Brian Convoy from Senator Javits' office looked. Phyllis Lessin from NIDA looked. Not a rock unturned.

Phyllis returned to Dr. Fine. "He's your best bet," she says. "He knows your case and he's a reasonable man."

"Phyllis, Dr. Fine has no interest is becoming a researcher for FDA and NIDA. He's made that very clear."

"But he doesn't have to be a researcher in the pure sense. That's the beauty of the special 'Compassionate Exemption.' " Phyllis and NIDA had a new idea. The agency would develop and hold the research license, minimizing the amount of paperwork the ophthalmologist would be forced to file. "Fine can treat you just as he always did but once a year he would need to file a report with the FDA outlining your situation. Nothing more than what he's doing already but with a copy to us. It's perfect."

I admitted that it sounded reasonable. "But Fine won't want to handle the stuff. The DEA says he'd need a 750-pound safe in his office to store the marijuana. Fine won't do that."

"Look, we can take care of that problem if Fine really objects. We can find a local pharmacy, maybe something at NIH." The young woman began to wander, thinking aloud.

"I don't know, Phyllis. I'm still worried about the DEA. They could make Fine's life hell."

Phyllis leaned towards me and lowered her voice. "You don't have to worry," she murmured, "You even have people there working for you. It really is an amazing thing."

It was a bureaucratic seduction scene. The temptress and the tempted. I wanted to believe the young woman but something gnawed at me, something wouldn't let me believe the friendly gesture.

Phyllis pressed on, explaining that a true evolution in government policy was at hand. If I could convince Fine to act as the physician and file the protocol, an entirely new precedent would be established. "That's the best part, Bob. Other doctors will be able to use this special exemption and the prototype we're developing allows for up to 50 patients per doctor."

It was an intriguing idea, one that appealed to me. The press coverage was prompting letters and phone calls from all around the country. I was already hearing from other patients who medically needed marijuana. Maybe the notion of helping so many others would appeal to Fine as well.

10 Decisions

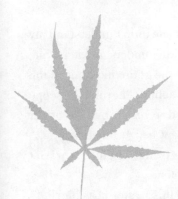

September 7, 1976
NIDA Headquarters
Rockville, Maryland

Phyllis Lessin's office was filled with many voices when I called. Her tone was tense and I got the immediate impression it had been a hard morning. Phyllis sounded abused.

"Look, I know we've worked hard to get Fine on line but it isn't going to work. The folks at the upper level here have vetoed the idea of NIDA holding the research license with Fine acting as the researcher. He has to sign an Investigational New Drug (IND) application."

I couldn't believe it. In the intervening weeks since I had met with Phyllis in August, we had crafted a proposition for the reluctant ophthalmologist and, to my amazement and his credit, Fine agreed. Four months of hard work was paying off. Everything was set. Now this.

"But he won't agree Phyllis, you know that. No one in town will." My voice was angry. "We've been through every ophthalmologist in

Washington. There's no one. Does anyone there understand I'm running out of time?"

I had been without marijuana for more than a week. The tricolored haloes and white-outs were coming with great regularity and I had begun to wonder if it wasn't the government's plan to force me into surgery.

"We know your situation, Bob." The agitation was extreme on both ends of the link. "You've made it very clear."

Phyllis was tired of my insinuations that she didn't understand my situation. From her perspective I clearly didn't understand hers. She had worked hard to resolve this, had spent the entire morning on the carpet taking a lot of heat for her perceived actions "beyond the scope of NIDA's mandate." She had even offered to resign but the upper level management at NIDA would not accept her resignation.

As she relayed all of this to me I felt a twinge of guilt. It wasn't good to attack your friends. I softened my tone.

"Is negotiation over NIDA's position in this matter possible?"

Phyllis conveyed the question to the mysterious voices in her office. There was indecipherable murmuring. "Maybe, but we're trying some other tracks. A number of us are meeting at NEI tomorrow to discuss the future of other requests such as this." It pleased me to hear they anticipated more requests but I held little hope for NEI. I wondered if Kupfer would also refer the delegation to the non-existent eye care program at the National Institute for Mental Health. Phyllis continued, "NIDA has got to observe its Congressional mandate in this area. We cannot extend into therapeutic evaluation."

"Phyllis," I began softly, "it is unwise for me to delay in moving toward medical control of my situation."

The NIDA bureaucrat understood what I was saying. Without some positive action by the federal government to release supplies of marijuana I was looking at a very risky surgical procedure, one that would likely blind me. Phyllis knew how tenuous my sight was. But there was little more that she could do.

The sense of tension lifted. "Yes, I . . . we understand that. We are moving with some speed . . ."

"Phyllis, is NIDA flexible at this point?" I pressed again. I needed to know if the avenue was closed or merely blocked.

"Look, the decision came from us . . . from very high up. But it has been a confusing day. I think there is some flexibility at policy level. Especially if NEI can enter at a future date and relieve NIDA of the administrative responsibilities."

"Would congressional intervention help?" I was thinking of Brian Convoy. A call from Senator Javits' office might be very persuasive.

There was more murmuring from Phyllis' office guests. "No, at least not today. Maybe tomorrow. It's good you informed us such a thing might happen. We will pass the information along."

"Phyllis, I won't allow this to go on much longer." It was close to a threat but I felt certain the young woman understood it was not aimed at her personally. Still awaiting the decision from Judge Washington and weary to the bone of waiting for government action on my petition, I was quite sincere. Things *had* to be resolved.

"I understand, Bob. Hold back another day or two while the dust settles a bit here. I'll call you tomorrow."

The phone went dead. The house was very quiet and the only sound was the whir of the air conditioner, working hard against the still warm air of early September.

For a moment I felt queasy and cursed myself for allowing the feelings of hope to build in the last few weeks. I should have known it was too good to be true. They were going to blind me. They were going to win.

I picked up the phone and called Paul but the attorney had little to say. John Karr was on vacation and Paul couldn't possibly take any action while John was away. "What you're talking about, Bobby, a civil suit, would be major bucks. How are you going to pay for that?"

I hung up the phone and stared straight ahead.

So close . . . We were so close . . .

I called Alice to relay the news. Her disappointment and concern was a welcome salve against a brutal day but it didn't alter the situation. "I'll see you in a couple of hours. I'll make some more calls. Maybe I can find some medicine." She was gone and I was alone again. I wondered how Alice would pay for whatever medicine—marijuana—she might be able to find. The rent had depleted the bank account. The lawyers were harping about cash. Fine and several other doctors were owed for visits. Even Johns Hopkins had been calling—the promised arrangement to pay for my week at the Baltimore facility appeared to have fallen through and collection agencies were being mentioned. How much longer could we keep this going?

The phone rang. It was Phyllis.

"I hope this excites you as much as it does me." Phyllis said. Her fatigue from earlier in the day was gone. She seemed genuinely thrilled.

"I called NEI and one of the folks over there told me about a new research application for marijuana and glaucoma. It's just been received so it's a bit behind yours but we can speed things along and I've talked with the doctor. He's willing to sign onto your request and treat you. It's unbelievable."

The young woman was talking very fast and I was having a hard time understanding why she was so excited. "Phyllis, I'll be honest with you. I can't afford to move somewhere else for eye care."

Phyllis stopped me in mid-sentence. "Bob, you don't have to move. The doctor is at Howard University. You know, up there on Georgia Avenue?"

I couldn't believe it. "Phyllis, are you saying you've found a doctor in Washington who is willing to treat me and prescribe marijuana?"

A giggle slipped from the other end of the line. "Uh huh. He's waiting for your call now. His name is John Merritt."

● ● ●

In the ancient Greek and Roman theater there was a device employed called deus ex machina—literally "the machine of the gods." Arriving on some form of stage machinery, either as a cloud from above the stage or, more likely, as a chariot from the wings, a deity would arrive to intervene in the action or neatly resolve a complex story line. John Merritt was my deus ex machina.

Initially I was skeptical. By this point I had spoken with countless doctors, visited with half a dozen or so, and discussed the case endlessly with whoever would listen. I felt trapped in a maze of countless dead-end turns. I wanted to believe John Merritt would work out but my hopes had been dashed too many times.

True to Phyllis' word, Merritt was awaiting my call. A meeting was arranged for the following day, September 8, 1976. We connected easily. He answered all my questions, and when I asked if I was asking too many he responded, "No, glaucoma is so unknown. The only way to learn is to listen." In my endless journey through the ophthalmology world there had only been one other doctor who had said such a sensible thing, Robert Hepler.

By Friday, September 10, Phyllis Lessin had John Merritt's signature on the IND she had originally prepared for Fine and NIDA. It was a crowning achievement. It was also her last act of kindness on my behalf. NIDA removed her from my case that afternoon and forbade her from participating in any future inquiries of a therapeutic nature.

Throughout the country the story of "Man asks for pot to save sight" was rippling across newspapers. The cat was out of the bag. Marijuana's medical use was no longer an abstraction buried in some dull governmental report. A real person was asking permission to use the illegal stuff and others with similar ailments were paying close attention. They were wondering if marijuana could help Uncle Harry's vision or Cousin Sue's chemotherapy. And they were calling the agencies, just as I had. NIDA was nervous, the whole of the federal drug establishment was nervous.

The removal of Phyllis didn't change any of this but it was the first step towards reestablishing the stone wall of silence, the initial effort to regain control.

Phyllis was removed from my case but not before she had stage managed an incredible deus ex machina moment. John Merritt became my doctor and the last impediment was removed. The formalities had been completed. The regulations had been observed. The ball was back in the government's court.

Not surprisingly the matter would drag on for several more weeks. By late September all was signed and sealed. The marijuana, Merritt told me, was in transit, arriving any day now via the U.S. Mail. This point was most remarkable. After months of jumping through hoops and hurdles to obtain this "dangerous" Schedule I drug, after Merritt was forced to purchase a 250-pound safe to securely store the "dangerous" substance, the "dangerous" drug would arrive by parcel post.

It all seemed terribly anticlimatic. But, that was, of course, an illusion.

October 5, 1976
8th St. SE
Washington, D.C.

I was floating comfortably on the waterbed, resisting the urge to awaken, when the phone rang. I could hear Alice sprinting up the stairs and raised myself up on one elbow. "Keith's on the phone. UPI is running the story about Howard."

I let go a curse and picked up the phone. "Keith, I thought we were going to coordinate this. I don't think you should have done this."

"It's not me Bob. UPI called me for your number. The reporter has government sources, knows everything about Howard. This is coming from the feds. I should get off the phone so UPI can get through." Click. Keith was gone. Within seconds the phone rang again. WMOD radio would like a comment, Alice yelled up the stairs. Jeez! What's happening?

I fed the local radio a morsel of a sound bite and asked where the reporter got the news. "On the wire," he said, implying that I might be slightly stupid to even ask.

The receiver barely touched the cradle before the phone rang again. I picked up quickly, hoping UPI was finally calling. "NBC radio here, is this Bob Randall?" Uh-huh. "Would you like to go live?"

"NO!" The response deflated the reporter. "Look, I don't have a clue as to what's happening," I said.

The NBC reporter was happy to bring me up to speed and read the wire story.

Acting on the appeal of a man who claims he needs marijuana to keep from going blind, federal drug regulation agencies have approved human clinical tests of "pot" for the treatment of glaucoma, government spokesmen said today.

The unusual "compassionate" approval for closely controlled studies by a Howard University professor may involve up to 50 patients, who either will be given marijuana capsules or be allowed to smoke "pot" to relieve pressure within the eyeball.

For now, however, the study has only one patient, Robert Randall, 28, who is fighting a criminal marijuana charge in a court case here.

The story went on to provide some background on glaucoma and my tests at UCLA and Hopkins. It also sang the praises of government agencies cooperating together. "It was a compassionate get-together. We responded to Randall's appeal and to his doctor's appeal."

I gave the reporter a "No comment" and promised to call back once I learned more details. I pressed the button to disconnect but left the phone off the hook. I needed a moment or two to think.

I had, undoubtedly, won. The petition was a success. By releasing the news the government agencies had cast the die. The contract was sealed.

I placed a call to Dr. Merritt. He should know about this. Maybe it was Howard who prompted the story?

"Are you trying to ruin everything?!" the physician began, "CBS, NBC calling! What in the hell . . ." Merritt's fury made it clear he knew nothing about the story.

"It wasn't me, Dr. Merritt. I'm getting the same calls and know nothing about it. The UPI is quoting government sources. It must have come from the agencies."

"No, it was supposed to come out tomorrow at 12. It was agreed on by everyone involved." Merritt was volatile and revealing.

"I knew nothing about such an agreement, Dr. Merritt. And I wouldn't do this without informing you first. All the news copy quotes government sources."

Merritt paused and absorbed the implication. If the government had released the story it was a major breach of trust.

We finished the conversation amicably and agreed to meet the next day.

Before the phone could ring again I quickly dialed Phyllis Lessin. "In my opinion you are ungrateful for all the help people have given you!" Her anger made Merritt seem calm. I was unprepared for the young woman's wrath. Her vocal intensity was extreme as she accused me of insensitivity on a monumental scale. "You don't care about your own sight. You want to save the world! You should be grateful. Instead you release this news and . . ."

"No, Phyllis. I didn't."

The words failed to register and her stream of anger continued. "I've worked for four months, so have others and. . . ."

Nature intervened and Phyllis paused for some air. I quickly seized the moment. "I've worked for fourteen months, Phyllis. I've jumped through hoops, I've submitted to dangerous, foolish tests in the name of science. The agencies have known since last December how critical marijuana is to my eyesight. Where was the 'compassion' then? I have not gone to the press when I should have gone to the press. I have respected your efforts and agreed to your terms. Now someone in the government has released this story without giving me or apparently you or Merritt any warning. I really don't think we want to get into a shouting match about who has put in the most time or effort here. . . ."

The words calmed Phyllis, but only for a moment. "And there's another thing," the tone of the introduction made me brace myself for the onslaught. "You'd better back off this idea of taking the marijuana home. The DEA and FDA have already agreed you can only be allowed to take home supplies if you agree to complete silence about it. No one must know . . . for your own security."

The source of the leak will probably never be known. Later Keith Stroup told me it was Bob Du Pont at NIDA. I have always suspected it was Ed Tocus at the FDA. We must also guess at the purpose of the leak but, with the hindsight of twenty years, I believe the intention was good. The bureaucrats who had worked hard to resolve my problem were attempting to lock things down before "others" could sabotage the efforts. My perceived role as someone out "to save the world" was undoubtedly worrisome to the bureaucrats. The entire effort could be sunk. Lock it down, preserve something, that was the goal.

As the weight of the now publicly confirmed IND settled across America's consciousness the very practical aspects of supply—where and how—began to command attention. Where would the government's marijuana be stored and how would I access it? This point would become the stickiest and nastiest of all.

My intentions were clear. I wanted to receive marijuana like any other drug, by prescription from a pharmacy. In the weeks of wrangling over the petition and the eventual IND, this point was constantly shuffled to the background. Whenever I would raise the issue I was instructed not to worry about it.

But now it had to be worried about and the DEA, the federal agency most concerned with the drug's security, became the principal actor in my evolving drama. They had already forced Dr. Merritt to purchase a 250-lb. safe that was bolted, from the inside, to the floor of his office. Here Merritt would store the supplies of marijuana used by the other patients in the research program.

My case was different. From the initial filing of the petition the intent had been to obtain marijuana for use as a conventional medication. Now, as the IND was approved, the hour of reckoning was at hand.

Initial alarms had been raised by Ed Tocus when he told Dan Greene in July that take-home supplies of the drug would never be allowed. Permanent hospitalization was discussed but quickly dropped when the obvious stupidity of such a suggestion was echoed back to the government officials who raised it.

The next scenario had me reporting to Howard University whenever my intraocular pressure needed control. The tests from UCLA had clearly demonstrated my need for ten marijuana cigarettes a day, most of them in the evening hours. The prospect of traveling to Howard ten times a day was as laughable as lifetime hospitalization. The DEA then proposed that I purchase a safe in which to store the marijuana. To demonstrate the extent of their flexibility I was offered two options: a 750-lb. freestanding safe or the sportier model chosen by Merritt, 250 lbs. bolted to the floor from the inside.

I made several points: 1) either model involved a considerable expense of money, 2) my landlady would probably not appreciate the damage that could be caused by installing either of the models, and 3) the only time marijuana had ever been stolen from me was when the police busted me in August 1975.

Now, in the emotion-laden conversation with Phyllis, the final gambit had been played. I could have the marijuana I medically needed but I must shut up, not tell a soul, keep quiet—"for my own safety."

I sought the advice of others about this latest offer from the feds. Several friends counseled me to take the marijuana in whatever way I could get it. Some said the government had the upper hand and was "looking pretty good." To refuse the offer and attempt to regain momentum via the media could jeopardize the entire arrangement.

Alice's counsel was chilling—accept the offer and become part of the myth that marijuana is too dangerous for rational use. She advised holding the line, confrontation if necessary.

The lawyers argued for patience and their suggested tack was reinforced by Creighton Burns, the reporter for *The Age* of Melbourne, Australia. Alice continued working for Creighton as a research associate and throughout the Bicentennial Year he had been an ad hoc advisor to our endeavors.

Creighton loved politics and saw, from the first, that this was predominantly a political question. His assessment was pragmatic and honed from years of political observation around the globe. With the wisdom of one who is comfortably detached, Creighton observed that the bureaucrats were "acting just fine" and noted he would "fire a damn bureaucrat that didn't make this difficult for you. They hire only 'safe people,' at least in the places you're being discussed. They'll never move as fast or as completely as a mindful person has a right to think. And," he added soberly, "they probably don't like you telling them what is and what isn't acceptable."

Creighton's ultimate advice was that of the lawyers—patience. But he added an important caveat. "Don't get publicly forced into anything. Someone wants this settled, that's obvious. Don't muck it up with public statements until you understand what's going on."

It was good advice. In the days following the initial release of the news story about Merritt and Howard University, my standard response became "No comment." Using the still pending criminal trial as an excuse, I was able to put off reporters from throughout the country. NORML had issued a press release following the unexpected UPI story and this had triggered an intense round of media interest including the return of Jim McManus from CBS, *Newsweek Magazine*, *The New York Times*, National Public Radio, *The St. Louis Post Dispatch*, *The L.A. Times*, and more. To each I said "No comment," citing the pending court decision, now scheduled for October 20th. It was easier than I originally thought. The news media, especially the print reporters, sensed a growing story and didn't seem to mind the delay. I encouraged the reporters to contact the government officials in charge of the case and promised "off the record clarification" of any confusing points. This proved an efficient way to glean important facts and better understand the dynamics of what was happening within the agencies.

The infusion of press inquiries only underscored how silly the government demands were, relative to the drug's security, as the reporters would sometimes laugh out loud at suggestions of lifetime hospitalization or daily reporting to Howard. Moreover, the simple fact of inquiring began to undermine the hoped for "silent solution." You can have it but don't tell anyone. How evocative of more recent government solutions such as gays in the military or the censure of abortion advice from government-financed health facilities. The government impulse to gag individuals is, sadly, an old and common theme.

On the 20th of October my lawyers informed me they had "gotten things a little confused." There would be no decision that day. It was, in fact, the day Judge Washington returned from vacation. Worse yet, the judge had returned from vacation and gone immediately to the hospital. A diabetic, the judge was having "some trouble." My heart plummeted at the news.

"Just wait a few more days, Bobby."

The days ticked by. The judge left the hospital but there was still no decision nor were there supplies of marijuana from the federal government. Inch by inch we seemed to be moving towards the final scene of Act I but in true theatrical style the most dramatic scenes were yet to come.

11 Giving Thanks

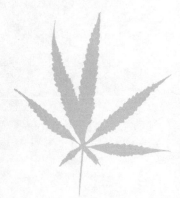

November 3, 1976
8th St. SE
Washington, D.C.

The gray drizzle of autumn made the roads slick and a slight fog settled across the streets. I stood at the window of the apartment and surveyed the scene, a harbinger of coming days that would be dank and cold.

Late on the previous day—a national election day that would see Jimmy Carter elected the 39th president of the United States—a reporter from WMOD radio had called with news that Judge Washington's clerk was hinting at a decision in my case by week's end. Now I punched in Paul's number hoping he could confirm this latest tease. After four months of anxious waiting I was more than ready to hear the verdict was in.

To my amazement, I was immediately put through to Paul and the lawyer was talking even as he picked up the phone.

"Bobby, we haven't double-checked this yet, it's being done now."

Not even a "hello." Paul was providing the correct build, the appropriate entry to the expected news. My adrenaline began to flow.

"Bobby, I don't know . . . on your court decision," the words were hesitant and, while still on track for possible good news, there was a tone that was very different. I began to reassess the conversation.

"From all we know, well, it's impossible right now. Bobby, all we really know is that Judge Washington had a diabetic seizure early this morning. He was on a flight of stairs at the time, collapsed, and broke his neck."

"Is he dead?"

"We think he's alive." These words were a jolt. My brain suddenly came alive with realization. Paul anticipated my next question. "We don't know the status of the decision. Something was said about dictation but we don't know if he had dictated it or was about to."

Paul, sounding sorrowful, rang off with the promise to call as soon as "anything new is learned." I replaced the phone on the hook and walked slowly to the kitchen to tell Alice the news.

The decision, in fact, had been dictated and was on its way to the typist. But an unsigned decision is no decision at all. If Washington failed to recover we would be back at square one. It had all become terribly maddening.

Meanwhile news reports about my case had begun to appear throughout the country. A story ran in *The L.A. Times* and was soon syndicated nationwide. *Newsweek* magazine featured the story in its November 8 issue under the banner of Medicine. *Jet Magazine* ran a small blurb about the Howard program and mentioned a "28-year-old man fighting criminal charges."

Momentum was building and the prospect of redoing the criminal trial was not a comforting one. Judge Washington had survived the fall but was paralyzed. Would it be permanent? Would he be able to certify somehow that his decision was done and would have been signed?

The other aspect of my case—legal supplies of marijuana—was

also stalled. Despite the public perception that my petition had been granted Dr. Merritt was still awaiting supplies of marijuana from the federal government.

November 12, 1976
Howard University
Washington, D.C.

I arrived early and found Merritt in fine form. The press stories were generating all kinds of interest and he was relishing the attention.

My pressures were high, 33/31. "Here, I want you to try this."

Merritt handed me a capsule, the color of oxblood. THC. I knew it well. It won't work, I wanted to say, but I realized Merritt had to play through the role of researcher. I quietly swallowed the pill.

"So, while you're hanging out here I'd like you to meet someone."

I followed the doctor to a room down the hall. As the door opened I was hit with the unmistakable odor of government marijuana. Merritt clearly had supplies of the drug. When would I receive them?

Sitting in the corner was an older man, just finishing a joint. Before I could ask about supplies Merritt launched into introductions and busied himself with taking the man's pulse. "170," he said clipply. Then he turned on his heel and was gone.

For the next two hours I would watch as Mr. Rupert, a 58-year-old research subject, coped with being stoned for the first time. We talked about glaucoma. He had already been through three surgeries—two filtering procedures and one cataract removal. Despite these operations Mr. Rupert was still experiencing pressures in excess of 45 mm Hg. Marijuana was his last resort. If it failed to work there would be a fourth operation.

Crammed in the small office with the hated fluorescent lights overhead, I wondered what it must be like to experience marijuana for the first time with such desperate measures at stake. It was, undoubt-edly, contributing to the man's anxiety. As we talked, I could see the tension begin to ebb. Mr. Rupert talked about his feelings, the "float-ing" of his mind, the small sounds that he found buried in familiar music coming from the radio.

It was a pleasant enough way to pass the time. I wondered what would happen with the man. Merritt came to retrieve me and we walked down the hall to his office. A quick pressure check revealed no change in my IOP. Once again THC had failed.

Merritt dismissed my inquiries about the older man and motioned me to a chair in the corner. For the next hour we talked about Merritt's plans in a frank and revealing fashion. Merritt was on the move. With the Howard program barely open Merritt was already making other plans. He talked about NEI, budgets, future research. There was a cockiness that was unsettling to me. There were refer-ences to "enemies" and some veiled comments on my behavior, my willingness to be "so insistent," to want things "my way."

It was all remarkably friendly but as I considered the young doctor before me there were warning bells ringing softly in the background. Merritt's intentions were not mine. For all the impulse of his emotion and his concern for patients, Merritt was willing to absorb method-ological constraints—double-blind studies, placebo doses—all in the name of science and goodwill with the upper echelon at NEI. Merritt was not only on the move, he was on the make.

It was late on Friday afternoon and the rambling talk had gone on too long. Merritt walked to his desk, opened a drawer, and handed me a clear, rectangular box filled with 45 marijuana cigarettes.

"Now look, Robert, the final clearances, certificates, what-ever, haven't come through yet. If you tell anyone about this take home . . . about this outpatient supply, it's my ass and your sight. You understand?"

I understood all too well. Taking the box from Merritt's hand, I looked the doctor straight in the eye. "But we're working on it, right?"

"You can be a real pain in the butt. You know that?"

"Thanks." I tucked the box into my pocket and extended a hand to the physician. "Thanks a lot."

As I exited Howard and hailed a cab I was awe struck with the stillness of the moment. More than a year after the saga began, here I was triumphant, and there was not a single camera, no waiting microphones, just a creaky D.C. cab finding one too many potholes and reminding me of my treasure each time my hip pocket hit against the vinyl seat.

I'd done it! I'd won.

Merritt was concerned about "no one knowing" but by the time I reached home, before I even told Alice, the news was filtering out. While I was at Howard, conversing with Rupert and Merritt, Jim McManus of CBS had called. "Was it true Robert was getting his medication today?" Alice promised I would call back.

It was close to 3:30 when I finally arrived home. Calls to Merritt and the attorneys pushed the hour to 4:30, too late for CBS. The glorious moment of triumph would remain—for the moment—a quiet victory.

November 18, 1976
Philadelphia, Pennsylvania

Arriving at Penn Station, Alice and I were met by a NORML representative who would escort us to the restaurant for the fundraising dinner. Planned more than a month ago, the trip to Philadelphia had come at a most inopportune time.

Yesterday morning, five days after I had received the first marijuana supplies from Merritt, Jim McManus and CBS had finally arrived at my home. They filmed the government's marijuana as well as a brief interview with "the nation's first legal marijuana smoker."

We were scheduled to see Merritt later that day so Alice could be trained to use the Schiotz, a pressure-measuring device that would allow us to track my IOP readings at home. I was led to a private room and given two marijuana cigarettes to smoke. Merritt had given me the take home supply of marijuana cigarettes the previous Friday but he had not yet observed my reaction to the drug. Today would be his first occasion to verify Helper's readings.

The resulting reduction in pressure was so dramatic that Merritt was ecstatic. It was a moment of conversion, a moment when all the abstract readings became crystallized in one tangible, quantifiable act. Intellectually converted by data, Merritt had now been witness to the extraordinary world of marijuana therapeutics.

That night Alice and I waited anxiously for the "CBS Evening News" with Walter Cronkite. Story after story flashed by and then Cronkite began, "Each year the United States spends $148 million to treat and aid the blind . . ."

Prepared for the Warhol-promised "15 minutes of fame," I braced myself for the story and watched as the report shifted to New York where blind protesters were demonstrating against the U.S. government for callous insensitivity and ill-applied aid.

I rationalized that two stories on the blind, or the near-blind anyway, would be inappropriate and assumed the piece, a "soft" story by news standards, would run the next night—the night we would be in Philadelphia at a NORML fundraiser.

That thought was bad enough but the call from Jim McManus in the morning made things even worse. There was "no visual backdrop" for the piece, McManus explained. Talking heads weren't enough and McManus wasn't sure the piece would ever be seen.

With a heavy heart I felt CBS was lost but there was little time to dwell on the disappointment. WTTG, a local station, was sending out Mary Tillotson to film a story about my legal access. The crew arrived on schedule and Tillotson deftly worked through a quick segment. Would I smoke? Nah, it wasn't time.

As the WTTG crew departed the phone rang with McManus. A CBS crew was already on the way. McManus explained he had realized that my "moment of medication" would provide the "visual background" needed. If I just happened to be medicating soon then the CBS crew could film it.

I groaned and accepted the inevitable. With silent apologies to Mary Tillotson I medicated for CBS news.

Two hours on the train to Philadelphia gave Alice and me a chance to slow down but the frantic pace resumed upon arrival in the City of Brotherly Love. Within an hour I had conducted two interviews for local TV stations and was locked into two studio shows for the next day. At the restaurant I fed comments and posed for pictures as an endless stream of reporters arrived and departed.

Keith arrived shortly after 7 p.m. He had flown in from Albuquerque and stopped by the hotel to freshen up. At 6:55, he reported, CBS ran the Robert Randall story. "Looked great, Bob." A young black man, overhearing the story, stepped forward to ask for my autograph.

We eventually saw the CBS piece, thanks to Jim McManus and a technician at the CBS news room. It was long before VCRs graced America's living rooms. The video clip was never captured for posterity unless it lingers in a CBS vault somewhere.

The anticipated media explosion was upon us. There was no reaction from the government. Smoking for CBS undoubtedly ruffled some feathers but buried the question of you-can-have-it-if-you-don't-tell, at least for the moment. The government had tried to draw a line in the sand but the uniqueness of the story was inescapable. "Bob Smokes Pot! And It's Legal" screamed one headline accompanied by a photo of me blowing smoke in the air. Photographers love smoke in the air, especially illegal smoke.

November 24, 1976
8th St. SE
Washington, D.C.

A light snow was falling when I pulled myself out of bed at 10:15. It was too early by my standards, but I would see Merritt at noon and the doctor wanted me to take 15 mg of THC at 10:30.

Alice was already up, planning a few hours at Creighton's after she dropped me at Howard. At 11:00 the phone rang.

"Bobby?" It was Paul. "John's secretary is on her way to the court-house. The decision is ready." The voice was triumphant and expectant.

"I'll see you at 2:00, Paul."

The lawyer was crestfallen. "You aren't coming down now? John has already called McManus and . . ."

I explained I was already 30 minutes into an experiment for Merritt and due at Howard in less than an hour. The lawyers will have to wait. So will CBS. After months of waiting I was amazed to hear myself calmly delivering this news. "Paul, I don't mind if I'm not the first to know the decision."

After arriving at Howard, Merritt immediately measured my eye pressure and discovered the THC once again, had done little to lower the fluid buildup. Merritt handed me two marijuana cigarettes, told me to "smoke as fast as you can," and left the room.

The next reading was dramatically different and Merritt chuckled. "The phenomena repeats itself, huh?" I delighted in the doctor's delight.

By the time I arrived at Karr & Graves I was, most definitely, stoned. Passing the receptionist with a wave, I rounded the corner and peeked into Paul's office. The lawyer was on the phone but handed the decision across the desk. Covering the mouthpiece he said, "Last page." Familiar with the office layout, I slipped away to the conference room.

I appreciated Paul's shortcut. The decision was hefty, twenty
pages of legal opinion. I flipped to the last page and read the final
paragraph:

> Upon the basis of the foregoing discussion, the Court finds that
> defendant, Robert C. Randall, has established the defense of
> necessity. Accordingly, it is the finding of this Court that he is
> not guilty of a violation of D.C. Code 33-402, and that the
> charges against him must be hereby DISMISSED.

Breathing a sigh of relief, I pulled out a chair from the table and
sat down. Quietly I began leafing through the pages, skimming the
section on "Facts" and moving quickly to "Opinion." My eyes darted
through the paragraphs snatching bits and pieces.

> Penalizing one who acted rationally to avoid a greater harm will
> serve neither to rehabilitate the offender nor deter others from
> acting similarly when presented with similar circumstances.

The words are an elixir. It was far more than I had hoped for. It
is a masterpiece.

Signed from his hospital bed, Judge James Washington had provided a detailed, cogent, perhaps airtight argument in support of his
decision. It was eloquent and seemed flawless. Each part of the argument resonated as the former law school dean carefully defined
the concept of necessity, an ancient seldom used common law tenet,
and then applied the concept to my medical need. Coining the term,
"medical necessity," Washington determined that I had a clear and
unequivocal right to use marijuana to treat my glaucoma. "The evil
he sought to prevent, blindness, is greater than that he performed to
accomplish it, growing marijuana in his residence in violation of D.C.
code."

Washington even went so far as to proclaim "Medical evidence suggests that the prohibition [of marijuana] is not well-founded."

I couldn't fully comprehend it in one sitting but I knew that an important precedent had been established.

I paused for a moment and looked out the window. A light snow was falling. The next day was Thanksgiving Day and the Fates had given me plenty to be thankful for. My thoughts slipped away to the judge, still hospitalized from his fall. "Thanks," I said quietly.

Robert Randall had won and the world was quickly finding out about it. John Karr and I gave several interviews to the local TV and radio stations. I then caught a cab for home where I found a pile of messages from reporters throughout the country. The UPI newswire was carrying the story far and wide.

Friends were notified and arrived with champagne and congratulations. Throughout the evening the phone rang with friends or press. Families were notified and there was much happiness.

By midnight the last guest was gone and the last call from the press answered. Finally alone, Alice and I settled into our own celebration.

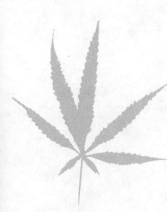

II

Changing Laws

12 Alone in the Lifeboat

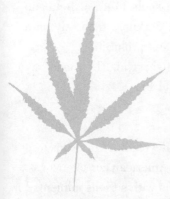

AS AMERICA'S ONLY legal pot smoker I felt like the only man to reach the lifeboat. I was the sole exception to a catholic and absolute prohibition. It was a position of great peril and possibility.

The Government sternly advised silence. If you speak, the bureaucrats warned, your small craft could be swamped by other souls seeking salvation. Better to remain still and be safe. It was not unwise advice. I heard unseen others struggling in the waters all round me.

It is a deeply moral question; to be safe and silent while others suffer. But more than moral motivations occupied my considerations.

The Government promised silence would bring security. But what security is there in silence? Who were we seeking to deceive? If I secretly agreed to the Government's scheme who would I turn to if my access to care was withdrawn? Besides, the bureaucrats would interpret my silence as submission. Most federal officials would be satisfied to intimidate me into muteness. But truly ardent drug warriors would fixate on the danger of my uniqueness. Understanding this threat, such men would not rest until I was erased from the scene.

There is no security in silence. Nor adventure. We were wandering into the last quarter of the first century of the Radio Age. Educated in rhetoric, Fate had conspired to provide me with a unique platform from which to pursue a matter of social merit. Could a lone actor alter the public mind? Would America listen? How might my fellow citizens respond? Six months ago medical marijuana was only mentioned in the backwaters of the federal bureaucracy. Now it was front page news across the continent.

Having won, why go mum? There were souls to save. Better to trust my fellow citizens and shout into the darkness than rely on a devious Government dedicated to a fraudulent prohibition.

Speaking out, I realized, was a matter of survival. The sooner my uniqueness became typical the safer I would be.

As the dramatic and eventful Bicentennial year was drawing to a close, my story virtually exploded upon the American consciousness. In addition to hearing from ordinary citizens with serious ailments I also heard from some celebrities. Cathy Douglas, the wife of Supreme Court Justice William Douglas, called to enlist my help in securing legal supplies of marijuana for a cancer patient. (The patient died before we could organize the effort.) I had some conversations with B. F. Skinner, the noted author and behavioral scientist. Dr. Skinner suffered from glaucoma and conventional medications were failing to control the disease. He tried marijuana, illegally, and felt it provided some relief. But the Harvard professor was uncomfortable using the illegal substance and could not find a way to adapt the substance into his rigid schedule of activities—a behavioral scientist unable to alter his own behavior.

The media blitz was intense and sustained. In the three months following my acquittal I spoke with countless reporters and radio stations. I traveled to New York to appear on "Good Morning America," gave a press conference in the fabled Playboy Towers Hotel in Chicago, posed for *People Magazine*, and taped numerous other TV segments. I was invited to several state legislative sessions where I testified about the medical benefits of marijuana and displayed my small plastic vials filled with government joints. Legislators would jockey to have their picture taken with "America's only legal pot smoker."

In February 1977 I taped a segment of "To Tell the Truth," a long-running TV game show in which celebrities ask questions of three panelists in an effort to determine which one has the unusual occupation or talent, in my case "Legal pot smoker." Not surprisingly I fooled no one. The celebrities, most notably Nipsy Russell and Peggy Cass, showed a sophisticated knowledge of marijuana. Even the elegant Kitty Carlisle was able to select me from the panel.

Robert Randall wasn't exactly a household word but my situation was well known. Invariably I would hear, "Oh yeah! You're that guy, that guy with the eyes." It became a running joke with Alice and me as we made our way through those incredible first months.

The atmosphere was bright with promise. Sanity, it seemed, could prevail. There was a new president, Jimmy Carter, whose young staff was peppered with marijuana smokers. Keith Stroup knew many of them and was optimistic that changes would come, and soon. He spoke in glowing terms of Carter's nominee for drug policy advisor, Dr. Peter Bourne. Throughout the latter part of my ordeal in 1976, Keith had often advised me to contact Bourne, who was then associated with the Drug Abuse Council, a D.C. think tank funded by the Ford Foundation. But I was already working with another individual at the Council, Jane Silver, and wasn't sure what Bourne could do for me in that turbulent year of 1976. Now, with such a contact well-placed in the White House, it seemed the possibilities for expansion of research and medical access to marijuana were opening like the petals on a rose.

This impression was reinforced by an editorial that appeared in *The Washington Post* just ten days after my acquittal entitled "Drugs and Public Policy." The December 6 editorial decried the lack of research into marijuana's medical use, cited my case specifically, and concluded:

"All this [uncertainty] is the clear result of permitting the criminal sanction to blind the rest of us to the fact that this substance needs a great deal of investigation in all aspects, hazards as well as benefits, so that we can protect ourselves from the former and gain what we can from the latter. None of this is happening now."

We were so overjoyed with our success, so confident of a new day dawning, that we didn't see the storm clouds gathering. Another editorial, this one across the continent, would issue a different opinion in the early days of 1977. Appearing in the Spokane, *Washington Chronicle* under the headline "Pot Users Try New Angle," the editorial noted, "Claims that use of marijuana retards glaucoma, an eye disease that usually leads to blindness, is the peg on which the National Organization for the Reform of Marijuana Laws (NORML) will hang its hat in a national campaign to decriminalize use and possession of the drug." The editorial would conclude with an ominous warning. "Opponents to decriminalizing marijuana should go to work immediately on building up a strong case against NORML."

Within six weeks of the decision in my case the battle lines were drawn in the war for medical marijuana. Those lines continue to this day, dug in like the weary soldiers of World War I facing an endless barrage of attack and counterattack. Caught in the no man's land between warring factions are the patients, still waiting for sanity to prevail.

On March 3, 1977, I appeared on the "Tomorrow Show" with Tom Snyder. The Snyder program, which followed Johnny Carson's immensely popular "Tonight Show" on NBC, had a loyal following, especially in the West where time zones presented the show at a more reasonable hour. Snyder was a skillful and playful interviewer. We connected well and the show sailed along smoothly. By that time I was accustomed to "Well Bob, how about lighting one up for the cameras?" I still rebelled against needless smoking but, under the glare of the TV studio lights, my pressures were climbing fast. When Snyder cajoled me to "light one up," I did so. It was the first time I smoked "live" on camera.

When I began my journey through the maze of federal bureaucracies I was focused on Robert Randall but as my story seeped into national consciousness in 1976 I heard from others with numerous afflictions. At first it was just a trickle of correspondence and phone calls. The dual victories of November 1976—legal access and acquittal—turned the trickle to a torrent. The Snyder show amplified the interest even more.

Alice and I responded to each call or letter with increased despair. There was a growing sense of obligation and responsibility to others, but what to do? The logical answer was to file more petitions, to try and do for others what had been done for me. But the circumstances were vastly different. Realistically we could not mount the type of effort that had been successful in my case. It was costly, time consuming, and far too dependent upon the petitioner doing an extraordinary amount of "legwork."

It would be better, we reasoned, if we organized the patients into a concerted effort. On April 26, 1977, we filed a petition with U.S. Attorney General Griffin Bell that was signed by 13 seriously ill individuals including a schoolteacher from Ohio, a craftsman from Missouri, a prisoner from Florida, and a cancer patient from Pennsylvania. Also among them was my old roommate from Johns Hopkins, Vincent Mustachio. We asked the Attorney General to schedule open hearings to consider the reclassification of marijuana and allow its medical use.

In the Spring of 1977, such an action by a diverse group of individuals generated another round of media attention and shifted the focus beyond me. Local news stories appeared wherever a petitioner happened to reside. In Kansas, *The Wichita Eagle* featured the story of 62-year-old Ara Cron, a glaucoma patient and retired schoolteacher, who lamented she was "too old to get the drug" but pleaded for an opportunity to try it. She left it clear the opportunity did not necessarily have to be legal. She cited a long family history of glaucoma and her concerns about risky surgery. Ara's story would, in fact, generate a "donation" of marijuana from a concerned citizen. She tried smoking the drug and her husband Gerald measured the results with a Schiotz. They were impressive, dropping from 40+ mm of pressure to readings in the high teens. This was enough to convince Ara's doctor who began pursuing an IND application of his own and was pleased with the cooperation promised by the FDA and NIDA. It seemed my case was opening the doors for others.

But it was also beginning to place me in some peril.

May 13, 1977
Howard University
Washington, D.C.

"You're not going to like this, but I can't give you any more marijuana." Merritt did not mince his words.

I was just back from California where I had participated as a panelist during the Medical Marijuana session at the National Conference on Drug Abuse (NCDA). The session was particularly well attended. There was a great deal of interest in America's Only Legal Pot Smoker, and the conference received a tremendous media push as a result of my presence.

Among the other panelists was Dr. Robert Peterson, the NIDA official who once told me "you'll never make it through the bureaucratic layers." The NCDA crowd was clearly sympathetic to me and I was highly critical of NIDA's failure to aggressively research marijuana's therapeutic applications. Peterson was forced to defend a policy that he obviously felt was shallow and stupid. After the panel, as I was being ushered away by a conference organizer, Peterson cornered me for an instant and asked how I could manage to travel to San Francisco on just a week's supply of marijuana. In fact, I had a nine-day supply.

Ever since my appearance on the "Snyder" show, there had been discussions about "Randall's take home supply" and increased mobility. High-up officials were annoyed with my public exposure and growing notoriety. The bureaucrats had ignored the initial press rush, assuming my celebrity status would fade. But now it was obvious that I was doing everything I could to feed the fires of interest in medical marijuana. There were those appearances on TV, game shows, travel to legislatures everywhere, and now I was appearing at conferences like an expert!

On May 12, as I made the press rounds in Los Angeles, a little known committee of the FDA, the Drug Abuse Research Advisory Committee (DARAC) was meeting in the Parklawn Building. It had "invited" Dr. Merritt to "discuss" his research program but the discussion quickly shifted to my personal conduct. After considerable talk, Merritt was asked to leave the room and a secret vote was held. Merritt was then informed that I would no longer be authorized to possess any more than a daily supply of marijuana. When Merritt protested that such a system would inconvenience him as well as me he was told, quite bluntly, that DARAC could revoke Merritt's research license if he failed to cooperate. Moreover, there were criminal liabilities that could be invoked. Merritt delivered the news to me the next day.

I immediately called Ed Tocus, my contact at the FDA. Tocus was not surprised at the call but he was taken aback at the extent of my knowledge. With the delivery of Merritt's bombshell, I had started putting the pieces together. While in California I had telephoned Dr. Hepler and learned of a "committee that was making some inquiries" about my "personality traits." Not surprisingly, Hepler refused to answer such inquiries. The committee had called Hepler shortly after the "Snyder" show.

I asked Tocus outright if it was the same committee that had met with Merritt and Tocus confirmed it was.

"Under the DARAC policy of daily supply I'd become a medical prisoner of the District of Columbia." I spoke slowly and with a measured tone. I wanted to be certain that Tocus answered the next question without any emotional overtones. "Do you expect me to stay in Washington until I go blind?"

There was barely a pause. "That, I believe, was the intention of at least some committee members in voting to restrict your supply."

Tocus' reply was delivered with such calm that it shook me to the bone. "Look, I have three joints left. That's enough for this afternoon. Today is Friday and Merritt has made it clear he will not be available this weekend. So, if provisions are not made to resupply me before this evening, you, DARAC, and the FDA will be in court on Monday morning."

I had no way of backing up such a threat. I was still in debt to my lawyers from the criminal case and there was little hope of finding anyone else on such short notice. But the bluff worked. My supplies were reinstated. DARAC had seriously overstated its power. As an advisory committee it could only "recommend" policy to the FDA, and the regulations did not allow such recommendations to become true policy until the minutes were published in the federal register and public hearing was held. That was months away. The FDA was acting in a totally improper manner by implementing DARAC's "recommendation" so quickly without review. Their braggadocio had been as bold as my own.

But the game was far from over. In mid-April, sensing that my days were numbered as America's Only Legal Pot Smoker, I had decided it was time to play the Bourne card. Since entering the White House Dr. Bourne's sensitivities to marijuana issues had been considerably lessened. As President Carter's drug abuse expert and special assistant to the President for Health, Bourne seemed to be leaning towards continued spraying of the herbicide Paraquat on Mexican marijuana plants. But he had remained silent on the matter of marijuana's medical use and this gave me some hope.

My purpose in writing Dr. Bourne in April 1977 was to inform him of our petition effort which Alice and I had organized with the other patients. I was careful with my words. "I have had limited desire to attack those agencies responsible for my access to marijuana." I wrote. "While the system of marijuana management itself seems ill conceived and mal-administered, I did receive a measure of justice. I had reason to believe, for a time, that adjustments would go forward."

Later in the letter I would write,

The present system pits public policy against human biology. The human reaction to this conflict of values cannot greatly enhance the authority of the law and creates the possibility of ill-informed individuals engaging in attempted medical self-treatment. The Schedule I prohibition has almost no benefits. It has been a failure in discouraging the recreational use of marijuana and a success at denying an expansion of our medical knowledge. It has the double disadvantage of denying millions of individuals the civil rights which are theirs and of denying additional millions of their biological well-being.

On June 6, 1977, Dr. Bourne responded. His letter was very clear.

As a physician, I understand and have great empathy with the issues you raised. I can assure you that my feelings are shared by hundreds, perhaps thousands, of physicians and researchers who have fought to bring relief and discover new treatments and cures. The responsible agency staffs and researchers in-

volved in the marijuana and glaucoma issue all share with me
a great feeling of compassion and are pledged to pursue the
question. However, this compassion cannot be allowed to over-
shadow the basic questions.

Bourne then elaborated on the need for research and the problems
with the cannabinoid eyedrop. Finally he got to the heart of the matter.

I understand that technical questions remain about your status
under the law in that you are not really legally authorized to
possess marijuana to treat your glaucoma. Under the law, the
researcher (Dr. Merritt in your case) is authorized to possess
and administer it. If you disregard some of the conditions of
the study, it may be jeopardized. I understand that the agencies
involved have not authorized your take-home supply but have
chosen to overlook it in their compassion for your case. Publicity in the case has forced consideration of tightening up the
dispensing of your supplies.

Dr. Bourne was threatening to use my medical need in an attempt
to constrain my right to speak. It was medical blackmail. Bureaucrats can threaten and bluster through procedures and phone calls,
but are seldom reckless enough to issue them in hard black and
white.

Within three days of the Bourne letter came a second blow. As
Bourne had noted, there was some concern about my status with
respect to legally possessing marijuana. My lawyers had appealed to
the U.S. Attorney General for a statement of immunity, and the appeal was forwarded to the Drug Enforcement Administration. The
drug agency refused to extend such immunity.

The warnings were now unmistakable. Either I could keep quiet and retain my marijuana or I could talk and my marijuana would be taken away.

My sight or my right to speak.

The research program at Howard University was becoming a battleground on which the government and I were playing out a game of constant escalation.

Seeking advice, and allies, I took the Bourne letter to NORML and showed it to their general counsel, Peter Meyers, who agreed the letter was a clear threat but advised that little could be done until the government rescinded my supplies. The letter was also shown to Keith.

Later that night I received a call from a reporter who worked with Jack Anderson, a nationally known syndicated columnist, renowned for breaking controversial stories on government officials. The reporter wanted me to comment on Bourne's letter! When I asked how he had obtained a copy of the document he mentioned Keith Stroup.

I pleaded with the reporter to hold the story. I had not discussed the matter with Merritt and I was very concerned about the potential ramifications of such a "leak" and how his study would be affected. Bourne had clearly stated the program could be in jeopardy. My pleadings were in vain. The next morning Jack Anderson reported Bourne's threats on "Good Morning America." The matter threatened to escalate even further when "Good Morning America" invited me to appear the next day to "explain this White House thing." I agreed, fearing that refusal to appear would further inflame the curiosity of the media. For slightly more than two minutes I answered questions on national TV, avoiding the mention of Bourne's name and attempting to defuse the situation.

It was a dangerous and revealing skirmish. Keith was willing to sacrifice my health care for an opportunity to watch Peter Bourne squirm. I learned to keep my own counsel. I learned that NORML's agenda was not necessarily my own.

In that reckless time there would be one more effort by the FDA to silence me, to force me from "patient" into "research subject."

June 20, 1977
Ohio Drug Studies Institute
Otterbein College, Ohio

The message light was blinking on my phone as I entered the hotel room. It was a call from Alice. I immediately dialed home.

"Merritt called. He sounds desperate. Something about a consent form."

I groaned and wondered what this latest crisis was about.

I put a call through to Howard University and found Merritt as Alice described him. The tension was palpable.

"Ten months, man! Ten months you've been receiving this stuff and *now* they want a consent form." Merritt was angry. "I swear, I don't understand those people, I don't understand them at all."

I understood very well. Consent forms aren't signed by patients; consent forms are for research subjects. By getting me to sign a form, the FDA would be codifying its control over my care.

After speaking at the Ohio conference, I flew back to D.C. where Merritt presented the form. I read it carefully. It was ominous.

By signing the form I would bestow on the FDA the following authority:

1. My marijuana could be replaced with placebo doses, regardless of the medical consequences.
2. The agency reserved the right to determine when "enough" research had been conducted.
3. The FDA had the right to determine which type of "THC vehicle" (smoked, pills, eyedrops) was appropriate.

The trap was transparent. "I can't sign this." I looked at the physician.

"You agreed to sign it last November." Merritt was not pushing, only making an observation.

"No. *We* agreed it wasn't necessary." Merritt said nothing but handed me my week's supply of medication. "I'll let the FDA know your decision."

I arrived home to a ringing phone. It was Merritt.

"Tocus made it very clear, Robert. Either you sign or I face criminal sanctions for supplying you with marijuana."

I promised to return to Howard. After hanging up the phone I entered my office, hastily typed a statement of duress, then headed back across town to Howard. Merritt watched as I reread the consent form, scratched through the offending paragraphs, and signed the document. "I don't think that will work, Bob."

"Well, maybe this will." I removed the statement of duress from my pocket and asked Merritt to watch as I signed it. I then asked Merritt to sign as a witness. Merritt shook his head as he signed the statement. "You're pushing it."

"No, they're pushing it, Dr. Merritt. I was clear from the first about my need for marijuana. I am not a research subject. I've been through research and it showed I need marijuana. I will not give up my rights to satisfy a bunch of bureaucrats who can't acknowledge the truth."

"Okay, okay." Merritt took the duress statement and stapled it to the consent form. "You stay here, I'll call Tocus."

It was a long fifteen minutes in Merritt's outer office. I *was* pushing, had been pushing. But I had never agreed to daily supplies and I wasn't about to backtrack now. NORML's general counsel had indicated there would be reason to sue if the government rescinded my supplies. If the statement of duress didn't work then I would go immediately to NORML from Howard. I didn't like the option but there were no others I could see at the moment.

The door opened and Merritt emerged, smiling slightly. "You

win," he said. "Tocus agrees to accept your edited consent form and your statement of duress IF you promise not to release either to the press or make any comments about this."

We smiled at one another.

"See you next week."

In that same week I would receive a call from Ara Cron. The news was not pleasant. Despite her doctor's willingness to sign the necessary IND papers, NIDA and the FDA bungled and delayed his request for permission to use marijuana in treating Ara's glaucoma. The anonymous gift of marijuana, sent as a result of her story in the *Wichita Eagle*, had lasted two weeks and was gone. Without marijuana Ara's IOP had risen to its old levels. She and Gerald didn't know where to buy more, didn't know who to trust, didn't know where to turn. For weeks they pleaded with Robert Peterson at NIDA and Ed Tocus at FDA. Senator Bob Dole intervened on her behalf but still the agencies stonewalled.

Trapped in red tape, Ara underwent surgery on June 1 for one eye and June 3 for the other. The operations were successful within the medical definition of success. Ara's IOP was under excellent management, but much of her sight was lost due to complications following surgery. Ara had been blinded by the same agencies that were demanding control over my own medical future.

Through a spiraling escalation of pressure and White House comment, the government had created a balance of terror. By reckless actions and statements I had been placed on notice. If I continued to talk my marijuana would be taken away. Like Ara, I would suffer irreversible damage before I could manage a response if I could manage one at all.

But the same reckless actions and statements were my best defense. That and the medical reality of marijuana's effectiveness. If my access was disrupted and I managed to pull together a court challenge the resulting damage to bureaucratic drug policies would be irreversible. Even if such an action finally lost in court the media lash would leave profound marks on future policy.

November 27, 1977
8th St. SE
Washington, D.C.

"There's a story on the wire," Dave Anderson at UPI said. "I'd like your comment."

The 3 p.m. wire story, dateline Wichita, carried Ara Cron's story to the nation. It had been triggered by my recent anniversary—one year of legal marijuana smoking.

Deep within the wire service copy was a passing mention of Dr. Merritt's study followed by a brief paragraph which read, "But he is phasing out the program until he moves to another city."

"Would you care to comment?" Dave Anderson asked.

"No," I said. "It's the first I've heard of anything like that. I've got an appointment tomorrow. It must be a mistake."

Dave doubted his wire service would make such a mistake. But when the UPI wire on Ara repeated at 5 p.m. the paragraph on Dr. Merritt's plans was missing.

The next day I traveled to Howard. The routine was typical. Pressures were taken, Merritt gave me my weekly supply. Then he drew me towards a small office. "We need to talk," Merritt said.

"Is it true you're leaving Washington?" I asked preemptively. "A UPI reporter called and. . . ."

After taking a deep breath Merritt said, "The UPI story is true. I was hoping to tell you first, but someone leaked the news. I've received a grant, a big grant, from the National Eye Institute to study marijuana's effects on glaucoma." Merritt nervously shifted. "But they won't give me the grant if I stay at Howard," Merritt said. "Instead, the NEI wants me to do the study down in Chapel Hill at the University of North Carolina."

"North Carolina. Like Research Triangle Park, North Carolina?" I asked.

"That's right."

"And they'd prefer that you give me up as a patient, right?"

"That's right. I mean, it would be impossible for you to keep up weekly visits if I'm 350 miles away." Merritt was trying to seem sensible.

"Maybe we could stretch out the time between visits." I was trying to remain calm.

"I don't think they'd allow us to do that," Merritt replied with the certainty of a man who had already explored the option.

"Well," I said, realizing my fate was sealed, "a big grant from NEI, and a promotion at a new school like the University of North Carolina is too good to turn down."

"It certainly is," Merritt smiled, self-satisfied by his coup. "It certainly is."

Having failed at numerous other attempts to "rein me in" the government finally found the weak link—Merritt. The bureaucrats at the DEA and FDA and NEI were willing to pay Merritt a very hefty price to disrupt my legal access—$95,000 per year for 3 years plus a professorship at UNC. With Hepler no longer involved in research, Merritt would have an exclusive right to explore marijuana as an ocular therapeutic. Generous federal funding, a new professorship, and all the professional credit he could handle. It was, simply stated, an exceedingly tempting offer. And Merritt, exceedingly tempted, had taken the bait, hook, line and sinker.

Merritt would continue his study of marijuana and glaucoma for a number of years at UNC, publishing numerous articles in scientific journals that underscored marijuana's ability to reduce intraocular pressure. He was genuinely interested in the medicinal properties of marijuana but I've always felt he erred in leaving Howard. In North Carolina he became part of the effort to develop synthetic forms of the drug that could be used instead of the natural substance. An admirable goal but one that does little for those with an immediate need, like myself and the countless others who contacted him for help when he was at Howard. Over the years we lost contact with one another.

As he began to prepare for his move to North Carolina Merritt promised to make some inquiries on my behalf to locate a new doctor. I'd been down that road before and didn't have much faith that things would work out. I was in serious trouble, again.

December 3, 1977
NORML
Washington, D.C.

Nationally interviewed, impoverished and, quite possibly soon-to-be blind, I walked into NORML with an agenda. The staff was deep into conference preparations. Everyone was friendly as I was ushered into Keith's office.

"What can I do for you, Bobby?" Keith said lighting a fat joint. Stroup took a drag, then passed it to me.

"I've got two problems, Keith. First, we need to make some money."

"You want a job at NORML?" Keith seemed receptive.

"No, I want you to give Alice a job so she can work on medical marijuana full-time." I was determined to keep myself out of NORML and NORML politics and, in particular, out of the "social" issue. Alice, on the other hand, was not publicly identified with the medical issue and already handling calls from patients on a regular basis at home. Her Aussie reporter, Creighton Burns, was headed home and she needed work. Moreover, many of the inquires we were receiving were being routed through NORML. Why not have someone working on the premises?

"Alice would like to call it the "Medical Reclassification Project," I added. It was better if Keith understood we'd thought it through.

"Well, Bobby. I'm not sure. We've had some husband/wife teams that didn't work out well." Keith was cautious. "What else is on your mind?"

"It seems my doctor's leaving Washington. He got a big grant to study marijuana in North Carolina . . ."

"But he can't take care of you, right?" Keith knew the score.

"So, I'd like your help in finding a doctor. Also, I need a good attorney," I said. "A really good attorney."

"Well, we couldn't possibly take this case in-house," Keith said protecting his assets. "And all the NORML lawyers are into criminal defense," Keith added, hedging his help. "But, we'll see what we can come up with. You all ready for the conference?"

I would be a speaker at NORML's 5th Annual Conference scheduled to open five days later at a posh Washington hotel. It would be populated by nearly 500 criminal lawyers, civil libertarians, Harvard professors, hippie activists, potheads, members of the press and other mildly psychotic types. Hunter S. Thompson was the keynote speaker.

NORML, which billed itself as a "public interest group" was, in fact, a legal referral service designed to deliver the victims of prohibition into the waiting hands of defense attorneys. A lucrative business operating under the guise of social outrage.

By late 1977, NORML's public image of working for the little guy—the "cannabis consumer"—was giving way to the grim rise of cocaine. Civil liberties for pot smokers was a nice abstraction. But the big bucks legal cases increasingly involved coke. Most NORML lawyers were long enough out of law school to be attracted by cash. And coke. They had built thriving practices representing people snared in small-time pot busts. In the process they got rich enough to afford cocaine. Needless to say, the conference was dominated by highly aggressive criminal lawyers en route to becoming cocaine cowboys. As a wag would later say, "Cocaine is God's way of telling people they have too much discretionary income."

We were mystified by cocaine: $100 per gram for an elusive "high" which lasted 15 minutes. Why bother? Why waste the money?

Regardless of our views the 1977 NORML conference was a "snowstorm." Everyone either had coke, or knew someone who had coke or was looking to score: big rocks, small rocks, razor blades and thin lines of finely chipped white power. People snorted coke in their rooms, in public bathrooms, at conference sessions, and during Hunter S. Thompson's incoherent keynote speech.

During the conference, we visited with friends made during the past year, met members of the press and spoke to a very small number of people actually interested in medical marijuana. By Saturday night we were so weary of cokeheads and coke-crazed crowds, we skipped NORML's notorious conference party and headed home to watch Mary Tyler Moore. It was, we would later learn, a very wise move.

13 Square One…Again

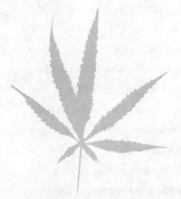

THERE HAD BEEN one bright moment during the NORML conference—Lynn.

Throughout 1977 we heard from many individuals who medically required marijuana. All had sad tales, nearly all were in desperate need of help. Most wanted Alice and me to help them. Lynn, initially, was no different.

December 1977
NORML Conference
Washington, D.C.

"Mr. Randall?"

I looked up from my chair in the lounge of the Capitol Hyatt to find a hairless young man—tall and thin as Lincoln—holding out a gigantic hand. "I'm Lynn Pierson. We spoke on the phone?"

Weary with conference fatigue, I invited the man to take a seat. Others departed as Lynn sat down, got introduced around, ordered a drink, and began to speak. "I was wondering if you could help me get medical marijuana," he said.

"Why don't you tell me something about yourself, first," I replied.

"We discussed this on the phone," Lynn was impatient.

"I talk to a lot of people. Refresh my memory." I vaguely remembered Lynn's call, but could not recall any specifics. "Tell me what you want."

"Legal marijuana," Lynn replied with a hint of annoyance.

"Everyone wants legal marijuana. Why do you want it?" After a year of listening to people I could be curt when I was tired. Lynn did not flinch.

"I have cancer," he said.

"And . . . ?" I didn't flinch either.

"And I need your help." Lynn was direct and, when challenged, mildly aggressive.

We could not have been more different. I was short, introspective, cynical and quick-witted. Lynn was tall, candid, and somewhat boisterous. More rodeo than redneck, he hailed from New Mexico, the Land of Enchantment. Lynn was a can-do creature of open spaces and grand vistas. We were an unlikely duo.

The outline of Lynn's story was written in his frame. At 25, cancer and chemotherapy had eaten his bulk and rendered him bald. A strapping young man riddled with a terminal disease, Lynn told us his tale.

Diagnosed in 1975 with testicular cancer, Lynn was being treated at the Albuquerque Veterans Hospital. He'd had surgery—"they cut off my nuts," Lynn explained—but the cancer had spread. So the doctors told him chemo was his only hope. The first dose of Cisplatin—then one of the newest, most highly toxic anti-cancer drugs available—left Lynn sick and vomiting for days.

"It was terrible," Lynn recalled. "I couldn't eat, couldn't even smell food without vomiting. There was constant nausea. I knew I wouldn't survive that kind of chemical torture. And it was real hard on my family too."

Lynn returned to the V.A. hospital and told his doctor "no way." He could not, would not tolerate the debilitating nausea and vomiting caused by Cisplatin. He bluntly told his doctor he would rather die.

The oncologist's reply shocked Lynn. "Have you tried marijuana?" The physician pulled out a recent issue of *The New England Journal of Medicine* and showed Lynn an article by Drs. Stephen Sallan and Norman Zinberg. "These Harvard doctors report marijuana can reduce the side effects of chemotherapy. You're a young man, Lynn. You can find yourself some of this stuff. Give it a try before you give up."

"It was a miracle," Lynn said. "A few puffs of pot took the nausea away. And there was hardly any vomiting. Then I got real hungry. Hell, I ate so much I actually gained some weight."

"So," I interrupted, "you know marijuana works, and you know how to get it. Why go through all the hassle of trying to get it legally, Lynn?" I listened to myself give advice that had made me furious in 1976. But I could tell by looking at the lanky New Mexican that chemo was tough enough. There was probably a good chance that, despite the chemo, Lynn was dying.

"Getting legal marijuana is not an easy thing to do." I continued. "I don't know how bad your situation is, but, to put it bluntly, you could spend the rest of your life trying to get marijuana legally."

Eighteen months ago I had bristled at such thinking but, with the 20-20 vision of hindsight, it was not such bad advice after all. This young man before me could spend his final days in better ways than chasing bureaucrats on the phone and waiting anxiously for distant authorities to make up their minds.

Lynn paused and chose his words carefully. "I have—had—a friend who needed help," Lynn said and went on to talk about an older man whom he had befriended at the Albuquerque V.A. Hospital. The two had much in common: the same diagnosis, the same mutilating surgery, and the intense negative reaction to chemo.

"I told my friend about how marijuana helped," Lynn said. "And his doctors urged him to try pot. But he refused. He was sick and afraid. He said he'd never broken any laws and wasn't going to die a criminal."

"So he suffered and died," I said. "And that's why you want to get legal marijuana?"

"Yeah." A silence fell across the table. I was lost in thought about Vince Mustachio and my days at Johns Hopkins. I understood what Lynn was saying.

"When did your friend die, Lynn?" Alice gently asked.

"About a month ago. Then I heard about this conference, and remembered seeing Mr. Randall when he came to Santa Fe to testify before our legislature. I thought maybe you could help me."

"Why didn't you talk to me after the hearing?" I asked, recalling the hearings in February 1977.

"You looked busy. There were a lot of people around. I was sick. It wasn't the right time," Lynn explained.

We continued chatting idly about family. Lynn was married but had no children. He was born in Kansas but grew up in New Mexico and had many connections, including some prominent friends in the legal system. Lynn had thought about going to court to receive marijuana but he wanted to do something bigger, something more inclusive.

"I was thinking about a study, like the one you're in." I resisted the urge to say I wasn't in a study. "That way others could get supplies, too. I know my doctor would help. He's the one who . . ."

"Lynn," I interrupted with a flash of insight. "You've got something I don't have," I said.

"What's that?" Lynn asked.

"A state legislature," I replied. "Maybe we should pass a law."

"Maybe we should," Lynn said smiling.

It was a "Eureka" moment, one of those split seconds in which things become crystal clear and a small part of your brain shouts, "Eureka!" In the animated cartoons from the 1940s and '50s, it is that moment when a light bulb materializes above the cartoon character's head.

Lynn returned to New Mexico and immediately began a two-track approach. He contacted a lawyer and explored the possibility of going to court to obtain marijuana. But he also began making phone calls to legislators and state government offices. Throughout the holidays we talked regularly on the phone, getting to know one another and outlining a political strategy. New Mexico state representative Tom Rutherford was interested and anxiously asked for legal language. I began working with the New Mexico's Legislative Council Services on the language for such legislation. While Rep. Rutherford's support was helpful, I advised Lynn to seek help on the Republican side of the aisle. New Mexico is fiercely conservative and I knew the legislation wouldn't fly without help from the Republicans.

NORML was skeptical about the chances of medical marijuana succeeding in New Mexico. When I mentioned the situation to Keith, the cagey drug reformer was categorical. "Bobby, don't put a lot of effort into this. There's just no way a state, especially a conservative state like New Mexico, is going to pass a medical marijuana law. No way." Two years before Keith had given me similar counsel about my own case.

And it was my own situation that received most of my focus during this period. Merritt was leaving and I needed to secure a doctor who could assume responsibility for my care. When Merritt first announced his departure I had held some hope that everything might work itself out but in my late December talks with officials at NIDA this illusion was quickly shattered.

"What's the problem?" Robert Petersen at NIDA asked. "You know how to get marijuana. And, believe me, unless you buy a psychedelic trip van and start selling pot to school kids no one in this town is ever going to bust you again. So, what's the problem?"

The message was clear. The bureaucrats did not care if I smoked pot but they were determined I would no longer do it legally. If I went blind, well, that's life. It was a risk the bureaucrats were prepared to take. It was a well-calculated assault based on the simple assumption that I could not assemble the considerable resources— the doctors, the lawyers, the funds—needed to challenge them. It seemed, at the time, a very safe bet.

Over Christmas Keith contacted Drs. Norman Zinberg and Lester Grinspoon at Harvard, but neither could provide any leads in the doctor search. Dr. Merritt was also running into a wall. None of his ophthalmic colleagues at Howard were willing to take responsibility for my unusual therapy.

Things were no more promising on the lawyer front. NORML, an organization awash in attorneys, could not find one lawyer willing to take what was certain to be a complicated, time-consuming, financially unrewarding case. There was, after all, no criminal charge. Instead, this would be a purely civil matter. Besides, no one was sure what kind of legal argument I could raise to compel the United States to provide me with medical access to an officially prohibited substance. Time was running out.

Alice got the job at NORML and started setting up the Medical Reclassification Project during the first week of 1978. While the job paid only slightly more than minimum wage it would pay the rent and transfer the growing costs of communicating with patients— phone calls and postage—out of our meager household budget.

As one of her first projects, Alice reprinted a report issued in October 1977 by the Hawaiian Public Health Service (HPHS). It was the first state-sponsored report on marijuana's medical use, a summary and bibliography of contemporary research. It would become a valuable tool in the coming months. Not surprisingly, the HPHS recommended more research but one recommendation was surprising.

Because glaucoma eventually results in blindness, the task force further recommends that persons suffering from glaucoma who are unresponsive to conventional medications not be prohibited from using marijuana to control their disease.

The report also provided a springboard for an unexpected trip. To capitalize on the HPHS report an attorney in Honolulu invited me to the Aloha State to meet with the Hawaiian legislature. In the dead of winter, with the gathering gloom of supply disconnection, I was more than happy to take an all-expense-paid trip to the tropics.

January 2-8, 1978
Honolulu, Hawaii

Hy Greenstein was an eccentric gentleman of advancing years who drove a flashy sports car, wore bright white suits and shiny green patent leather shoes. "It helps clients remember my name," Hy explained. Hy had lived in Hawaii for decades, knew the important players, and was well regarded by the locals—a Don Quixote character who defended the weak.

I found Hy easy to like. The man had style. Upon our meeting, he presented me with a beautifully hand-painted T-shirt featuring an all-seeing blue eye in the middle of a huge green marijuana leaf. Very handsome. I wore the shirt once and then had it framed.

Hy—who had made his fortune long ago—treated me to first class accommodations on the beach at Waikiki. In return, I spent my days working the Hawaiian legislature. I also blanketed Honolulu media with multiple press and TV interviews and loads of radio talk. The incoming chatter was all positive. People knew about the HPHS Report and widely accepted its conclusion that marijuana should be legally available to the seriously ill.

One evening, after the legislature closed and the media quieted, I was invited to dine with Senator Anson Chong, a young Hawaiian of Chinese descent and the member of a powerful family.

Senator Chong drove me into the hills above Honolulu to watch the sunset and see the city lights come on. Following an excellent Chinese dinner we wandered among the Japanese tourists on Waikiki, then stopped at an elegant piano bar for drinks overlooking the beach. After an hour of pleasant talk, Senator Chong—now Anson—said, "Robert, it's time you see the real Hawaii. You're with me, so it will be safe."

We drove to a neighborhood dive where tourists feared to tread. Anson returned with a huge man in tow.

Though only an inch or two taller than me, the man was utterly, massively square in that way Samoans can be. "This is my friend," Anson said. "Show him your marijuana, Robert."

Without much thought I pulled out my brown prescription bottle, popped the lid and showed the man my government-rolled pot. "That's marijuana?" the large man said with a slight slur.

"Yes," I said, putting the cap back on the bottle.

Without comment the man reached across, plucked the bottle from my hand and headed out the door. Anson had disappeared into the crowd and was unavailable to help. I was just intoxicated enough to follow the massive man into the street. "You can't have that," I said.

The huge Hawaiian abruptly stopped and turned causing me to slam into the massive man's rock hard stomach. "Marijuana is wrong," he said.

There was no way—no way—I was going to force this man to give back the pot. I fumbled for words. "I need that marijuana," I said.

"No. I won't give you it."

"Why not?"

"I fought in Korea for freedom. Pot is wrong. You are a criminal."

"You fought in Korea?" I was confused. The man seemed too

young to have participated in the Korean conflict but the bar had been dimly lit and I had barely focused on the man before my bottle was snatched away.

"Yes. I was fleet wrestling champ," the massive man said proudly. There was no reason to disbelieve him. "Then I lost my eye."

"You're blind in one eye?"

"Yes. Blind from shrapnel. No more wrestling."

"But that's why I need marijuana," I said. "I'm also blind in one eye. And marijuana helps me keep the sight in my other eye. It's medicine."

By this time Anson had caught up with us on the dark street. "What he's saying is true," Anson told his massive friend. "This man came here to help us, to educate us. You should not treat him like this. He is our friend. Please, give him back his marijuana."

The huge Hawaiian studied me carefully with his one good eye and then, without warning, enveloped me in a crushing embrace. "I am sorry," he said. "I misunderstood."

The simplicity of the statement was heartfelt and sincere. Driving back to the hotel I wondered why the government could not be as kind as my huge Hawaiian friend.

January 13, 1978
Howard University Hospital
Washington, D.C.

Dr. Merritt's office was cluttered with cardboard boxes. The photos were off the walls, the file cabinets emptied, the desk cleared. The pressure check was anticlimactic; perfectly normal.

"I'm giving you all the marijuana I have," Merritt explained as he cleaned out his safe and counted out the last joints in the last tin. "Just over 100. If you smoke carefully this should get you through the end of the month. After that . . ."

I'm on my own, good luck, I thought. As Merritt handed over the pre-rolled joints, I reached into my coat and pulled out a ten-page document. "I've worked on this over the last two weeks," I told Merritt. "I'd like you to read it, make any corrections, then sign it. How long before you leave town?"

"I leave in two days," Merritt said as he flipped through the typewritten pages. "What is this, anyway?"

"It's an affidavit. It reviews my last 14 months of treatment, describes how marijuana is medically used to control my eye pressure, and reaches some conclusions about the nature of my care. I think you'll find it very matter-of-fact," I said. It was, of course, a test. How far had Merritt defected?

"This is to help you if you have to go to court?" Merritt was wavering.

"That's right," I replied. "We can refine it when—if—I get an attorney. But I thought it would be wise to make a clear record before you leave town. I don't want to have to track you down in North Carolina."

"That makes sense," Merritt said. "And I don't see anything in this affidavit I disagree with."

"Fine. But give it a careful read. I'll call tomorrow to correct any mistakes or get a signed copy. Oh, if you sign it make sure there's a notary. This has to be notarized," I was insistent.

Merritt looked up from his desk, smiled. "I'll see you tomorrow, Robert."

Merritt signed the affidavit and vanished into his new world. I was truly sorry to see him go. He'd appeared out of nowhere, offered help when no one else would and been a very good doctor. For over a year Merritt had protected me from the most blatant bureaucratic abuses but, as his departure drew near, some part of me wanted to protect him. I couldn't understand why he was surrendering his secure position at one of the nation's leading universities for a pocketful of promises.

Merritt believed, somewhat näively, that he could outsmart the bureaucrats: believed he could take their money and prove marijuana really did help people with glaucoma. If he played his cards right he could secure his career, make a name for himself and save the world.

With Merritt's defection I realized the bureaucrats were willing to pay nearly any price to shut me up. I was causing too many waves. Doubtless, Merritt had even used me as leverage to secure the best possible deal from NEI and FDA. In the end it was simply too good to turn down.

"You'll look me up if you come to North Carolina?" Merritt had asked.

"If I still have my eyesight," I promised.

In 1976 I had learned a valuable lesson: when confronting danger speak loudly. With any luck someone will hear. The press had been my salvation on several occasions and now, with increasingly bleak options, it was time to make noise. But how?

For more than a year I had made news. Big news, little news. The story was featured in national magazines, reported on national news broadcasts, repeated on local TV outlets and enhanced by hours of radio talk. But it was episodic and opportunistic. I would attend a legislative hearing in New Mexico or Iowa and make news. Or do a press conference in Chicago arranged by *Playboy* and make news. Or help someone like Ara Cron and make news.

But, since the end of my trial there had been genuine national news only once, when Alice and I organized the thirteen other seriously ill patients and publicly petitioned the DEA to end the medical prohibition.

NORML could have made news but I did not want to be NORML's news. Besides, the leak of Bourne's letter to Jack Anderson had made me wary of NORML.

The nation's only legal marijuana smoker was about to be cut off by bureaucrats trying to control his speech. Surely, I thought, this is news.

For a week I typed and retyped a press release. The final result was a lumpy, all-too-wordy four-page diatribe. Less than satisfied, I made multiple copies, mailed many, then delivered others by hand to the National Press Building.

Silence.

I learned getting legal marijuana was news. Losing it was being just like everyone else. Being like everyone else ain't news.

It was looking grim, I thought, as I smoked my way through the last government joints. Very grim.

January 24, 1978
8th St. SE
Washington, D.C.

I reached for the ringing phone.

"This is Dave Anderson at UPI. We spoke last year about the DEA petition and more recently about Ara Cron? I've just been handed this release. Is it true—is the government really trying to take away your pot?"

We met that afternoon. Dave Anderson was the UPI reporter assigned to cover religion. But his editors occasionally allowed him to do other stories. A bearded fellow in his early thirties, Anderson was a rumpled walrus of a man—the Hollywood stereotype of a wire service reporter. No dash. No glamour. Just the facts.

After listening to the story, Dave reviewed the facts—"this press release certainly contains a lot of information," he noted—then said,

"I think my editors will be interested in this story. Have any other outlets picked it up yet?"

"Not yet," I said without trying to seem anxious.

"Fine," Dave said. "By the way, what are you going to do when your government pot runs out? Are you going to go back to the streets to buy pot?"

An obvious, but dangerous question. After a few seconds, I replied, "I'm going to do what any sane person would do. I'm not going to go blind."

Dave jotted down the quote and smiled.

January 25, 1978
Washington, D.C.

Shortly after noon Alice phoned from her new office at NORML's Medical Reclassification Project. "I have good news. Hawaii has introduced legislation."

My friend, Senator Anson Chong, had finalized his legislation which would authorize the medical use of marijuana for treatment of glaucoma, cancer chemotherapy, and asthma. The proposed legislation, the first to be introduced in the United States, authorized the establishment of a system for manufacturing, distribution, and dispensing of the drug through the state's health department. Extensive hearings were expected.

"But there's more than that," Alice was excited. "There's another legal smoker. A cancer patient."

In California, Judge Don Work of the El Centro Superior Court had issued an order allowing the release of confiscated marijuana supplies to a 21-year-old cancer patient named Craig Reichert. The young man, confined to the Scripps Clinic in La Jolla, was terminally ill. For more than two years he had battled a rare tumor, which was cancerous and had developed near his kidneys. Like young Lynn

Pierson, Craig had been told to try marijuana to help with the nausea and vomiting that resulted from his cancer treatments. When his parents saw how much it helped their son they took steps to secure the drug legally by meeting with the local judge.

Following the meeting, and after speaking with the doctor, Judge Don Work, sitting on the bench for the Superior Court for Imperial County, issued a string of unprecedented orders immunizing Craig, his family and medical caregivers from arrest and authorizing the local sheriff to deliver confiscated supplies to the hospital.

A stupendously gutsy decision.

I was elated. A genie, once released, cannot be put back. Even if the bureaucrats cut me off, public awareness of medical marijuana was spreading. The knotted lie at the heart of the medical prohibition was, however slowly, coming undone. Judge Work had signed the landmark order on January 23, my birthday. A swell present. And, I wondered, perhaps a route to my own salvation?

Ironically I was making my way through the last of the marijuana cigarettes from the government when I heard the news. It seemed like an omen. In an odd gesture I found myself taking the last joint and placing it safely in a wooden engraved box.

Later that afternoon Alice phoned again. "Go buy a copy of *The Washington Star*," she said gleefully.

Dave Anderson's UPI story burst over Marble City like a distress rocket arcing across the black media void. *The Washington Star*, the capital's only evening newspaper, gave the story Page 3 prominence. Accompanying Dave's article was the now infamous photograph of me puffing legal marijuana. The caption under the photo said it all. "Robert Randall: 'I'm not out to pick a fight. I'm out to save my sight.' " Then the media machine kicked into high gear and the phone started ringing as reporters looked for comments on the Reichert case and, later, my own situation.

The next morning Lynn called. *The Albuquerque Journal* had picked up the Dave Anderson story about me. "Good story," Lynn said. "And it seemed to really spark some fires under the legislative counsel office. I had a call this morning and they are planning some hearings."

Indeed, the UPI wire was everywhere. Reports flooded in from around the nation. These reports were immediately followed by a rush of radio as stations across the country locked onto the story: Boston, Des Moines, L.A., St. Louis, San Francisco, ABC and Mutual Radio Networks.

Sitting in my Capitol Hill apartment, I threw my voice around the continent. A year of hitting local markets, doing local press and radio talk made my story seem local. Reporters I had not spoken with in months phoned for comment. From early morning through late afternoon I lit up the ethers; fielding calls, doing "actualities" and on-air interviews, and scheduling future radio talk.

In the midst of this flurry of calls, Peter Meyers, NORML's in-house lawyer, managed to break through. "Robert, I've been trying to reach you for hours." I explained it had been a busy afternoon.

"Look," Peter rushed on, "I received a call from an attorney at one of those legal factories on Connecticut Avenue. He saw *The Star* story and has an interest in your situation. But," Peter said, "he won't call you because it would be unethical to solicit a client. So he asked me to call. If you're interested I've got his number."

I was interested, very interested.

14 Steptoe Steps In

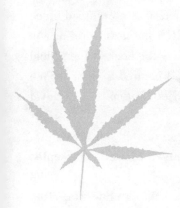

January 27, 1978
Steptoe & Johnson
Washington, D.C.

It was almost 6 p.m. when Alice and I found ourselves staring at the directory in the marbleized lobby of a modern building on Connecticut Avenue. Over a hundred attorneys were listed under the firm's name, Steptoe & Johnson. Peter Meyers wasn't kidding about a "legal factory."

Tom Collier was on the sixth floor.

The paneled elevator opened onto a large foyer. The walls were stark white, the woodwork simple, but elegant, the marble floor covered by a thick-pile oriental carpet.

A minute later a side door opened. "Are you Mr. Randall?"

"Yes. And this is Alice," I said.

Tom Collier and I each seemed surprised by the other.

We were approximately the same height—which is to say short—and same age—which is to say young. I had moderately long hair and was dressed in a Marine overcoat, bulky knit sweater, well-worn cords and aging hush puppies. Collier had curly blond hair longer than expected and was in a rumpled white shirt rolled up at the sleeves. His tie was loosened. He was eager and engaging.

It was my age more than anything which seemed to astonish Tom Collier. When glaucoma is mentioned senior citizens come to mind. I had just turned 30. And when corporate Washington lawyers are mentioned older, grayer men come to mind. Tom Collier was actually several years my junior. Should I trust my fate to someone so young?

Collier led us through a maze of corridors into a cramped office where a single window faced the back wall of the next building. As we entered the small room it became obvious the floor was a critical part of Tom Collier's filing system. He had cleared a chair for me already, but Alice's presence forced a hurried, but careful, removal of additional paper from a second chair.

For the next two hours Alice and I recapitulated our adventure. After we finished, Tom told us something about himself and Steptoe & Johnson.

"Steptoe thinks of itself as a conservative southern law firm," Tom began. Misters Steptoe & Johnson started the firm in West Virginia in 1913. During World War II, Mr. Johnson served as Assistant Secretary of War and later as Secretary of Defense under President Harry Truman. The Washington office of Steptoe & Johnson was established in 1945. Over the years Steptoe & Johnson had grown with the government and was now one of the top five law firms in Washington with a string of wealthy corporate clients and more than 150 attorneys on staff.

Tom Collier was a small-town Mississippi boy with big ambitions who always wanted to be a lawyer. After graduating from the University of Virginia, where he was president of the student body, Tom received his law degree from the University of Mississippi where he graduated with honors. He was a clerk for an Appeals Court judge in the 5th Circuit before he joined Steptoe as an Associate.

Tom was a 3rd year Associate, midway through a seven-year apprenticeship. At the end of that time the Steptoe partners would review his work and promote him to junior partner or throw him out of the firm. A brutal system.

Having survived three years so far, Tom Collier was looking for a case he could control. Steptoe, he explained, prided itself on providing select clients with *pro bono publico* legal assistance.

"That means 'for the public good?' " I asked. "Without charge?" My heart had begun to race a little faster at the prospect.

"Yes, that's right." Tom Collier was looking for an interesting *pro bono* case which would appeal to the senior partners and excite the interest of other Associates. He thought my case was interesting.

"Clearly," Tom said, "the government is manipulating your medical care to curb your free speech rights. And, clearly, they are willing to blind you to achieve their goal. This could be an important case. But it would require a great deal of effort."

I tried to rein in my excitement. This young attorney had hit the nail on the head and was extending the possibility of a major Washington law firm coming to my aid. Steptoe & Johnson was altogether different from anything I had experienced. I had grown accustomed to freewheeling criminal lawyers who worked in small practices on small cases. Steptoe was light years beyond—buttoned-down and top drawer. Perched at the pinnacle of the legal profession the firm was huge; rich, well-staffed and deeply connected. Steptoe was a bastion of the capitalist system. It represented Fortune 500 companies. Eager young novice lawyers who survived at Steptoe were slowly transformed into powerful players on the national stage. How, I wondered, would a corporate, well-connected, obviously conservative "southern" law firm respond to the idea of medical marijuana?

Tom seemed to be reading my thoughts as he carefully explained the need to propose my case to a committee which could reject the idea. The young attorney was honest and straightforward, offering hope but making no promises.

By the end of the two hour meeting Alice, Tom and I were comfortable with one another and there were good feelings as we parted.

As the elevator car began its descent Alice turned to me and uttered one word: "Wow!"

It would be two weeks before Steptoe & Johnson agreed to take my case. Like any corporate entity, Steptoe & Johnson had its own bureaucracy and Tom's request would make its way through the corporate structure.

But from the first we had a powerful ally at Steptoe. *The Washington Star* article had been first seen by a senior partner, Jane McGrew. It was Ms. McGrew who had pointed it out to Tom.

Jane McGrew had served as counsel to the Shafer Commission and gone on to specialize in pharmaceutical regulation and law. It was the second time in my adventure that a graduate of the Shafer Commission would come to my aid. The first had been Brian Convoy in Senator Javits office.

Coincidence? More of Alice's cosmic circles? Another deus ex machina? Who can say? Regardless of what you might call it, the entry of Steptoe & Johnson upped the ante and leveled the playing field considerably. I was still without a doctor and my government marijuana—save for one cherished joint—was gone. But I had new allies and they were very powerful indeed.

February 2, 1978
Washington, D.C.

I stared at the cookies on the counter. I couldn't do it; I couldn't eat another chocolate chip, marijuana-laced cookie.

In late January some friends had come to dinner bringing with them more than half a pound of very green, uncured marijuana. The couple, who lived in posh Chevy Chase, Maryland, had grown the plants as a lark. During the previous summer I had posed for pictures amidst the bright green foliage. "We're not sure about the quality," Jack said, "but we thought it might help."

The Chevy Chase chartreuse—as I dubbed it—smelled moldy, smoked rough, and produced less high than headache. So I put some of the marijuana in a vat of boiling water and butter, reclaimed the butter, then made some excellent, albeit slightly green, cookies. Not perfect, the cookies produced a better high than smoking the low potency weed and helped lower my eye pressures. After a few days of trial and error I had settled on an appropriate cookie dose and had been swallowing cookies on a regular basis. Now they stared up at me and I couldn't bring myself to lift one more to my mouth.

Reasoning that someone at NORML would have a joint, I traveled downtown to smoke and generally hang out. Towards evening Keith stopped by Alice's office. "Some people downstairs to see you, Bobby."

Keith introduced Alice and me to a young backwoods couple with thick Ozark accents. They were dressed in ragged hand-me-down clothes and looked like impoverished sharecroppers. And, in a way, they were.

"It's a real honor to meet you, Mr. Randall, sir," the young man said displaying southern manners and an uneven hillbilly grin. "Our friend Frank said you was having trouble with the govr'mint." Frank, an extremely talented Arkansas farmer, had presented me with a sample of his product during the NORML conference in December.

The young man nudged his girlfriend who pulled a large mason jar from her burlap purse. He handed the jar, packed with buds, to me. "Bet you won't get anything this good from Uncle Sam," he said with unalloyed pride. "That's Ozark grass, right out of the hills of Arkansas. That there jar is from Frank, with compliments. We—me 'n my girlfriend—we grew this stuff ourselves." With that the young man pulled out another jar, slightly smaller, and opened the lid. The pungent perfume of really fine pot instantly filled the room.

The young couple, having cared, cured and manicured their crop were making their annual post-harvest sales trip to the Northeast, returning home through Washington. "Do you think you could put us up a day or two?" the girlfriend asked. "We'd like to see Washington."

They were much welcomed guests who stayed two days. In addition to the mason jar packed with primo buds from Frank, the couple, on leaving, gave me a large cardboard box filled with less well-manicured buds, lots of shake and a mass of fragrant leaves. "This stuff's not fit to sell—not up to our clients' standards," the young man explained, "but we'd be plenty pleased to give it to you. It might help get you through a dry spell. And," he added, "it'll be better than your cookies."

Salvation! Ark grass with an Ozark accent. It was one of my first encounters with a highly secretive guild of premium pot growers who serviced wealthy tokers willing to pay top prices. The Ark grass would save me from blindness. And, from that day on, Groundhog Day would be my favorite holiday.

15 New Mexico

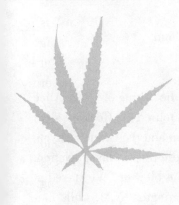

January 28, 1978
8th St. SE
Washington, D.C.

"Man seeks legal marijuana as balm," the headline read. It was the first press account of Lynn Pierson and was, in my opinion, outstanding.

Just a month before, shortly after Lynn returned to New Mexico from the NORML conference, I had painstakingly outlined my views of the media in a three-page letter to my new ally. I warned Lynn against "the fast and splashy route" or "the folk hero trip." I counseled the young New Mexican to stay focused. "The media is after a story—you, as the story focus—have a great deal to do with the type of focus received." I reminded Lynn of Andy Warhol's oft-quoted comment that everyone gets fifteen minutes of fame but admonished the New Mexican that, "The issue of marijuana therapeutics cannot be resolved in fifteen minutes. Keep yourself in a good position and don't worry, the media will come because it is NEWSWORTHY."

Now I was reading the results of Lynn's first encounter with the press and it couldn't be better.

"There was little hesitation in Lynn Pierson's voice," the story began, " 'I'm not supposed to be alive,' he said, his voice revealing a trace of pride in a wave of humility."

The article, which appeared in *The Albuquerque Journal*, was a relatively "soft" newspiece, an interesting story about a man with a problem. There were no inflammatory comments, no heroics. A simple, homespun story about a local fellow who had some ideas about passing a law.

"A damn quick study," I mumbled out loud.

I had been to New Mexico three times. In the Spring of 1972, Alice and I drove her VW beetle to the Far West, toured the Rockies, slept on snow under starry skies, saw Bryce, Zion and the Grand Canyon. We were headed home when—in the middle of the Navajo Nation, just east of Four Corners—the VW's engine blew up. We stayed at the curiously named Encore Motel in Farmington, N.M. while mechanics repaired Alice's car. Five days later, and a thousand dollars poorer, we headed home in the newly rechristened "Encore."

Later that summer, I was back in Washington, driving a Red Top cab, when I picked up a fare at National Airport who happened to be the campaign manager for a Republican House candidate in New Mexico. After a brief conversation the manager hired me to be the campaign's Research Director. The wrong party, but it was a job— an experience.

And what an experience. For six weeks, I lived between Albuquerque, Silver City and Las Cruces. I nearly died in a flash flood and flew around the state in a private plane, meeting Indian chiefs and local sheriffs. Among my chief responsibilities was learning where to drop off the money on election day. The campaign manager, as might be imagined from his hiring practices, was an inept novice: the candidate was unfit for dog catcher. I finally told the candidate I wanted $500 cash and a plane ticket to anywhere in America or

I'd go to the press. Within an hour both my requests were granted and I blissfully flew out of harm's way. It was a good move. Despite the Nixon landslide, the New Mexico House candidate lost by a huge margin. Which proves people will vote for a crook, but not a fool.

It was my first and last venture into electoral politics. But the experience taught me a great deal, generally about politics and specifically about New Mexico. In the early part of 1978, I could put that knowledge to good use.

New Mexico, despite its immense geography, is a very small place. People actually know people, and politics is personal. There was only one media market—Albuquerque—with small outposts of print in Santa Fe, Silver City and Las Cruces. Blessed with vast distances and a small population, New Mexico was one of the first states in America to be wired for cable TV. So electronic media generated in Albuquerque covered the entire state. In political terms New Mexico was a compact, comprehendible place—a community.

My third trip to the Land of Enchantment came in February 1977. I smoked legal marijuana for the media in Albuquerque, then spoke before a committee of the state legislature in Santa Fe. On that day, somewhere in the back of the room, was Lynn Pierson.

Now, less than a year later, Lynn was approaching the same legislature for help. Lynn was a native son—which counts for a lot. After our meeting in Washington, Lynn returned home, continued chemo and, despite terminal illness, drove almost daily from his home in Albuquerque to see legislators in Santa Fe.

Open, engaging, and obviously in need of help, Lynn walked—some would say "stalked"—the halls of the state capitol building. The New Mexico legislature was comprised of nearly 100 Senators and Representatives. Lynn spoke personally to nearly every one of them.

His dogged determination captured their attention and his obvious need would soon win their trust and affection. "It's wrong," Lynn would tell them, "that cancer patients are throwing up because our government won't admit marijuana has medical benefits." They could find no way to disagree.

At the outset it was a message Lynn delivered alone. Soon his doctors realized Lynn was serious about passing a law and quietly, behind the scenes, began phoning legislators to confirm Lynn's observations and express their support of his goal.

I advised Lynn to seek help from both Democrats and Republicans. That advice was soon amplified by a more illustrious voice— the Governor. Lynn had easily won the support of Senator Manny Aragon, a Democrat who had sponsored the unsuccessful decriminalization bill in 1977. Senator Aragon discussed the issue with New Mexico Governor Jerry Apodaca and the Governor told Aragon that if he and Pierson could win the support of Senator John Irick, a staunch anti-marijuana hard liner, then they could almost be assured of success in the legislature.

Without hesitation Lynn descended on Senator Irick and explained how marijuana had prolonged his life and helped him tolerate the dreadful chemotherapy treatments. Senator Irick, initially skeptical, was clearly moved by the young man's courage. He told Lynn "If you get over 50 % of the Judiciary Committee we'll figure out something."

The Committee met at the end of January and heard from several witnesses including Lynn, his doctor, a pharmacist from Albuquerque, and Rev. M. Buren Stewart, Lynn's minister and senior pastor from St. John's United Methodist Church in Albuquerque. Rev. Stewart told the committee, "Lynn is trying to help himself and humanity. He is not asking for decriminalization but that [marijuana] be reclassified for doctors to give it for treatment." The proposal sailed through the Committee and Lynn secured Irick's support although the Senator fell short of cosponsoring the bill. For Lynn, and the Governor, it was enough to have Irick's vote and silence.

Nearly all of this was accomplished without much public comment. But, once the Judiciary Committee endorsed the concept in late January Lynn became a bona fide celebrity in the compact media world of New Mexico. He was a natural interview—likeable, determined, absolutely certain he was right. In the press Lynn's quest quickly became a Don Quixote story—dreaming the impossible dream, tilting against windmills. Lynn captured hearts and minds easily. New Mexicans embraced his cause with an almost mystical fervor.

New Mexico politicians were not Washington bureaucrats. They rushed to Lynn's defense and Lynn, suddenly very unalone, became the public face of a State that was absolutely certain compassion could overrule regulation. New Mexico entered the medical marijuana issue with all the hope and optimism that marked the opening of the American West. New Mexicans were accustomed to large and grand accomplishments, carving town and villages from wilderness, mining ore and precious metals from harsh terrain, taming the vast open spaces for use as ranches and farms. When a people can do all this how hard can it be to craft some words that will allow the ill and dying to smoke some weed?

After the Judiciary hearings the real work began on the bill. In order to get the initial hearing, Lynn and Aragon had borrowed the recently introduced Hawaiian bill and submitted it to the Judiciary Committee. The bill flatly recognized marijuana's medical value in treating life- and sense-threatening diseases like cancer and glaucoma. It ended the medical prohibition and authorized marijuana's licit medical use under a physician's supervision. It was a start and marked a radical departure from the absolute prohibition of marijuana. But it was merely a broad sketch. It lacked the fine detail necessary for conformity to state and federal law.

It also failed to identify a source of supply for the drug. For Lynn this was the critical point. Without a legal source of supply he knew that other cancer patients, like his friend from the V.A. Hospital, would never be provided with marijuana.

The bill was sent to the New Mexico Legislative Council Services for fine-tuning. It was unlike anything the Council had ever seen. Many questions were raised in staff meetings. The staffers, intent on helping Lynn and others in New Mexico, turned to Washington for guidance, Expecting sympathy and understanding, perhaps even kudos for this "groundbreaking legislation," the New Mexicans were surprised at the reaction they received.

The bureaucrats in Washington were myopically focused on getting rid of America's Only Legal Pot Smoker and were slow to realize the erosion that was taking place throughout the country. Their initial responses to New Mexico's Legislative Council Services were blunt and abrasive. New Mexico, the bureaucrats asserted with a haughty certainty, could not abandon the medical prohibition. It was not allowed. Besides, they added with smugness, where will you get the marijuana? Going for the obvious, New Mexico officials noted marijuana was grown by the federal government so couldn't they just get some of the government's pot? No, said the feds. Government marijuana would only be given to government sanctioned "research programs." New Mexico did not have the authority to use the government's marijuana. It couldn't be done. Period.

This was really nothing new to New Mexicans; they were accustomed to "going it alone" and weary to the bone of government intrusion. If Washington wouldn't help then they would help themselves. The Legislative Council Services turned to Lynn for guidance. He seemed to know a great deal about all of this and, after all, it was his request they were trying to honor. But Lynn was too ill. He did know what he wanted but he had little patience with bureaucrats—state or federal—who told him marijuana couldn't be gotten legally. He advised the Council to speak with his friends Robert and Alice.

For two weeks we conversed regularly with the folks in New Mexico, raising possibilities, brainstorming ideas. It was new territory for us, too. We didn't have an answer but we were at least willing to explore the options, which was more than the federal bureaucrats had been willing to do.

For a few days we explored the Reichert model, the California judicial decision that released confiscated stocks to a cancer patient. Supply was not a problem, the Council reasoned, because there was plenty of marijuana in New Mexico sitting in the offices of sheriffs and local police. Instead of burning it as contraband why not meet urgent human medical needs and devise a system of drug "destruction" via authorized use?

The Albuquerque Journal seemed to agree when it weighed in with an editorial entitled "The Case for Marijuana" which concluded, "As a civilized society, we should do what we can to help make those who suffer from dread diseases more comfortable. Denying Pierson marijuana thwarts that ideal."

It was a wake-up call to Washington.

The feds began to realize that something was afoot—big time. As the idea of using confiscated marijuana was floated publicly, the Washington bureaucrats who had been so rude just a few days before suddenly were initiating calls to "their colleagues" in New Mexico. They offered the opinion that the use of confiscated marijuana might be illegal. It certainly was unsanitary. After all, how could New Mexico possibly know if contraband pot seized from slimy drug criminals was contaminated? God knows, the DEA was spraying illegal marijuana fields with Paraquat—a deadly herbicide. What might happen if a cancer patient got hold of Paraquated pot? Consider the liabilities?

Employees from the Legislative Council Services began making calls about testing marijuana for contaminants. For the first time doubt began to set in. It became obvious that the use of confiscated marijuana *did* carry some risk. Testing supplies would be an arduous, and expensive, proposition.

Attention then turned to the possibility of growing marijuana in-state but DEA officials quickly squelched that idea pointing to the need for licenses and the expense of securing, harvesting, and preparing the plant.

For the first time since returning home from Washington in December 1977 Lynn became disheartened. The federal effort to reimpose fear began to have an effect. For a while there was talk of simply authorizing Lynn to legally use illegal marijuana via a legislative "memorial." For nearly a week it seemed the bureaucrats would block New Mexico's drive to legalize medical marijuana.

Things were falling apart when, through a series of brainstorming sessions with a friend at the Legislative Council Services, we hit upon a simple question: "Why couldn't New Mexico authorize a statewide research program that provides federal supplies of medical marijuana to cancer patients?" After all, the bureaucrats in Washington insisted the government wanted research. So, why not give them research? New Mexico could help Lynn *and* help the nation by answering some of the critical questions about marijuana's medical effects.

The compromise position made Lynn nervous—"How can we trust the federal bureaucrats, Robert?" I had no answer. I knew the bureaucrats could not be trusted, but, in the final analysis, it was the only plan that could work.

The compromise bill, now entitled the New Mexico Controlled Substances Therapeutic Research Act (CSTRA), swept through the necessary committee hearings in both assemblies. It sailed to the floor of the House on February 11th where it was enacted by a lopsided vote of 53-9. Three days later it arrived in the Senate where the vote was even more impressive: 33-1.

"It was a rout," Lynn shouted into the phone. "We whipped 'em good." Lynn was loving it. "I bet I get government marijuana before you do," he told me. I declined the bet—bad luck to tempt Fate.

To underscore the urgency of their historic measure the Legislature forwarded the newly enacted bill to the Governor Jerry Apodaca for his immediate signature. It was the first "emergency legislation" enacted since the outbreak of the Korean War. Lynn, the legislators felt, should not have to wait for care.

Ignoring the threats of faraway bureaucrats, Governor Apodaca invited Lynn to the bill-signing ceremony on February 21, 1978. After signing the measure, the Governor turned to Lynn and said, "Okay Lynn, you can start smoking it legally now."

It was just ten weeks since Lynn and I had decided to pass a state law. Cameras flashed, wires ran, and, all across America, ink and megawatts proclaimed that the end of marijuana's medical prohibition had arrived in that most unlikely and conservative of states, New Mexico.

The New Mexico law was a dagger thrust into the heart of federal policy. A near-blind man in Washington and a terminally ill cancer patient in Albuquerque had dealt a mortal blow against the medical prohibition. Lynn's crusade created a landmark law fully supported by inhabitants in the Land of Enchantment. Seemingly without reservation the people of New Mexico wanted Lynn to get his government pot.

"We done good," Lynn said.

"We've done very good," I replied. "Now, all we have to do is get the feds to hand over the marijuana."

That's all.

16 Back in the Lifeboat

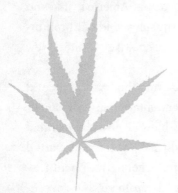

WHILE GOVERNOR JERRY Apodaca was signing the New Mexico Controlled Substances Therapeutic Research Act into law, I was seated in one of Steptoe & Johnson's impressive conference rooms overlooking Connecticut Avenue and the city of Washington. The firm had agreed to take my case on February 10th and Tom Collier immediately began to coordinate his legal strategy. After one or two preliminary meetings I was called in to meet the "team."

February 21, 1978
Steptoe & Johnson
Washington, D.C.

"This is a huge case," Tom said. "Unless they agree to a settlement we'll have to sue three federal agencies—the DEA, FDA, NIDA—and two cabinet Departments—Justice and Health, Education & Welfare. This is going to take weeks organize."

While dismayed by the prospect of a long delay, I was more than pleased with what Tom had accomplished thus far. Seated around the table were five bright, young, and highly aggressive attorneys who, after years of laboring to advance corporate power, were eager to apply their talents to aid an afflicted man in search of justice.

"This is John Bates—constitutional law, Jim Young—bureaucratic procedures . . ." Tom made his way through each one. I quickly learned Tom was an exceedingly competent lawyer but his true talent was in coordinating the talents of others. This was the first real test of Tom's ability to marshal Steptoe's tremendous resources and direct the crafting of a large, important case. The firm's partners would closely monitor Tom's progress. Success was his only option.

When the band of young attorneys left the room Tom turned to me. "Impressive, huh? But," Tom advised, "I don't want you talking to them. Too confusing. You talk to me. I talk to them."

I did not object. But I also wanted to be part of the team, not merely its excuse for being. "How can I help?"

Tom had read as much of the criminal case as he could extract from the record. "Who wrote these affidavits?" he asked.

"I did. They okay?" I asked.

"Plenty okay," Tom said with admiration. "You know the doctors, you know the important medical facts. So, you write the affidavits. That will allow the lawyers to focus on legal questions. Let's get to work."

It was agreed that Dr. Fine's 1976 affidavit would suffice but new affidavits for Drs. Hepler and Merritt were needed. I was delighted to be put to work, especially on the affidavits. It gave me control over how the facts were articulated.

Soon we decided to expand the affidavits to include the stories of other patients who had found marijuana helpful in treating glaucoma. Tom reasoned that such affidavits would demonstrate to the

Court the extent to which government restrictions were harming the public and the difficulties faced in trying to obtain marijuana. I drafted affidavits for some of my first allies—Vince Mustachio and Ara Cron—as well as some new friends including Jim Ripple of Arizona, a 65-year-old retired cowboy whose wife, Mildred, had called Alice in early January.

The Playboy Foundation agreed to provide some funding for "out-of-pocket" expenses that might be associated with the case, just as they had with the criminal trial.

Despite all this progress one critical element in the case—a doctor—was missing. Without a physician to supervise my use of marijuana there was no case. I returned to Dr. Fine and once again began the slow dance of persuasion. The good doctor waffled, as usual. It was, in the immortal words of Yogi Bera, déjà vu all over again.

In New Mexico, meanwhile, work began on implementing the historic legislation and across the nation other patients had begun to wonder if their states could pass a law like New Mexico's. At the Medical Reclassification Project Alice would receive calls from legislative research services in Arkansas, Pennsylvania, Maryland, and California.

In late February, Hy Greenstein invited me back to Hawaii for hearings on the Hawaiian therapeutic bill and on March 1st I would arrive in Honolulu for the second time in two months. The Hawaiian legislature, near adjournment, would not enact the medical marijuana bill. But the trip did provide me with an opportunity to meet Dr. Tod Mikuriya who, in 1969, established the nation's first publicly acknowledged program of marijuana. He did not last long. At the outset Mikuriya näively suggested government-funded research should neutrally explore marijuana's harmful effects and therapeutic benefits. The government had no interest in neutral scientific discovery. In a matter of months this politically motivated research compelled Mikuriya to leave government service.

After being removed from his federal post, Mikuriya retired from government service, moved into private practice in Berkeley and wrote a book which compiled historical information on marijuana's therapeutic uses—*Marijuana Medical Papers*.

While I toured Hawaii with Tod, Alice was having her own adventure.

March 2, 1978
State Capitol
Annapolis, Maryland

The small room was hardly filled. Just a few members of the Judiciary Committee and a handful of witnesses had bothered to attend the hearing on hastily proposed legislation which would reclassify marijuana to recognize its medical utility in the State of Maryland. Alice had spoken briefly and submitted the Hawaiian Report as evidence of the drug's therapeutic potential. She also had mentioned the recent signing of the New Mexico bill and focused on the drug's ability to help cancer chemotherapy patients.

Alice's testimony was followed by that of Meredith Sykes, a lovely 25-year-old woman whose composure gave little clue to the disease, multiple sclerosis (MS), that was beginning to ravage her body. Meredith had been making some headlines of her own by publicly discussing marijuana's beneficial effects on the unwanted muscle spasms that are a hallmark of that illness. She had persuaded Dr. Denis Petro, a neurologist and FDA scientific review officer, to backup her claims of therapeutic utility. Petro had reviewed the current and historical literature, determining that "Ms. Sykes' anecdotal observations seem to be rooted in science."

The trio's testimony was followed by a second panel comprised of law enforcement officials and a representative of the U.S. Labor Party, a right-wing organization backed by Lyndon LaRouche. All spoke forcefully and with great animation against the measure to reclassify marijuana, using inflammatory language and farfetched projections of imminent harm.

The chairman warmly thanked the second panel and quickly moved to table the measure. His motion was seconded by an aging Representative who declared, "If this bill is enacted hippies will go out and get cancer just so they can smoke pot!" The appalling nature of the statement, coupled with the spiteful delivery, left Alice numb. The car ride back to Washington was a silent time of grim reflection.

Later that day, in the Scripps Clinic at La Jolla, California, Craig Reichert lost his battle with cancer. In the news accounts of his death, Reichert's family publicly confirmed that legal access to marijuana had made Craig's last days easier, helping to quiet the violent attacks of nausea that followed his chemo.

Several hours before he died he confided to his fiancée that one of his last wishes was to thank the man who had made his final days so much easier, Judge Don Work. "He always said he couldn't believe it had happened," his fiancée told the press. "But that afternoon he told me he wished he could get out of bed and go out there and talk about this."

It would be four days later that Alice learned about the young man's death. Upon hearing the news her thoughts flashed back to the Maryland legislator and his absurd contention that "hippies will get cancer just to smoke pot." The cruelty seemed almost overwhelming. She had never met Craig Reichert, and had spoken only briefly with his mother. Nevertheless, it seemed as though a friend had died. For nearly six weeks Reichert had been America's Only Legal Pot Smoker. Now he was gone.

Ides of March, 1978
FDA Headquarters
Rockville, Maryland

The joint, two-day meeting of the Controlled Substances Advisory Committee and the Drug Abuse Research Advisory Committee (CSAC & DARAC) was called to order at 9:00 a.m.

A year earlier, in a private meeting, DARAC had been plotting to restrict my access to care, curtail my travel, and limit my speech. I had been barely aware of their existence, let alone the impact they could have on my life. The FDA was packed with little committees of this sort, "public" advisory groups that the public knew nothing about.

Things were changing, however. It was the era of sunshine-in-government and the FDA had been forced to make public the meetings of its "public" advisory committees. There was some grousing about this but the law was the law.

When Tom Collier first learned about the meeting he felt it was important for me to address the committees and begin laying the groundwork for the lawsuit. It was, Tom explained, one step in the process of exhausting administrative remedies. "The court will insist we try every possible avenue of resolution." I wasn't pleased but I prepared written testimony and made certain I had enough copies for the committee members and the press.

The nearly 20-member combined panel met in an airless room in the bowels of FDA's Parklawn Building—second in size only to the Pentagon. During one break I ran into Ed Tocus, the FDA bureaucrat who supervised government approved marijuana research. Tocus was jovial and tried to be friendly. But I was in no humor for social give and take. I had no patience for Tocus' efforts as Mr. Nice Guy and did little to conceal my contempt.

"My job is to protect you," Tocus asserted.

Without thinking I tartly replied, "If I let you protect me, I'll go blind. And you know it." The arrow found its mark. Tocus winced and turned away.

The meeting droned on. The tedious talk, the long delay, the glaring florescent lights, and herd-like hypocrisy took its toll on me. I was frugally making my way through the Arkansas gift and had brought only one joint to the hearings. Anticipating that the committee would take up the issue of marijuana therapeutics at the appointed hour, I had used the medication far too early in the day and by late afternoon I was white blind, totally unable to read my own testimony. It was nearly 5 p.m. before my name was called.

"My client," Tom Collier began, "is experiencing some difficulties. We request his testimony be postponed until tomorrow morning."

A simple request. But, after a brief discussion, the panel rejected any delay. My heart sank. I could barely see Tom's face let alone words on a page. I conferred with Tom and suggested an ad lib presentation but Tom was insistent on sticking with the prepared testimony. There was little I could do. "This is my attorney," I began. "He will read my testimony for the record."

While Tom read, I tried to imagine the panel's reaction. I thought about Alice's story of the Maryland hearings—"hippies getting cancer to smoke pot"—and realized these committee members probably had similar feelings. They did not—could not—view me as a person in danger of losing my sight. It was too real and harnessed them with too much responsibility. They, after all, could change things.

Instead, the panel saw me as a 'drug reformer,' a troublemaker anxious to injure their precious prohibition. The panel's inability to accept me on human terms left me with no doubt about the outcome.

Tom finished reading the testimony and received a terse "Thank you" from the chairman. There was an immediate flurry of not-so-hushed talk from the panel members and I could hear terms like "media trick" and "outrageous" float across the room in my direction.

It was clear some members of the combined panel viewed the episode as a staged affair, designed to milk sympathy from the assembled press members.

There was no way to dissuade the thought. With Tom's help, I found my way to the exit and left the room.

Things were about to get very rough.

After three weeks of waffling, Dr. Fine, true to form, got cold feet and withdrew from the case. Tom was very angry, feeling that Fine was cowardly and unethical. But I was surprisingly calm. I never expected Fine to reach the finish line with me. It would be my last encounter with the doctor who, in a very real sense, saved my sight by playing straight. By not rushing me to surgery he saved me from the fate of Vince and Ara.

On March 24th, the day after Fine's final defection, the heavens opened once again and brought forth a new doctor. He was a friend of Merritt's. Tom spoke with him in the morning and arranged an appointment for me in the afternoon. I was skeptical but, then again, I had been skeptical of Merritt.

March 24, 1978
Columbia Road N.W.
Washington, D.C.

Dr. Richard North was in private practice and had no opinion regarding marijuana's medical use in glaucoma therapy. But, he was intrigued by the possibility, and disturbed by the ethical implications of what Tom Collier had told him.

Dr. North's office was on Columbia Road in Adams Morgan, the most lively, ethnically diverse neighborhood in Washington. The early spring day was warm and the street was packed with people speaking foreign tongues, listening to jazz, African, and Caribbean rhythms as I arrived at the doctor's office.

Dr. North was about Merritt's age, but they were very different men. Unlike Merritt, who had excessive nervous energy, Dr. North had an easy, pleasing manner. Merritt was intense and guarded. Richard North was open and loved to laugh. He seemed to enjoy my cynical wit. We immediately liked one another.

Just like every physician who first examined my eyes, North winced at the damage he found.

"You have hardly any sight," he said. "Just a rim of healthy tissue."

"Tell me something I don't know," I replied.

"Your pressures are very high—over 30," North continued.

"Didn't smoke. I wanted you to see how things really are."

"You're on your standard meds?"

"Yes. And my pressure will go higher towards evening. Now," I asked, "would you like to see the difference marijuana can make?"

"I thought you didn't have any government marijuana," North said.

"I'm out of government pot. But I have some high quality marijuana. Would you like to see it work?" I knew I was tempting North.

"Where could you smoke?" North said without hesitation.

"Oh, I'll just go out in the street. No one cares," I said.

Dr. North cared. He was uncomfortable with the idea of a patient—his patient—wandering around Adams Morgan smoking a joint. "Why not out back?" He led me to a fenced yard behind the office. "No one will bother you here. I have another patient coming. Why don't you relax, smoke out here.

I sat on a small brick wall, enjoying the warm sun and took my time smoking two of the Arkansas joints. Then I returned to North's office and had my pressures checked.

"This is amazing," Dr. North said recalibrating his tonometer, then rechecking my pressure. "There's been a 50 % decline in your eye pressure! It's now normal. In just over an hour. Does marijuana always work this well?"

"Always," I said. "If it didn't I'd be blind."

"Impressive."

"So," I asked, "will you be my doctor? I have lots of attorneys and a good legal case. But I need a doctor to monitor my condition, make reports and write script. Are you willing to help me?"

"I'd be pleased to be your doctor, Robert," North said without equivocation. "You understand I can't say much about marijuana—this is the first time I've seen it work. But having seen this . . . to deny you care would be unethical. Downright unethical."

Dr. North, I learned, was an ethical man who responded to facts, especially facts he could measure on his tonometer.

By the end of March the affidavits were done and the last legal briefs were being evaluated.

The legal argument, Tom explained, was tricky. "There is no constitutional right to sight," he said. "But that does not mean such a right does not exist."

"You clearly have a right to speak. The government cannot take that away from you. And," Tom said, "just as clearly—as the Bourne letter plainly shows—the government is trying to manipulate your medical care to control your speech. That's a start."

At this point, however, the law became theoretical. "Do you," Tom wondered, "have a constitutionally protected right to your sight?"

To me the answer seemed obvious. If "medical necessity" could be used as a defense to criminal charges, certainly the Constitution must, in some way, recognize the right of an individual to protect his sight—his biology—against government interference.

"Yes," Tom reasoned, "but does that mean you have a constitutionally protected right to see? Or, more specifically, to compel the government to provide you with a legally prohibited drug to retain your sight?"

This legal question deeply intrigued the Steptoe Associates and multiple briefs were prepared in an attempt to locate and articulate a legal "right to sight."

The consensus was that by implication the Constitution must afford protection against undue government interference in medical care. A "right to sight" must exist somewhere between the right of parents to teach a child German (*Meyer v Nebraska*, 262 U.S. 390, 399 (1923)) and the Supreme Court's recognition of a woman's right to abort a fetus (*Roe v. Wade*, 410 U.S. 113, 152 (1973)). "Certainly," Tom argued, "if a woman can elect—based on her innate privacy and biological rights—to abort a fetus, a man can elect to smoke marijuana to preserve his vision."

Having settled on this interpretation, of an implied right within an already accepted spectrum of rights, the Associates returned to their law books to obtain citations to sustain the claim. "It is," Tom admitted, "less than certain how this might turn out in court. But, I think we can demonstrate the Constitution protects you from government actions that seek to control your speech by jeopardizing your sight. I'm fairly sure," he continued, "the government does not have a right to blind you for your speech."

The case was coming together and by the first week in April the suit was ready to be filed. Before rushing to court, however, Tom Collier decided to make one last "good faith" effort to resolve the case. So he began another round of calls into the bureaucracy.

April 7, 1978
Steptoe & Johnson
Washington, D.C.

"I have bad news," Tom said with apprehension. On the other end of the phone I began to tense.

Ed Tocus, at the FDA, was suggesting an alternative to marijuana. A new, unapproved drug called Timoptic was in final Phase III testing. If research went well Timoptic could be approved by October. "Perhaps," Tocus suggested, "this new drug could help Mr. Randall retain his sight short of smoking marijuana."

Tocus provided Tom with the name of the company that produced the drug and a list of ongoing studies. "Perhaps we could get Mr. Randall into one of these studies? That might solve everybody's problem."

I was livid. Marijuana controlled my glaucoma—that was a well-documented fact. A doctor was ready to monitor my care. Hundreds of hours of research had gone into refining a credible legal argument. "I'm not going to become a government guinea pig!" I said.

"I'm not certain we have a choice," Tom replied.

The team of Steptoe Associates quickly assembled. All agreed: if a legal alternative to marijuana existed then questions of rights diminished into issues of preference. I could not "prefer" an illegal treatment over a legal therapy.

"But marijuana works. What if this new, unapproved drug doesn't work?" I protested.

"Then we have an even better legal argument," Tom replied.

Steptoe researchers scoured D.C. medical libraries for information on Timoptic. It was derived from timolol maleate, a beta-blocker used in heart care. Merck, Sharp & Dome had developed a topical timolol eyedrop under the brand name Timoptic. The results were outstanding.

On paper, Timoptic looked like a wonder drug. It lacked the myopia-inducing properties of most glaucoma drugs, and reduced intraocular pressure in 8 of 10 research subjects. Phase I and II testing revealed no alarming adverse affects. Now Timoptic was in final, Phase III testing. If no serious problems were detected, Timoptic would receive FDA marketing approval by fall.

"There is a 14 % failure rate which cannot be explained," Alice noted, reading through the reports from Steptoe. "But it looks like a promising drug."

After prodding from Tom and cajoling from Alice, and after speaking with Dr. North, I reluctantly agreed to be a guinea pig, even agreeing to stop my marijuana use during the test. This was not difficult; the Ozark grass was fast running out.

It was all chillingly familiar and images of Johns Hopkins were looming in my head. But, unlike Paul Smollar, Tom made no decisions without me. This was not a question of Tom conspiring to satisfy some intellectual curiosities. His logic was sound and there was no choice except which particular research site I wanted to travel to.

The closest test site was, ironically, at Johns Hopkins. I had burned my bridges there and was refused admittance. The next closest Timoptic test site was at Duke University in North Carolina, just up the road from the Research Triangle Institute where the government processed Mississippi marijuana into pre-rolled cigarettes and where Mario Perez-Reyes had infused me with pure THC.

Yogi Berra time—again.

April 18, 1978
Duke University Eye Center
Chapel Hill, North Carolina

The Timoptic study was being conducted by Dr. R. Bruce Shields, a middle-aged man who wanted me to view him as a compassionate healer. Instead, I viewed R. Bruce Shields as FDA's coconspirator, an impression underscored by Shield's opening comment.

"I understand the FDA has a particular interest in your case."

The first exam was routine and my pressures were high, just under 40mm Hg. Shields splashed Timoptic into my eyes and did another pressure check an hour later.

"Excellent. Already responding," Shields triumphantly said. "Almost down to 20."

With that I was given a week's supply of the drug and sent home to Washington. The four-week plan called for me to travel to North Carolina once a week where Shields would evaluate the progress. The Playboy Foundation agreed to pay the travel expense. During the intervening days Dr. North would assess my condition daily. This would eliminate questions regarding controls and provide an early warning if something went wrong.

For the first few days all was well.

"This is astonishing," Dr. North said. "Your IOP is 8. Just amazing."

The news, which at any other time would have been greeted with glee, deepened my sense of impending loss. Was modern science about to steal my legal case and save the medical prohibition?

The next day my IOP was 12. North was pleased. My gloom became overwhelming. On the third day my IOP was 18. "I don't like the looks of this," Dr. North said, noting the increasing IOP readings. "We may be seeing a trend."

On the fourth day my IOP was 22—above normal, in the danger zone. By the fifth day it was clear things were not quite right. My IOP was 26. "This could be tachyphylaxis, a rapid onset of tolerance to a drug's therapeutic effect," North explained. "You're developing a tolerance to Timoptic. If your IOP keeps going up we'll have to stop this study. These elevated pressures are endangering your sight."

Dr. North notified Tom Collier of the creeping IOP elevation. Both agreed to continue the experiment. "It's important," Tom explained, "to give Timoptic a fair trial."

On my second visit to Duke, with pressures slowly rising, I hoped Shields would recognize the problem and terminate the experiment. But the doctor would not admit defeat. "This is a surprising result.

You're taking the Timoptic every 12 hours as instructed?" he questioned.

"Yes," I replied. "Dr. North suggested tachyphylaxis?"

"Oh, I doubt that," Shields said, ignoring the evidence in front of him. "We had a case or two like that, but we shouldn't jump to conclusions. I'll see you next week."

I returned to Washington, continuing to see Dr. North daily. During the entire second week my IOP was above normal, constantly creeping higher. Dr. North became alarmed. "You can't tolerate much more of this without permanently damaging your sight," he said.

When Dr. North informed Tom Collier of the disappointing results, the Steptoe Associates—distressed as I was by the unexpected Timoptic test—were galvanized into action. "We're prepared to file as soon as Dr. Shields determines Timoptic has failed," Tom Collier said.

By the third trip to North Carolina things were seriously out of control. "Your IOP is over 40," Shields said with mild alarm. "You are not responding properly to Timoptic." Shields' tone was accusatory, implying it was the patient, not the drug that had failed. "Are you taking your doses properly?"

"Yes. And Dr. North has administered many of the doses," I said, weary of the game being played with my sight. "I'm not the problem. Timoptic simply does not work. Does it?"

"No, it isn't working," Shields admitted. "But, I cannot allow you to leave with these pressures. You're in grave danger of losing your sight." He called in a nurse, spoke to her in hushed tones, then returned to me. "You'll be staying here tonight." It was not a question, but a command.

"Why?" I asked with confusion. "Why would I stay here?"

"The nurse is arranging for the first available operating theatre. We'll do your surgery this evening, and keep you here a few days for observation." Shields spoke the words with remarkable detachment.

"The hell you will," I replied. My tolerance for R. Bruce Shields' arrogance was exhausted. "I am not going to have any damn operation. Not here. Not now. Timoptic has failed, right?"

"Yes," Shields sighed. "If Timoptic doesn't work nothing will work. If you don't have an operation—an immediate operation—you could be blind in a few days, maybe a couple of hours."

His scare tactics increased my fury.

"I am not—repeat NOT—having an operation," I was emphatic. "I am going home to smoke marijuana and get these pressures under control. My attorneys will contact you for a written statement."

R. Bruce Shields sneered at the mention of marijuana, then tried once more to compel me into a surgical procedure I had avoided since diagnosis in 1972. As Shields continued to press, I abruptly stood up and headed for the door. "Thanks for your help. My attorneys will be calling."

It was time to file the lawsuit.

Three days after my return from North Carolina, May 8, Tom filed the case.

It was, as Tom predicted, immense. The factual record, including affidavits, research reports, and correspondence ran more than 150 pages. The mean-spirited dialogue between me and the bureaucrats— including Dr. Peter Bourne's inartful threats—hung like a fuse at the heart of the brief. If the case went to trial the President's chief adviser on health and drug abuse, the DEA Administrator, and high-ranking FDA officials would be hauled before the court and compelled to publicly explain their threats. The press would flay them alive.

If the fact case was dense, the legal argument was equally thick, with a lean commentary interlacing constitutional claims to cites of federal statutes and relevant case law.

The final product was a handsome, intimidatingly large package

held together by binding rings. The last piece of evidence was Dr.
R. Bruce Shields' statement confirming Timolol's failure. Shields,
however, omitted any written reference to his dire warning of my
imminent blindness.

For two years I had been bullied and threatened. Now, when their
evil deeds were about to be publicly exposed, the government folded
like a house of cards. Within 24 hours of filing suit I was conferring
with Tom Collier and the other associates to craft a settlement to the
case.

I wanted to fight the bastards! To hell with a settlement.

Tom wanted to fight too. But Tom Collier was learning to be a good
attorney and a good attorney knows a settlement—on your terms—
is better than a protracted courtroom battle fought to an uncertain
outcome.

"If we force the government to publicly give you legal access to
medical marijuana your sight can be saved and your public position
could not be stronger," Tom advised.

In crafting the settlement we agreed on a simple formulation: my
access to marijuana would be treated as any other medical prescription. The script would be written by my private physician and honored by a pharmacy. Beyond these elemental demands the settlement
would strictly prohibit my involvement in future research. There
would be no more Timoptic episodes. Finally, the bureaucrats could
not use medical access to marijuana to restrict my right to speak or
freedom to travel.

The proposed settlement compelled federal agencies to accept an
anathema: A private physician writing script for marijuana and a
pharmacy responsible for obtaining and dispensing supplies. I asked
for this in hopes of avoiding the anxiety and fears Dr. Merritt experienced when bureaucrats arbitrarily delayed shipments or came to
account for supplies. I wanted Dr. North insulated from marijuana
and bureaucratic pressures.

The traditional patient-physician-pharmacy arrangement seemed so simple but it undermined the entire regulatory scheme. I was certain the government would reject the idea.

But in filing the lawsuit we had moved beyond the bickering of agencies. A U.S. Attorney was now in charge of the government's case and he accepted the settlement the next day. Tom then began hammering out the specifics with the various agencies. We can only imagine the scene at the FDA, NIDA, and DEA. Profound interagency frictions were at work and there was much unhappiness, especially at the DEA.

Tom was skillful and resolute, demanding the best possible agreement for his client. Regulations that had seemed rigid and intractable fell away before the awesome power of the case.

To satisfy the FDA, Dr. North agreed to be an Investigational New Drug (IND) researcher. The usually complex, months-long IND process for marijuana vanished before the pressure exerted by Steptoe & Johnson. North received automatic FDA authorization to write script for marijuana.

A settlement was sealed before the weekend. As NIDA began processing a shipment, DEA, brutalized in the bargaining, rushed to identify a federal pharmacy in Washington.

Ed Tocus, when asked what the FDA would call this unusual process said, "Oh, it's a 'Compassionate IND' which allows for the medical use of a nonapproved drug."

"Compassionate IND"—it was a term that had first surfaced briefly, in the summer of '76 but "compassion" had been dropped as hard-liners got the upper hand during that long summer of trial and negotiation.

It was, in fact, the first time the FDA authorized the medical use of an unapproved drug. The fact that marijuana was legally prohibited was ignored. It was a crack in the FDA structure with profound future implications.

May 16, 1978
Washington, D.C.

Eight days after the case was filed, I went to Dr. North's office. Dr. North took my pressures, then carefully wrote out a prescription for 70 marijuana cigarettes. He handed the script to me, then we shook hands and laughed. For the first time in 40 years a private physician had written legal script for marijuana.

In a block of aging government buildings on the Federal Triangle I found the pharmacy, run by the Public Health Service (PHS), just a few blocks from the U.S. Capitol.

Bob Golden, resplendent in his white PHS uniform, greeted me with ease, and said how pleased he was to perform his role in the drama. I handed over the script. "I don't suppose I could keep this?" I asked.

Mr. Golden, a tall, church-rounded man, chuckled. "Afraid not," he said. "After DEA certifies it this script will probably be sent to the National Archives."

I watched as Mr. Golden's excited PHS staff unsealed a large round tin packed with NIDA pre-rolled marijuana cigarettes and carefully counted out the prescribed dose. "How'd you like these packaged?" Mr. Golden asked.

We settled on large brown prescription bottles big enough to hold 20 joints. "How should the bottles read," Golden wondered, perched over a typewriter. After some thought he typed, "Marijuana Cigarettes—Smoke as directed."

"The pharmacy's phone number is on the label," Mr. Golden said. "If you run into difficulty, have the authorities call this number so we can verify you're legal." He reached through the small window and shook my hand. "Good luck, son."

With a small brown bag filled with prescribed marijuana, I left the pharmacy and walked home, past the gleaming dome of the U.S.

Capitol building. I walked quickly, anxious to be home and eager to employ my regained medicine.

I had won a smashing victory against astonishing odds. My sight was secure. My rights assured. After two years of strife and months of unyielding stress I was, at last, safe.

I was also, once again, America's Only Legal Marijuana Smoker.

17 Suffer to Their Deaths

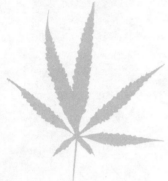

May 25, 1978
Albuquerque, New Mexico

"I'm glad you declined that bet," Lynn said, sounding weak. "I woulda lost big time. I'm still waiting and things don't sound too good."

Lynn was confirming what Alice had already told me. Earlier that day she had talked with Anne Murray, her contact in the N.M. Legislative Council Services Office. "It's all falling apart, Alice," the woman sounded very frustrated.

For three months officials in New Mexico had been working to obtain federal supplies of marijuana for Lynn and other cancer patients. They approached FDA in good faith. When the Washington bureaucrats asked for a "research protocol" the physicians at the University of New Mexico quickly complied. But the FDA found the proposal lacking. A second draft was submitted. And then a third.

Like hamsters running in a wheel, New Mexico officials could not satisfy constantly expanding federal demands. Most frustrating was FDA's refusal to directly address the "problems" in the protocol.

"You're not going to believe this, Alice." Anne went on. "When

one of our doctors tried to clarify a point of procedure the reply from
FDA was, 'You're getting warmer.' They treat this like it's a game."

Of greatest concern to Lynn was the attempt by FDA to impose
"double-blind" testing. Under this plan fewer than half the cancer
patients in New Mexico's would actually receive marijuana. Others
would be given placebo cigarettes or synthetic THC pills.

Lynn was furious. "I didn't fight so half the cancer patients in New
Mexico would be tricked into getting phony pot."

Lynn's powerful friends in the legislature, the Department of
Health and the media agreed. The law entitled cancer patients to
receive medical marijuana. New Mexico did not intend to turn desperately ill cancer patients into U.S. government approved guinea
pigs.

As Lynn had feared, the bureaucrats in Washington could not be
trusted. Despite federal assurances of providing supplies of marijuana, bureaucratic resistance stiffened as other States began exploring New Mexico's historic legislation. If federal drug warriors
could block New Mexico's request for supplies, other States would
be less inclined to follow New Mexico's lead.

And there was ample reason to be worried about other States. On
May 10th, as the Steptoe lawyers hammered out the last pieces in
my settlement, I was in Tallahassee, Florida, testifying on behalf of
a New Mexico style marijuana-as-medicine bill. Similar legislation
was moving along in Illinois and Louisiana. All three bills had a
chance of passage in 1978.

July 5, 1978
NORML Headquarters
Washington, D.C.

"Are you sure, Mildred?" Alice was having trouble comprehend-
ing what she had just heard.

"That's what Mr. Tocus said." The elderly woman was sure. "He said the FDA has destroyed its marijuana and only has enough for Bob Randall."

Mildred and Jim Ripple, like Ara and Gerald Cron, had obtained some marijuana and discovered it worked on Jim's glaucoma. Now Mildred was determined to get Jim legal access. She had spoken with the officials in New Mexico about joining that neighboring state's program once it was authorized. Officials there, frustrated with the FDA's refusal to approve the state's program, had sent her to the FDA. Let them speak with real people who have real problems, they reasoned.

Now Mildred was calling with this odd news. "The FDA doesn't have any marijuana," Alice said, trying to explain the difference between the FDA and NIDA.

"Not any more they don't!" The Arizonan woman was dead certain about what Tocus had said. "I don't know why they just don't grow more. But Mr. Tocus said Bob Randall was getting it all and they'd have to send pills to the New Mexico folks. Do you know if the pills would work for Jim?"

Alice still couldn't make any sense of it but she was sure it was a warning flag.

It was, perhaps, the first glimmer of the "supply problem." New Mexico expected several hundred patients in its program . . . once it was approved. Other states began passing laws. Florida's bill passed 96-6 in the House and by overwhelming voice vote in the Senate. It was signed into law on June 26th. In Louisiana, the final measure was passed in July and would become law on September 8th. Illinois would become the fourth state to enact therapeutic legislation on September 9, 1978, when conservative Governor "Big Jim" Thompson signed legislation. These three states had higher population numbers than New Mexico. Surely they would require a comparable amount of marijuana, most likely more.

More worrisome yet was the growing number of states that were preparing legislation for the 1979 legislative sessions.

The federal government was facing an awesome possibility— thousands of patients needing marijuana cigarettes. Ed Tocus' odd comments to Mildred Ripple will never fully be understood but they were, perhaps, like the canary in the mineshaft, the first whiff that something was wrong. The bureaucrats were nervous.

July 19, 1978
Washington, D.C.

Alice picked up *The Washington Post* at the bottom of the stairs and began scanning the headlines.

"Carter Aide Signed Fake Quaalude Prescription," screamed a headline. The three-column story was accompanied by a picture of Dr. Peter Bourne.

"Holy cow," Alice whispered to the empty hallway. She began reading:

Prince William County police have arrested a Washington woman who attempted to buy the drug Quaalude with an alleg- edly illegal prescription signed by President Carter's chief ad- viser on health and drug abuse, Dr. Peter G. Bourne.

On the following day, the Bourne story had moved from the bottom of page one to the top, just under *The Post* banner. Bourne was put on paid administrative leave while the Quaalude caper was investi- gated. The physician was attempting to ride out the storm of contro- versy. But then reporters got hold of another bit of news. Peter

Bourne, it was said, had been seen snorting cocaine at the NORML party in December 1977.

R. Keith Stroup, chairman of NORML told *The Post* he wouldn't "deny" that Bourne used the illegal drug and then, coyly, added the refusal to deny "was significant."

The illegal Quaalude scripts combined with Keith's too clever comment sparked a political firestorm that consumed Bourne. Several reporters who attended the NORML party had been in the room— and in some cases snorted cocaine with—Dr. Bourne. These reporters now acted as background "sources" for other reporters. The story mushroomed and things got crazy.

"This is Christine Russell of *The Washington Star.*" I glanced at the clock. It was 2 a.m. "Is it true you saw Dr. Bourne use cocaine at the NORML party?"

"No," I told Ms. Russell. "I did not go to the NORML party. Instead, I came home to watch Mary Tyler Moore." The phone line went dead.

Within 24 hours of the first story on July 19, Dr. Peter Bourne imploded, resigning in well-deserved disgrace. Liberals, elitists and drug reformers wailed they had lost a true friend but I knew better. Bourne had learned the dangers of kowtowing to everyone and supporting no one. I was delighted to see the pompous creep thrown out of office.

R. Keith Stroup fared little better. He had trusted Bourne too much, become too chummy, crossed too many lines, then refused to lie. Keith's jealous rivals in NORML demanded his head. By year's end Keith resigned.

As NORML spun out of control, reformers squabbled over spoils. Alice's Medical Reclassification Project became NORML's only viable enterprise. With reformers preoccupied by petty concerns, she moved to reorient NORML's resources.

Mark Heutlinger, NORML's business manager, guided her efforts. "Stay out of the fight; keep doing your job," he advised. Mark was loyal to Keith but he was even more loyal to NORML. As Keith faded, Mark worked closely with Alice, shifting resources, providing critical guidance through the intrigues tearing NORML apart. A good friend.

July 20, 1978
Los Angeles, California

"I met Johnny Carson!"

Lynn Pierson's voice was filled with excitement. He was calling me from Los Angeles where he had just taped the Tom Snyder "Tomorrow" Show. It was good to hear Lynn so upbeat.

Things were moving in New Mexico. At least that's what Lynn thought. On July 13, the State of New Mexico certified Lynn as the first patient in the statewide program. News accounts, including a story in *The New York Times*, reported that "the FDA was expected to approve the program and it could start in a little more than 30 days."

The news account was picked up by the "CBS Evening News" which featured Lynn in a July 15 report. Two days later the Snyder show had called and Lynn was flown to L.A.

I tuned in the show and was shocked at Lynn's appearance. I had met Lynn only once, at the NORML conference in December 1977. Now, seven months later, Lynn had the look of a concentration camp victim. He was gaunt beyond words and there was a sallowness about his eyes that even the TV makeup couldn't erase.

I looked at my friend and realized Lynn would not live to see his legal marijuana.

• • •

Within 24 hours of his return to Albuquerque, Lynn was admitted to the V.A. Hospital in critical condition, suffering from internal bleeding. Transfusions would help for a short while and he was able to go home.

On August 11, Lynn collapsed at his home and lapsed into respiratory failure. The emergency rescue team worked frantically to revive him but by the time he was admitted to the hospital Lynn was comatose and brain dead. For the next four days Lynn's family would agonize over what to do. Lynn's brain waves were flat, his breathing controlled by a respirator. Finally, on August 15, Lynn Pierson died.

He was 27.

August 17, 1978
St. John's United Methodist Church
Albuquerque, New Mexico

The memorial service was packed with state government officials, friends, and family. Officiating was the Rev. M. Buren Stewart who, just six months before, had testified on behalf of Lynn's proposed legislation.

I flew to New Mexico for my friend's funeral and was startled by the emotions I encountered. State officials made a point of seeking me out, thanking me for all the help I had given Lynn, and then venting an absolute contempt for the endless delays, the incompetence and sheer brutality of federal bureaucrats. Lynn died without ever receiving legal marijuana from the federal government and New Mexico was furious about it.

On the day of Lynn's death this rage was expressed to Washington in no uncertain terms. Sensing a PR nightmare, federal agencies moved quickly to blunt the impact. Within three hours of learning about Lynn's death, the FDA verbally approved New

Mexico's application for a statewide medical marijuana program. Mourners at Lynn's service talked excitedly about this news. Too late for Lynn, they sadly noted, but at least he had not died in vain.

The day after Lynn's memorial service the FDA "clarified" its verbal approval and New Mexican officials realized they had been had . . . again. For a while New Mexican officials again considered confiscated stocks of marijuana but finally, with resignation, realized the use of such stocks posed immense legal liabilities.

It would take several more months and eight more patient deaths before New Mexico reached the end of its patience.

On October 27, 1978, Dr. George Goldstein, New Mexico's Secretary of Health, wrote a scathing letter to HEW Secretary Joseph Califano. If New Mexico's request was not approved, Goldstein promised to hold a press conference to publicly denounce the FDA delays as "neither morally nor ethically defensible. If DHEW's desire is to prevent programs such as ours from being implemented, please state that position publicly rather than prevent their implementation through indirect action and prohibitive procedures, while well-meaning citizens submit applications and suffer to their deaths wondering why they have not received the marijuana which they expected."

Finally, on January 26, 1979, New Mexico would receive its first shipments of marijuana and the long-anticipated research program would get under way. A few days later the New Mexico legislature would convene. Among their first acts was to name the statewide program The Lynn Pierson Therapeutic Research Program.

Lynn died without ever receiving his first legal joint but Lynn did not fail. Despite terminal illness he had been a powerful ally. His valiant efforts produced the New Mexico model for medical marijuana, a standard that would be taken to other states and adopted overwhelmingly.

There would be new allies. The fight would go on. But Lynn was special. Pathfinders always are.

18 Committees and the Ripples of Change

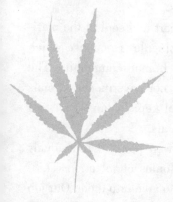

THERE HAD BEEN two sudden departures—Peter Bourne and Lynn Pierson. In the weeks that followed I reflected long and hard on these absences and the contrasting reactions to them. There were lessons to be learned.

Lynn represented the tremendous power of a lone actor able to shatter conventional wisdom and generate genuine change.

Peter Bourne preached change and became a darling of the drug reform community. At his confirmation hearings in May 1977 Bourne would acknowledge past marijuana use and argue the illegal substance was far less harmful than tobacco. Less than three weeks later, fully confirmed and in place at the White House, Bourne would write his shocking June 6 letter to me. Later that year he would publicly support paraquat spraying. Bit by bit he squandered his integrity in hopes of appeasing the federal bureaucrats, especially hard-liners at the DEA.

But straddling a fence can have painful consequences, as Bourne learned in the summer of 1978. Peter Bourne went down in a blaze of media-fueled immolation and the bureaucrats and reformers lined up on both sides to throw on the gasoline. He had no support. In less than a week he was gone, and drug reform in America was set back twenty years.

The people of New Mexico had no interest in drug reform. Probably fewer than one in ten could have told you who Peter Bourne was. They simply wanted to help Lynn get the medical care he required. These public motivations were not political, but personal. Lynn was a neighbor in need of help. They willingly gave him their support because they trusted his intentions.

This, I began to understand, was the heart and soul of the marijuana therapeutic issue. It is an issue of singular resonance which strikes a chord deep in the center of the human community. The stark realization was that neither activists nor government officials held the key to change. Patterns of thought kept looping back to a single refrain—the power lay with individuals.

As we entered the last half of 1978 there were plenty of individuals in need of help and the states—those colonies of salvation established by our forefathers—seemed willing to give it to them. Our job was to focus the energy, keep the information flowing, and try to stay one step ahead of the feds.

It would require some fancy footwork.

August 28, 1978
31-NIH, Conference Room 9
Bethesda, Maryland

Alice and I settled in for our first meeting of the Interagency Committee on New Therapies for Pain and Discomfort. The huge, 32-member committee, chaired by Dr. Seymour Perry, had been meeting since late 1977 but the feds had not been eager to publicize its existence. The group "was formed in response to the expressed interest of the White House and Dr. Peter Bourne . . . in the problems of pain and other discomforts of the dying and in fostering research on the possible pain-relieving characteristics of abused substances not approved for treatment in the United States."

The Committee had numerous subcommittees, including the Subcommittee on the IND Process for Schedule I Drugs.

Alice had learned about the Committee from Judith Quattlebaum, an articulate and well-connected woman from Potomac, Maryland who had formed the National Committee on the Treatment of Intractable Pain. Quattlebaum's group was attempting to reinstate heroin in the U.S. Pharmacopoeia as a legitimate drug for pain relief.

Judith had been warned by federal officials to "keep her distance" from the drug reformers "like NORML and Randall." As time passed, however, Judith realized the feds were not entirely trustworthy. She and Alice began communicating on a regular basis. By midsummer of 1978, Judith was encouraging Alice to attend the Interagency meetings. "There's a lot more talk about marijuana," Judith said. "You're missing some interesting stuff."

The Committee had all the usual suspects—the FDA, NIDA, DEA, NIH, NIMH, NCI, NEI, HEW, DoJ—and some new faces from the Dept. of Defense. Unacknowledged but undoubtedly present, was the CIA. The old MKDELTA crowd plotting how to stop medical marijuana by pretending to explore compassion as a bureaucratic option. Great cover.

The meeting droned on for two hours before we heard anything worthwhile. An official from NCI referred to the "Current Status meeting of last May" and the very promising results of Nabilone, a chemical similar to delta-9 THC but totally synthetic. Nabilone, it was reported, was heading for the final phase of approval at the FDA and officials expected the last of the paperwork to be filed by the first quarter of 1979.

From the smiles and nods that went around the table it was clear to us that we should learn more about Nabilone.

• • •

We were beginning to understand that a great deal of information could be gleaned from committee meetings and Alice became more conscientious in tracking the agendas of the endless number of government committees that seemed to have their finger in the medical prohibition pie.

DARAC, the committee which had plotted my comeuppance in the first half of 1977, was experiencing its own comeuppance as Alice doggedly attended their meetings and forced the members to confront a levelheaded, likable young woman who could be very persistent about marijuana's beneficial therapeutic effects.

In September 1978, perhaps hoping to escape the increasingly public meetings in Washington, DARAC members headed south for a meeting at the University of Mississippi. Close on their heels was Alice.

September 28, 1978
"The Pot Plantation"
Oxford, Mississippi

On her 31st birthday, Alice stood in the middle of five acres of land affectionately referred to as Uncle Sam's Pot Farm. DARAC was taking a "field trip" and Alice was brushing shoulders with an elite group of farmers—the legal marijuana farmers employed by the U.S. government.

The 1978 crop was mostly gone, harvested just a week or so earlier. All that was left was a field of dark delta mud littered with broken stalks drying on black plastic tarps in the hot sun. In the center of the plot were a few plants of the indica variety, shorter and more bushy than their sativa cousins.

"Specialty items," noted Carlton Turner dryly. The director of the University of Mississippi Research Institute of Pharmaceutical Sciences (RIPS) was giving the DARAC members the grand tour. Turner, a thin, oddly behaved fellow, referred to all marijuana not in his 5-acre fiefdom as, "Cannabis which has escaped from cultivation." There was not a hint of amusement at such a notion. Marijuana, in his mind, is "a crude drug."

The farm was surrounded by a double fence of barbed and razor wire. Between the two fences was a path for guard dogs. Watch towers with searchlights stood at the corners of the barren enclosure, empty because the pot had been harvested.

Looking about the acreage Alice was astonished at how small five acres could be. The cute references to the Pot Plantation had implied a huge operation, but it was tiny. Much of the land wasn't even tilled. "How," she wondered, "could this farm grow enough marijuana for New Mexico, Florida, Louisiana, and Illinois?"

The small group scuffed about in the dirt, posed for some pictures and then returned to the RIPS facilities where Alice was introduced to an aging southern gent; a professor of Botany with a mane of snow-white hair and gracious Mississippi manners. Unlike Turner, who greeted inquiries with a tinge of paranoia, the old botanist was delighted by Alice's interest in his arcane endeavors. Without hesitation he pulled out a large scrap-book to show her his favorite marijuana leaves from past harvests.

Officially, the Mississippi "pot plantation" began its work in the late 1960s. It was obvious to Alice that the farm had been in operation much longer. The elder Botany professor with his treasured book of long-ago harvested leaves suggested the pot plantation was decades old.

September 29, 1978
Ole Miss Campus
Oxford, Mississippi

The farm had been an interesting sideshow but the real item on the agenda which had captured Alice's attention was "Discussion of proposed protocols for Schedule I drugs."

The Ripples had become regular correspondents with both Alice and me. Jim Ripple's protocol had been submitted several months before and Alice was certain it would be part of the presentation. Mildred was feisty and determined. She was not going to let Jim go blind if there was something that could help him. Jim's family had a long history of glaucoma. His mother and a brother had been blinded by the disease, their eyeballs literally rupturing from elevated pressures. Mildred would not let that happen to Jim.

The elderly couple lived in the southernmost deserts of Arizona, three hours from Tucson, not far from the Mexican border. Their doctor was sixty miles away. Their remoteness seemed daunting but Mildred had painstakingly put together the necessary pieces to apply for permission to use marijuana. In July, Jim's doctor had submitted an IND protocol, copied almost word-for-word, from my approved Compassionate IND.

To make certain that compassion prevailed, Alice discussed the case with Tom Collier who, in turn, discussed it with a friend in Arizona. Before long Mildred and Jim had the high-powered, Phoenix-based legal firm of Brown & Bain at their disposal.

Once Brown & Bain got involved the FDA became more helpful. Ed Tocus did not want a replay of my case. A glaucoma patient— an aging, retired cowboy—suing the government for marijuana was certain to attract media attention and garner public sympathy.

Mildred lined up some political support by contacting Senator Barry Goldwater and asking for his help in expediting Jim's request. She also enlisted the support of Senator Muriel Humphrey, widow of former vice president Hubert Humphrey. There had been rumors that Mr. Humphrey had used marijuana during his chemotherapy treatments.

Now, in a sterile room in Mississippi, Jim Ripple's fate was being discussed and it was tying Alice's stomach in knots.

There was grousing from some committee members about letters from a lawyer and the Senators. Repeatedly the committee returned to regulatory procedure and the inappropriateness of releasing an unapproved drug to a "single patient" who was clearly not part of any "viable research." There was worry about precedents and not much concern about an ailing cowboy who had exhausted all conventional routes of treatment.

Finally Alice could contain herself no longer and raised her hand. "I am not sure it is appropriate for members of the public to make comments," Alice began politely, "but I think you have got to realize that marijuana is unlike other drugs that go through the IND process. I know this case you are talking about. I know the individuals involved and I know that the man has used marijuana illegally."

The committee listened respectfully as Alice continued. "You've got to remember that marijuana is available to people, and that is the big difference between it and the other drugs you are dealing with. I think it is far better for this man to receive marijuana through his doctor than to find it on the street."

"You say you know this specific case, the 65-year old man?" the DARAC chairman asked.

Alice explained the human side of a case known to DARAC as Protocol K and the members listened, some with open amazement. Protocol K would survive DARAC. Jim Ripple's protocol would be approved in early October. But the Arizona cowboy would not get his legal marijuana any time soon.

Alice's excursion to the "pot plantation" raised many questions. Indeed we had a growing list of questions. There was Mildred's recanting of Tocus' curious claim that "all the marijuana has been destroyed." There were the references to Nabilone at the Perry Committee. What was that? And now there were these curious hints of a long established marijuana farm in the Mississippi Delta.

We decided to file a freedom of information request to see what we could learn about the government's production of marijuana and, while we were at it, we asked for minutes from any committee meetings at which medical marijuana had been discussed in the past two years.

The FOIA materials arrived very fast. The large packet contained detailed information on annual production, stockpiles of raw material and a complete inventory of finished, pre-rolled marijuana cigarettes. There was enough budgetary information to calculate the cost of production: Uncle Sam spent about 90 cents per ounce to grow marijuana, with two-thirds of this cost going to security. The actual price of production minus security came to 30 cents per ounce.

Given these figures, is it any wonder pharmaceutical companies promoting expensive synthetic drugs have little interest in pursuing marijuana's therapeutic utility? Sure, marijuana might aid the afflicted. But how could a pharmaceutical company profit from such a cheap, easy-to-produce product? This was a bottom-line question that animated the prohibition. Beyond dogma there were dollars.

Also in the materials were pages of minutes from various government agencies that had been discussing marijuana's medical use, including the mysterious "Current Status" meeting which had taken place, we learned, in May 1978, about the time of my legal suit against the government. The minutes, which were no more than two pages in length, summarized the day-long meeting and provided us with information on Nabilone as well as some other tidbits which would become extremely critical in the coming year.

The FOIA materials would also give Alice an unexpected opportunity to travel to the Southwest. Her knowledge of the price of marijuana production—gleaned from the FOIA-obtained reports— legitimized her status as an "expert witness" at a trial in New Mexico involving a rather unsavory individual who was an informant for the government and was trying to collect his bounty following the arrest of some major drug smugglers. Not exactly the type of case with which we wanted to be associated but the attorneys were convincing and there was a large expert witness stipend.

Further rationalization came when Alice reasoned she could use the opportunity to meet people in New Mexico and Arizona with whom she had been working for almost a year.

So, in December 1978, after testifying in Las Cruces, Alice flew into Albuquerque and met Lynn's family who lent her Lynn's car for her travels to Sante Fe. There she met with officials to discuss the still inactive state research program. New Mexican officials were hopeful the marijuana would arrive soon.

Then she traveled to Arizona and spent an afternoon with the Ripples. They too were still waiting for the promised marijuana.

In the great Southwest there was much anticipation for the New Year.

19 Critical Mass

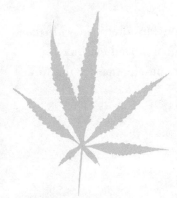

March 22, 1979
NORML Headquarters
Washington, D.C.

Alice was weary. She had returned to NORML after another committee meeting, her third of the week. Her desk was cluttered with phone messages and mail. The medical marijuana issue was exploding.

She swiveled her chair around and looked at the map on her office wall which was cluttered with many small pins of different colors, some very large black pins, and a sprinkling of handmade, marijuana-leaf "flags."

The small pins represented patients, individuals with serious ailments who had contacted NORML for information on marijuana's medical use. There were many, many pins. Alice had begun the exercise to judge how my travels, which had been extensive in the first quarter of 1979, impacted the requests for information. For a while there seemed a clear correlation. But in recent weeks the requests were mushrooming at an incredible pace. There was no discernible pattern, just sheer momentum.

The large black pins, a total of sixteen, indicated a medical marijuana law had been introduced and was in some stage of consideration: committee hearings, house or senate vote.

The flags were Alice's favorite symbol. They meant a law had been passed. There were seven flags on the map, the four original states from 1978—New Mexico, Florida, Louisiana, and Illinois—plus the recent successes from 1979—West Virginia, Washington, and Virginia.

Sixteen states considering plus seven laws passed: twenty-three! Almost half the country actively considering medical marijuana! And that didn't even begin to include the indications of interest from other states, proposed or active lawsuits, and people like Jim Ripple, who were willing to fight the long battle for individual access to marijuana. Jim's supplies had arrived in mid-January, just after New Mexico received its shipment. The retired cowboy had been using the legally supplied marijuana for two months with great success. His glaucoma was well controlled. Mildred was delighted. "This is really incredible!" Alice thought, staring at the map. "They'll have a hard time getting the lid back on."

Earlier in the week Alice had attended yet another of the monthly meetings of the Interagency Committee on New Therapies for Pain and Discomfort. The Committee had lost their champion when Peter Bourne resigned in July 1978. There was an evident weariness. Medical marijuana dominated the discussions. There was no longer the patina of humanitarian concern or discussions of "helping the states" and "facilitating research." The darker forces, which had advocated a tougher stance against marijuana therapeutics, were beginning to prevail. The focus was now on stopping the firestorm of medical marijuana legislation that was sweeping across the country. Words such as "discourage," "deactivate," and "defuse" were freely used. There was no effort to conceal the bureaucratic contempt for the States efforts.

Alice was reflecting on these events when Mark Heutlinger, NORML's business manager, stopped by to say hello.

"I hear Iowa could be next," he said, following Alice's gaze to the large map on the wall.

"Um, could be. The Washington and West Virginia bills get signed next week."

"I can't believe Dixie Lee Ray is signing." Mark said, shaking his head in wonderment. Governor Ray, a staunch conservative, was a darling of the Republican Right. "It's like Goldwater helping that cowboy get marijuana. It's just unbelievable!"

"Believe it, Mark. This isn't decrim," Alice said, alluding to the NORML policy of decriminalizing possession of small amounts of marijuana. "It's a lot bigger than decrim."

Mark smiled. He had grown accustomed to Alice's assertion that medical marijuana would dwarf the personal use issue.

"Well, once the research data comes in from New Mexico and a couple of these other states they'll have to legalize it for medical purposes." Mark said, turning to look at Alice. "What do you think? Three, maybe five years more?"

Alice quickly did the math in her head. "1984? Orwell's 1984? The year marijuana is re-legalized for medical purposes?" Alice laughed with delight at the idea. "Don't count on it. They're plotting right now to stop this thing."

Throughout 1979 the medical marijuana issue gathered more and more steam smashing ideological and cultural divisions which had long acted as barriers to drug reform. NORML's amazement at the support of conservative politicians was echoed in the actions of Washington bureaucrats as they attempted, and failed, to activate conservative opposition. Conservatives get cancer, too. Dixie Lee Ray, the Washington Governor who signed the nation's fifth marijuana-as-medicine bill, was one of them.

Indeed, it was conservatives—arch foes of centralized power— who became medical marijuana's most ardent proponents. After 50 years of federal encroachment, conservatives were ready to reclaim state power, and defend the sovereign rights of citizens to medical care.

And citizens were ready to demand it. In every state that considered a marijuana-as-medicine bill in 1979 the effort was propelled by a human interest story. Some were small and lacked notoriety. Others blazed across the media skies, capturing attention, inspiring change. It is not necessary to catalogue each of these battles. But it is illuminating to explore the various ways in which people, media and politicians worked to end the medical prohibition.

- In Washington state the doorkeeper to the House of Representatives made it a point to tell every legislator about his wife's successful use of marijuana in combating the side effects of cancer chemotherapy. Washington legislators also took testimony from dozens of cancer patient who vigorously endorsed marijuana's medical usefulness.

- In Nevada legislators heard testimony from a 23-year-old woman blinded by the side effects of diabetes. She testified that marijuana helped ease the ocular discomfort she experienced and it stimulated her appetite which was helpful in controlling the diabetes. The Nevada bill, enacted in June 1979, was initially requested by a Mormon judge who suffered from cancer. In testifying for the bill the judge said, "I, myself, because of my cultural background, would be reluctant to smoke marijuana. However, I might reconsider that cultural opposition if it appeared to be medically appropriate."

- In California, Patrick Mayer, a cancer survivor, would spearhead the campaign for that state's medical marijuana bill. Mayer, whose leg was amputated as a result of cancer, was an articulate young man who claimed to be one of the anonymous patients to first report marijuana's medical usefulness to the Boston oncologists in the early 1970s.

- A 50-year-old farmer's wife named Elva Emry inspired action in two states, Nebraska and Iowa. The cancer patient, a resident of Nebraska, asked her neighboring state of Iowa for help in obtaining legal access to marijuana because medical facilities across the border were closer to her home. The request sparked legislation in both states. Iowa's bill would pass in June 1979.
- In Louisiana, Michael Pobuda, a 24-year-old victim of Hodgkin's disease, spent his final days of life struggling to implement the Louisiana bill enacted in 1978.
- In Wisconsin a former alderman, Donald Murdoch, credited marijuana with his survival. "Marijuana can help. I know from my own experience," Murdoch told legislators. He had used the illegal substance during radiation and chemotherapy treatments.*

In that extraordinary year of 1979 there were many individuals who came forward to support medical access to marijuana. Many more quietly worked in the background, writing letters and making calls. But from our personal point of view the most compelling story of 1979 was Keith Nutt, a young man from Michigan who had the misfortune to contract cancer in his 22nd year of life but was blessed with fine parents who helped make his final days of life expansive and triumphant.

Like Lynn Pierson, Keith Nutt had testicular cancer. It was diagnosed in the spring of 1978. At the time he was living in Columbus, Ohio. His parents, Mae and Arnold Nutt, were living in Beaverton, Michigan. Keith had surgery to remove the cancerous testicle but, unlike Lynn, Keith did not immediately begin chemo. The doctors felt they had successfully removed the cancer. Keith tried to get on with his life but was unable to maintain his

*The Wisconsin bill would not pass for several years (April 1982).

energy and, in the fall of 1978, he moved back home with his parents.

On January 1, 1979, Keith told his parents the cancer had returned. His remaining testicle was hard and enlarged. He saw a doctor the next day and was hospitalized that afternoon.

The second surgery was followed by extensive chemotherapy. Keith received cisplatin and there were severe problems with nausea and vomiting. His parents watched in horror as chemo took a rapid and devastating toll. Keith couldn't eat, couldn't bear to even smell food. His weight dropped dramatically.

For Mae and Arnold it was all too reminiscent of another son's illness. Keith's younger brother, Dana, had Ewings Sarcoma and suffered grievously during his short nine years of life. Keith told Mae he did not want to suffer like Dana. He vowed he would take his own life rather than waste away as Dana had. Keith extracted a promise from Mae that she would help him when the time came.

These were dark days for the Nutt family. Keith lost more than thirty pounds and grew weaker by the day. Mae was concerned she would be called upon to fulfill her promise to her eldest son.

Mae read in a local newspaper that marijuana could help cancer patients endure chemotherapy. Initially she scoffed at the idea but when she mentioned it to Keith he confirmed that other cancer patients talked about it. Mae needed no more encouragement. She began making calls to obtain more information, including packets from Alice's Medical Reclassification Project.

Mae and Arnold read it all and were convinced. They began making inquiries to obtain marijuana for Keith's next chemo session but there was none to be found. Finally, they would "score" through an unlikely source—a Presbyterian minister who listened carefully to their story and arrived at their house late in the evening on the night before Keith's chemo with a small baggie of marijuana.

The next day, with some anxiety, Mae and Arnold watched Keith smoke the marijuana just as the nausea began to well up inside him.

It was, they would later say, "miraculous." There was no vomiting, no nausea. Quite the contrary, Keith's appetite improved. In fact, his entire being improved. The aches and pains diminished. He was able to join his family for dinner—an act of sublime simplicity made possible by an illegal weed.

As Mae watched her son improve she became enraged at the prospect of breaking the law to help him. She and Keith became vigorous and vocal advocates for the New Mexico style legislation that had been proposed in Michigan. Despite his improvement, Keith was still very ill but he wanted others to know how helpful marijuana could be. Like Lynn, Keith was thinking of others.

On March 11, 1979, in the local *Bay City Times*, the Nutts went public:

Keith Nutt of Beaverton doesn't care who knows he uses marijuana. It is the only thing that relieves the terrible nausea that follows chemotherapy treatments for cancer, says the 23-year-old man. Right now, Keith is still able to drive to his sources of marijuana. If the time comes when Keith can't get out of the house to buy the illegal drug, his mother, Mae Nutt, 58, says "that's where I come in! But it shouldn't be necessary to break the law to get help for a child who is very, very ill."

The story of Keith Nutt resonated across the Michigan countryside, invaded every nook and cranny of the state, gave focus to legislation which would easily pass in early October (House: 100-0, Senate:33-1). When Keith was too ill to travel to the State Capitol, Mae and Arnold would go alone and speak not only for their son but for all the sons and daughters who needed legal access to marijuana.

On the evening of Sunday, October 21, 1979, Mae and Arnold went to say goodnight to their son. They told the young man that Michigan's medical marijuana bill, the nation's 18th such law, would be signed the next day in Lansing. Keith was very happy that his efforts had made a difference. He smiled and said goodnight.

Early the next morning Keith Nutt died. That afternoon the bill was signed.

Mae and Arnold could have easily "retired" from the medical marijuana issue. No one would have criticized them for doing so. But they remained committed to Keith's goal of helping others and they were ever-mindful of the difficulties they had had in obtaining a drug that gave so much comfort. Before Keith's death, supplies of marijuana would arrive in all kinds of ways—the mailbox, the front door stoop, small bags passed along by friends. There was more than Keith could use so Mae began giving it to other cancer patients. She became known as Grandma Marijuana and her "delivery service" became the Green Cross. Mae would continue this work for several years after Keith's death, providing some comfort to cancer patients while Michigan's state program became mired in the same swamp of government red tape that entangled New Mexico.

But, we're getting ahead of ourselves.

It was late 1979. There were now eighteen state laws. Another ten states were considering similar measures with passage likely in more than half of them during the 1980 legislative season. Keith Nutt was gone but new recruits had seized the standard. A cancer patient in Pennsylvania, Anne Guttentag, had been relentlessly pursuing legal access via the IND process. Her case would now move to center stage.

In Georgia, a young woman was shaking off her first layer of widow weeds. Before his death, Harrison Taft had found great medical benefit from marijuana. He and his wife, Mona, had talked about the states that were passing laws. It would be nice, they thought, to do something like that in Georgia. But Harrison was too ill. After his death in late June 1979, Mona took some time to rest and then set out to preserve his memory by passing a medical marijuana bill. One of her first calls was to Alice at the Medical Reclassification Project.

Meanwhile, the bureaucrats were sweating bullets. The demand for legal quantities of marijuana was steamrolling across the nation. There seemed to be no way of stopping the states from enacting these laws but the bureaucrats knew they had the upper hand: they controlled the supplies of marijuana. By controlling access they could, ultimately, control the outcome.

20 The System Comes Unstuck

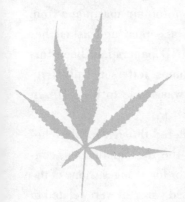

ANNE GUTTENTAG WAS 57 and suffering from ovarian cancer. She had been battling cancer for more than three years. In 1976 she had a radical mastectomy and hoped the cancer was stopped. It wasn't. In early March 1979 she had a second surgery for ovarian cancer. This procedure was followed by chemotherapy. Anne was given cisplatin and adriamycin. It was a nightmare.

"I vomited until there was nothing left. Then I retched until my ribs and my back and my chest ached. Then I vomited again . . . Hours of tortuous, degrading vomiting, feeling your insides tearing . . . My thoughts turned to death and how peaceful I could be."

Regular medications failed to stop the vomiting, and when Anne learned marijuana might help she lost no time in trying to obtain the drug. She began making calls to everyone she could think of including the police chief in her home town of New Hope, Pennsylvania, trying to learn how the drug could be obtained legally. When no one could help her she called the press. A reporter from *The Trenton Times* (NJ) was happy to visit with her.

Anne was determined, publicly declaring. "I demand [marijuana] and I'm going to get it one way or another."

The article, which appeared in March 1979, was comprehensive and obligingly provided the address of Anne's doll store in New Hope. She and her husband, a law professor at Trenton State College, lived above the store.

Alice immediately wrote the woman, offering assistance in helping Anne's doctor apply for permission to obtain marijuana from the federal government. Anne quickly accepted and asked her doctor to cooperate. By mid-April the IND papers had been forwarded to Anne's physician at the Thomas Jefferson University Hospital in Philadelphia. Application was made to the FDA in June 1979.

For the next five months, as Anne suffered through regular chemotherapy sessions, the FDA nit-picked the IND application, constantly returning the document to the doctor for changes. None of the changes related directly to Anne's proposed care, all were related to administrative matters or reporting procedures. Finally, in November, just in time for her last scheduled chemo session, Anne's doctor received supplies of the THC pill. The FDA insisted she try the THC before using marijuana. She tried the synthetic and complained bitterly about the dosage form and the effect. She had used natural marijuana, illegally obtained, with great success. But the THC pills "were nothing like the cigarettes" she told Alice. "I feel so heavy, like I've been on a binge."

Her doctor immediately reported to the FDA that Anne had great difficulty keeping the pills down, a common problem. Both doctor and patient were hopeful, however, that the chemo sessions were finished and there would be no further need for THC pills or marijuana.

But the cancer wasn't gone. In January 1980 Anne was back for more chemo. The THC continued to fail but FDA insisted Anne's doctor try the pills six times "before deeming it a failure." Anne even agreed to give up her illegal use of marijuana during this tortuous round of "research."

"It was," she would later say, "a living hell."

In mid-March 1980, exploratory surgery was performed and though the cancer had shrunk it was still present throughout Anne's body. More chemotherapy was administered in April. Once again the vomiting was awful. But Anne's doctor had good news. He had called FDA again and told them of THC's failure. FDA promised she would have the marijuana cigarettes she needed before her next treatment in May.

While Alice monitored the condition of her friend in New Hope we also followed the remarkable progress of a Georgia woman—Mona Taft.

With raven hair, an engaging style, and an absolute sense of righteousness, Mona had little trouble in swaying the political consensus of Georgia to accept marijuana's medical usefulness. She began her crusade a few weeks after her husband's death from Hodgkin's' disease in June 1979. She was careful and methodical in her approach, first lining up the support of her parents, then calling Alice at the Medical Reclassification Project for information. She read and studied the data, then approached her husband's doctors. Having won their support she set her sights on the Capitol Building in Atlanta.

An attractive young woman, Mona quickly found her legislative champions. Representative Virlyn Smith was a kindly, conservative Republican and a cancer survivor. Virlyn was a legend in the Statehouse and his support on any piece of legislation gave it great weight.

On the "other side of the aisle," Mona enlisted the powerful Democrat Senator Paul Broun. Senator Broun's wife was battling cancer and he openly embraced the proposals for a marijuana-as-medicine bill.

Throughout the Fall of 1979, Mona would work through Smith and Broun's offices to collect more data and prepare a bill for the 1980 legislative session. It was introduced immediately in the New Year and barreled through the Georgia legislature faster than Sherman's march to the sea. In the House it passed 158-6. In the Senate 50-0.

On February 22, 1980, Governor George Busby signed the bill into law. It was the nation's twentieth medical marijuana bill.

For Mona, who was invited to attend the bill signing ceremony, it was a bitter sweet moment. It was the anniversary of Harrison Taft's birthday. He had been dead for eight months.

April 17, 1980
NORML Headquarters
Washington, D.C.

"Ms. O'Leary, this is Bob Hundley with the Select Committee on Narcotics."

The call was unexpected.

"Ms. O'Leary, the Select Committee has convened a task force on the therapeutic use of marijuana and other Schedule I drugs. We would appreciate your assistance in identifying potential witnesses and providing any information that might be pertinent."

Medical marijuana could no longer be ignored. Since the enactment of Georgia's bill in February four more states had passed medical marijuana laws—South Carolina, Ohio, Minnesota, and Arizona. Another half dozen were considering measures.

It was not a surprise the Congress was considering hearings. The surprise was that it had taken so long.

Alice learned the hearings would be chaired by Rep. Stephen L. Neal (D-NC). Other members of the task force were Lester Wolff (D-NY), Billy L. Evans (R-GA), and Larry McDonald (R-GA). Alice found the inclusion of two Georgia Congressmen to be of particular note.

Hundley was friendly and professional. He was particularly interested in any patients who "had used or were using marijuana for medical purposes, especially cancer patients. Do you know someone who might want to testify?"

"Well, there is a woman named Anne Guttentag."

Select committees offer Congress a wonderful way of engaging in activity that looks great in the hometown newspapers but does little to actually alter the course of events. Select committees cannot legislate. They are "fact finders."

Task forces are even lower than select committees. With nearly half the States endorsing a citizen's right to legally access marijuana for medical purposes, it seemed more appropriate for hearings to be held before a justice or health committee—a committee that could actually resolve the conflict between federal regulations and the desire of the states to help their seriously ill citizens. But no such committee came forward.

Anne was invited along with another cancer patient, Richard Csandl, also from Pennsylvania. Richard had also tried to obtain marijuana through the IND process and experienced great frustration. Ultimately, Richard abandoned chemotherapy after nearly a year of treatment. He credits illegal marijuana with helping him survive the oatcell and small cell carcinoma that he was told in April 1978 would claim his life in 4–6 weeks. After tolerating eleven months of chemo he simply walked away from the grueling medical treatments and began an aggressive program of diet and exercise. In 1995 he was still alive and active in drug abuse counseling in Pennsylvania.

I completed this panel of "patients." The Task Force listened

respectfully as each of us told our story. There were a few questions
focusing on the difference between THC and natural marijuana.
There were also some specific questions from the Select Committee
Chairman Lester Wolff about my attitudes towards general drug legalization. It was clear Rep. Wolff had been briefed about my case,
most likely by DEA.

We were followed by a panel of physicians, including Dr. John
Merritt who was still teaching and researching at the University of
North Carolina. All of the physicians on the panel expressed concern
about the THC pill. The oncologists noted the absurdity of having to
give an oral medication to a vomiting patient. Beyond that, however,
they were concerned about the formulation of THC, its erratic performance and disturbing side-effects.

Then the Task Force heard from the government's representatives.
Seven bureaucrats sat at the table to give testimony. It was the representative from NCI, however, who dropped the bombshell that day.
Dr. John MacDonald, associate director for Cancer Therapy Evaluation, Division of Cancer Treatment, quietly announced that THC
would be moved into the NCI's Group C program. "Under Group C,"
Dr. MacDonald explained, "a compound is considered to have doc-
umented medical efficacy for a specific indication and not be a research drug per se, although it remains investigational."

Group C drugs can be distributed to community/regional/compre-
hensive cancer centers as well as medical school affiliated hospital
pharmacies. "This would amount to 500 to 600 separate pharmacies
scattered around the country at these institutions." The drug would
then be available to nearly 3,000 oncologists.

It was the first public indication of the government's strategy to
end-run the unceasing drive by the states to enact marijuana-as-
medicine bills. Group C had been occasionally referenced during the
Perry Committee hearings but we had no concept of the scale—500
to 600 pharmacies! 3,000 doctors! This amounted to virtual approval
of THC.

MacDonald's testimony was followed by Dr. Richard Crout, director of the Bureau of Drugs for the FDA. Crout's bombshell was even bigger.

"We have agreed with NCI that THC may be a candidate for Group C investigational status. NCI has therefore prepared an application for this classification which we received on May 12. In anticipation of this, we had already scheduled a discussion on placing THC in the Group C plan for FDA's Oncology Advisory Committee meeting to be held on June 26, 1980."

Still later in the hearings the representative from NIDA would put the icing on the cake when he told the task force that "NIDA, in collaboration with NCI, is preparing to manufacture 500,000 THC capsules by July 1 of this year. And plans call for another 500,000 to be manufactured by January 1, 1981."

It was a done deal. The meeting of the Oncologic Advisory Committee in June was a mere formality. For more than two years the bureaucracies had been bombarded by constant demands to release marijuana for medical purposes. They had been stuck in the mire of ideological drug policy masquerading as science. The agencies had now found a way to extend the masquerade. Marijuana, they were saying, had no medical value. THC, just one of its components, did.

The country would soon be flooded with THC and the government would happily blur the distinctions between marijuana and its synthetic component. In short time THC would become known as the "pot pill," and the states were told they could have all the pot pills they wanted without having to pass those nasty old laws.

But there were two problems—THC didn't work and the states wanted marijuana.

After the Congressional task force hearings, Anne Guttentag returned to New Hope with some new hope of her own. On June 6 she arrived for her scheduled chemotherapy expecting the marijuana cigarettes.

They were not there. She had been disappointed in early May but accepted it. Now, after her appearance before the Task Force and listening to the promises of bureaucrats who had said marijuana was easy to obtain by qualified researchers, now Anne Guttentag was very angry.

After resting for two days, Anne sat down to write the Task Force Chairman on June 8:

My dear Mr. Neal:

Once again that I thank you for permitting me to speak before your committee on Narcotics Abuse and Control, May 20.

To bring you up to date, a prescription was issued for the marijuana in cigarette form in April. I have not received them as requested. I was treated again on June 6 with only the pills (THC) and Compazine. Needless to say both failed.

I'm about ready to give up. The fight to live is not worth going through this anymore. I feel no one cares, nor will any one do anything to help. Not when it took months to be given a pill that common sense tells you will be thrown back up. And then to be made to wait months for the cigarettes that are known to work. I wonder if anyone realizes the anxiety that goes on?

I have stopped buying the marijuana illegally. My friend who got it for me and whom I felt confident would only supply good marijuana is dying from cancer of the brain. How's that for a finale? The government won't help and the one person that was helping is now a statistic—that one-out-of-four in this country dying from cancer.

Where is the group who told your committee that there was no problem with the paperwork and that marijuana was now easy to get? Show them this letter, for someone is telling an untruth.

Very truly yours, Anne Guttentag.

On July 24 Anne received her legal marijuana cigarettes—thirteen months after she asked for them. She called Alice to say "they made a BIG difference." Her voice was weary but triumphant.

Anne would have her marijuana cigarettes for the remainder of her treatments but the chemotherapy could not save her. Nevertheless, she spoke out often in the press and on TV, advocating legal access to marijuana.

She would speak to Alice for the last time on February 26, 1981. It was a painful conversation for them both. "I'm going down, Alice. My mind is sluggish. I can't be sure of what I'm saying anymore."

Her last months were a nightmare of medical and physical complications. Alice kept in touch with her husband, David, but Anne would not speak with Alice any longer—she was letting go bit by bit. On August 23, 1981, the sixth anniversary of our "bust," Anne Guttentag died.

III

Synthetic Solutions

21 Let 'em Eat THC

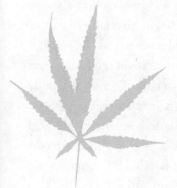

WITH THE MAY 20, 1980, announcement
at the Neal Hearings of the Group C inclusion of THC, the bureaucrats had, at
last, found their footing after enduring a
groundswell of change. It was just 27 months after New Mexico enacted the first state law recognizing marijuana's medical value and
there were already 24 state laws passed! It was just 3½ years since
I had first received legal supplies of marijuana and became "America's Only Legal Pot Smoker." It had been an extraordinary period
of rapid change and nothing worries a bureaucracy more than rapid
change.

For more than forty years the FDA and DEA had enjoyed a free
ride of escalating restriction. No serious challenge to the increasingly
strident control of drugs, legal and illegal, had ever been mounted.
Even the pharmaceutical companies, with their wealth and vast resources, had capitulated to the growing power of the FDA, especially
after the Thalidomide debacle of the early 1960s.

Now, in the face of an unexpected national plebiscite on medical
marijuana, the bureaucrats had been forced to engage in their own
capitulation. It is doubtful any of the agencies ever anticipated the

wide-scale distribution of delta-9 THC but that is what had been forced upon them by the medical marijuana movement.

The federal agencies could not stop their ongoing political rout in the states but they could maintain some control through their absolute monopoly over the U.S. marijuana supply. Trapped in a public mask of "encouraging research with Schedule I drugs," the FDA freely promised federal stocks of marijuana to each state. This prevented the States from adopting extreme measures such as the use of confiscated stocks or exploring state-based cultivation programs.

The strategy worked very well in New Mexico but as the number of state laws increased the gap between static federal production and expanding state demands created a supply crisis. There was simply not enough federal marijuana to meet the demands from the States. Even the Council on Scientific Affairs for the American Medical Association (AMA) could see the writing on the wall. In a report issued in the first half of 1980 the Council advised, "It may become necessary to place additional acres under cultivation."

There were only two solutions: 1) NIDA could expand federal marijuana production to meet accelerating patient needs, or 2) a synthetic, pharmaceutically prepared solution could be released.

Expanding U.S. marijuana production was the rational option. But this solution was bureaucratically unacceptable. The consequence of expanding marijuana production was obvious. Increasing U.S. marijuana supplies would increase state demands for supply. If this supply-demand dynamic took hold the government would, in effect, become the de facto pharmaceutical manufacturer of marijuana.

This outcome would challenge the very core of the drug control complex; it was unacceptable and dangerous to expand cultivation so the bureaucrats turned their attention to the synthetic solution.

By mid-1978, Alice and I were aware of the shortfalls in marijuana production and the pressure this situation would apply to the agencies. The only question was which option the government would choose. We began tracking the closed-door activities of the bureaucrats through the keyhole of the increasingly dysfunctional Interagency Committee on New Therapies for Pain and Discomfort.

It was here that the scrambling efforts to locate a synthetic alternative to marijuana first emerged. Numerous companies, including Abbott Laboratories, Pfizer, and Eli Lilly, were investigating marijuana-like agents. The most promising of these, Nabilone, was a patented THC-analogue developed by Eli Lilly. As federal agencies lost the political struggle in the states, the FDA accelerated Nabilone development, allowing Lilly to "double-track" experiments. In effect, the FDA permitted human testing to begin before animal toxicology studies were completed.

Double-tracking seemed reasonable. Marijuana and THC were safe. FDA assumed Nabilone, a close chemical cousin to THC, would have a similar safety profile.

On May 9, 1978, as the rebellion in the states was picking up steam and New Mexico was filing its IND, the Interagency Committee heard from a Lilly representative who spoke enthusiastically about Nabilone trials involving more than 100 patients. The minutes of that meeting note, "They [Lilly] anticipate being able to file for an NDA in the first quarter of 1979." (NDA stands for New Drug Application, the final step before marketing approval by FDA.)

We suspected the delays encountered by New Mexico were, in part, based on FDA's hope of substituting Nabilone for marijuana. A bureaucratic bait 'n switch.

Throughout 1978 there was a general feeling the situation was under control. This was evident in the relaxed manner of the Perry Committee, the friendly banter, the knowing smiles. True, the bureaucrats had to endure some rough verbal abuse from "those folks" in New Mexico. But, all in all, things were well contained. Preliminary Nabilone results were encouraging and there was a surprising amount of pre-release press coverage for the drug. Eli Lilly was anticipating prompt approval, brisk sales, and expanded applications well beyond cancer chemotherapy. The drug was being touted as "the

new Valium." One article heralded the synthetic as "The Tranquil-
izer for the New Age." Scientists at Lilly were even working on an
eyedrop formulation.

While Lilly was licking its chops at the prospect of a profitable
new drug, the bureaucrats believed Nabilone would extinguish medical marijuana's political fire, dampen public demands, and save the
medical prohibition. Then the dogs died.

Beagle dogs to be exact, caged at the University of Arizona and
part of Lilly's "long term use" studies. Some of the animals, given
Nabilone regularly for close to one year, began to experience "unacceptable neurological toxicity." More indelicately, the dogs seemed
perfectly normal until they slammed into a wall of toxicity that caused
profound spasticity. After hours of uncontrollable shaking the dogs
collapsed, then expired.

Eli Lilly informed the FDA and promptly halted the studies. It
was January 1979. Nabilone's nearly instantaneous evaporation occurred as a dozen states were preparing hearings on marijuana-as-
medicine bills. Federal agencies panicked.

With Nabilone returning to the drawing boards, drug warriors frantically renewed their search for a synthetic substitute for marijuana.
Suddenly the Perry Committee hearings were decidedly more tense.
Instead of relaxed banter there were terse comments. There was a
palpable strain to the meetings and a marked increase in participa-
tion by DEA representatives. Knowing smiles were replaced by fur-
tive looks.

The only other possible substitute was THC. But there were problems with THC. The bureaucratic notion that THC and marijuana
are precisely alike was, of course, deeply flawed. Marijuana is a mild
euphoriant. Pure THC is a major hallucinogen. But federal bureaucrats, fixated on marijuana's "high," simply assumed that what got
you high got you well. This assumption persisted even after it became
obvious that the two drugs were dramatically different.

I knew this first-hand from my THC experiences in North Carolina, UCLA, and Howard. THC did not lower my eye pressures. Nor did it help Jim Ripple's glaucoma or the score of patients studied by Dr. Merritt. It wasn't much better for cancer patients, as Anne Guttentag and others had learned. The problems had first emerged in early cancer studies, as Perez-Reyes explained to me in North Carolina.

The studies were conducted at the Sydney Farber Cancer Institute by Drs. Stephen Sallan and Norman Zinberg of Harvard University. Federal agencies refused to provide marijuana, insisting on synthetic THC instead. The Harvard researchers found THC could reduce vomiting in some patients but there were complaints about the erratic absorption and performance of the synthetic. The investigators determined the 'high' was essential to attaining the proper therapeutic outcome, i.e. no vomiting. But oral THC absorbed so slowly and at such a different rate among patients it was difficult to arrive at a proper dose. This could easily lead to over-dosing.

In follow-up evaluations, Zinberg learned 25% of the cancer patients in his study obtained marijuana off the streets. Why? Patients said marijuana worked better, faster, and with fewer side effects than THC. This research was published in *The New England Journal of Medicine* in 1975. Sallan and Zinberg noted, "Theoretically, smoking might be the preferable route [of administration] since it may result in less variability of absorption. . . . Moreover, smoking provides greater opportunity for individual patient control by permitting the patient to regulate and maintain the 'high.' "

Synthetic THC presented an entirely different profile. Individuals given a standardized dose of THC experienced inconsistent, highly unpredictable results. THC is the most psychoactive agent in marijuana but its therapeutic value is very questionable. In pure form THC has the consistency of pine pitch and is not water soluble. When swallowed, THC is irregularly digested. If the synthetic dissolves it is slowly taken up by the intestines and delivered to the liver. The liver filters out much of the THC, then releases what is left into the bloodstream. Once in the blood, THC finally makes its way to the brain.

This indirect route of drug delivery means it takes THC a very long time to work. And it works differently each time it is taken. On one occasion a patient may obtain relief in an hour. The next dose, however, may take two or even four hours to become bioavailable.

In May 1978, when Nabilone's approval seemed assured, NCI reseachers candidly discussed the merits of marijuana and THC. Minutes from the May 9 meeting concluded, "The oral absorption of THC is erratic, and the current formulation of THC was felt . . . to not be acceptable." The report went on to note, "[A]ll in all smoking the [marijuana] cigarette may be the best means of administering the drug." Nevertheless, research with THC continued, most notably in an NCI-sponsored study conducted at the NIH campus in Bethesda, by a young researcher, Dr. Alfred Chang. Ultimately, his research yielded the same erratic, unstable results with THC.

In January 1980, the Lynn Pierson Therapeutic Research & Treatment Program issued its first report. Significantly, New Mexico's findings mirrored the NCI/Chang study. Cancer patients given THC reported high anxiety and uncertain benefits. Ninety percent of cancer patients smoking marijuana, however, experienced reliable relief from vomiting. This astonishing result was repeatable and predictable. Little wonder New Mexico cancer patients preferred marijuana over THC.

The bureaucrats knew all this but it didn't matter. From their perspective they had no choice. Large population states were rushing to adopt the New Mexico model. In rapid order Texas, California, Michigan, and Georgia joined in the chorus for the limited federal supplies of marijuana. A month after the Neal Hearings, New York would enact marijuana-as-medicine legislation, another populous state that would need enormous supplies of federal marijuana.

The decision was made to divert THC into the NCI Group C program. NCI wasn't particularly happy about it. They had always viewed themselves as "above" politics. But in the end they caved in to the intense bureaucratic pressure to "stay with the policy." The FDA could not admit a mere weed was more effective than modern synthetic chemicals. The DEA would not allow medical marijuana to erode its enforcement powers. To help their sister agencies maintain the medical prohibition NCI officials would condemn a generation of cancer patients to debilitating vomiting, uncertain relief and unnecessary suffering. "We're just the scientists," they would say.

In the battle of institutional interests the welfare of mere mortals is unimportant. Having settled on synthetic substitution the drug warriors emerged from the bunkers and went on the attack.

We also went on the attack.

We began with a press release a week after the Neal Hearings that outlined the federal shortage of marijuana and summarized the problems with the bureaucratic plan to substitute synthetic THC. I expanded the attack in a full-length article that was submitted to *The Washington Post.*

On June 23, 1980, just three days before the FDA Oncologic Advisory Committee meeting that was scheduled to approve the Group C program for THC, we issued another press release, accusing the FDA of pushing "phony pot pills" to disguise a marijuana shortage.

By the time the Advisory Committee met, our news was picked up by the wires and reprinted in hundreds of newspapers, sparking a rush of radio talk as a thousand stations across America repeated the alarm. In states where patients were awaiting promised federal supplies the reaction was intense and sustained.

The FDA watched tensely as the Oncologic Advisory Committee narrowly approved the Group C program by a vote of 5-4. There were strong objections raised by Dr. Edmund O'Brien of California's Research Advisory Panel who asked that the release of THC "be delayed until data is accumulated determining a generally recognized safe and effective dose and characterized effect." O'Brien's comments were underscored by Dr. Charles Moertel of the Mayo Clinic who said "it is premature to release THC to the cancer patient population."

But, in the end, the FDA got what it needed.

Just three days later *The Washington Post* ran my article in the Sunday op-ed section. "Medical Substitute for Marijuana Won't Work" read the headline. The article pulled together the various bits of information we had collected in the intervening two years—quotes from the NCI memo which praised the marijuana cigarette and condemned THC, a review of the Chang study and New Mexico reports, and a sobering analysis of the number of patients who would be denied relief by the refusal of the government to increase marijuana production. I concluded by accusing federal drug bureaucrats of sacrificing seriously ill Americans on the altar of the drug war. *The Post* article was picked up by other press outlets around the country.

Suddenly I was extremely visible once again. The issue—legal access to quality-controlled medical marijuana—had what it needed to combat the upcoming federal publicity assault: a national spokesperson.

The tripwire was pulled by California, which had enacted a marijuana-as-medicine law in July 1979. The state had been negotiating for IND approval with FDA but concern over uncertain federal supplies caused California to leapfrog other states by publicly requesting 1 million marijuana cigarettes before the FDA approved their state protocol.

This amount exceeded NIDA's entire inventory. The California request and our sudden, sustained press assault on THC ignited a supply scramble. Other states rushed to secure their FDA-promised marijuana. It was like watching a run on a bank. The supply crunch, so long hidden, hit with a vengeance.

States demanded answers. Congressmen were called. Editorial writers and radio talk hosts spoke of "bureaucratic betrayal" and "a government too dumb to grow weeds." The rising rage was appropriate. Dying people were being deceived, scientific data was being altered, state laws were being ignored. Throughout the summer the assault intensified. As the story ricocheted around the nation, public and press took up the attack and soundly whacked Washington bureaucrats and the medical prohibition. People were damn mad and wanted answers; wanted to know who made the silly decision to promote phony pot pills.

We also wanted to know. Had one man deep in the bowels of some sinister state-within-the-state decided to push THC? It is seductive to believe a villainous cabal directs evil events. But it is doubtful the demonic, moronic decision to push THC reflected any intelligence whatsoever. Bureaucrats kill people in committee. No one is responsible.

Released from the restraints of law and logic, bureaucrats, as Orwell predicted, become savages. The nation accepts that marijuana has medical value and, in a two-year plebiscite, determine to make it legally available to the seriously ill. Democracy in action.

Then, a congealed clump of unelected men and women conspire to evade public demands and overturn state laws while plotting to deceive the sick by promoting phony pot pills deemed "not acceptable" for human use. This is a descent into madness—the American nightmare of unrestrained government come to life.

From my own perspective, which was unique and highly personal, I sensed a demented aspect in the bureaucrats' barbarous behavior. Like the child who tells lies, federal agencies had progressed from petty assaults to monstrous results. In 1978, when the government tried to deny my legal access to marijuana, the bureaucrats did so with the uneasy apprehension of men who knew they were doing wrong. When legal action threatened to expose this wrong they flinched.

Now, a mere two years later, these same bureaucrats were planning to deceive entire states and deprive whole classes of people of legal access to appropriate care. It was a breathtaking leap from small crimes to crimes against humanity. The institutional inclination to conform had overwhelmed compassion.

Our anti-THC assault exploded before federal agencies could implement their strategy of synthetic substitution. The intense media barrage outflanked the agencies, threw off their timing, and further complicated interagency planning. While federal agencies coped with the chaos of escalating state demands, we used the media to educate America on the differences between THC and marijuana.

We knew we could not stop the strategy of synthetic substitution. But we trusted that Americans, when given the facts, would quickly grasp the game and reach the right conclusions. The American people did not disappoint us.

Mona Taft had attended the Neal hearings and returned to Georgia with an uneasy sense. She wasn't quite sure what all that talk about Group C meant and the dire warnings from Alice and me about "subversion of the intent of the states" had seemed a bit too strident for her taste. She was confident the state of Georgia would prevail. Besides, she was weary and needed a break.

By midsummer Mona was revived enough to reengage. She had been following the news about synthetic THC and staying in touch with the various officials in Georgia who had been assigned to implement her state law. She was increasing dismayed at what she heard.

The FDA had attempted to force the THC solution on the Georgia Patient Review Board, the group established to implement the Georgia law. To their credit, the group refused to be intimidated. But the

FDA was relentless and it was quickly wearing down the Board, all of whom had other full-time jobs. A full-time, paid employee was needed to help keep things on track and, in early August, the State of Georgia asked Mona Taft to accept the job.

It did not take Mona long to comprehend that federal officials had no intention of providing Georgia—or any other state, for that matter—with legal supplies of marijuana, despite the assurances she had heard at the Neal Hearings. She also realized she would need political help in Washington if she was to secure Georgia's fair share of the limited marijuana supplies.

She returned to her original source of support, Rep. Virlyn Smith, and asked if he knew of any members of Congress from Georgia who might intervene with the FDA and the NCI. Rep. Smith suggested she meet with his young friend, U.S. Representative Newt Gingrich.

Newt Gingrich, serving his first term in Congress, was considered by many a conservative bomb thrower. Gingrich was already making waves. Many members of Congress felt he was immature and too aggressive; even reckless.

Mona arranged to meet Smith and Gingrich in Washington in late September to generally discuss the issue. She also asked me to attend the meeting.

On September 10, 1980, the federal government formally announced the inclusion of THC in the Group C program. It was hoped the announcement would begin to dampen the clamor for medical supplies of marijuana. It was far too late. Our efforts had worked and across the country there was a highly sophisticated understanding of the difference between natural marijuana and synthetic THC. *The Atlanta Constitution*, which strongly supported Georgia's medical marijuana law, editorially fumed over the government's phony pot pill scam.

Gingrich was intrigued. He expanded his scheduled meeting with Mona and others to include representatives from the NCI, NIDA, and DHHS.

On September 26, we all met on Capitol Hill in Gingrich's office. Prior to the arrival of the federal representatives, Mona and I outlined the facts to Gingrich. Virlyn Smith spoke about political realities "back home." Gingrich proved to be a quick study. Locked into conservative concerns over irrational federal power, he readily understood the problem. A bunch of bureaucrats in Washington were blocking a Georgia law. Cancer patients were suffering. After an hour's discussion, the representatives from the agencies arrived.

The Deputy Chief Counsel of HHS and her two staffers entered the room with confidence. Gingrich sat them on a sofa, offered them a coke, listened to their trite explanations, then unloaded.

The FDA had promised Georgia marijuana. If Georgia did not get marijuana, Gingrich would call for a congressional investigation. Rough, direct, demanding.

There was a sense of awe in the room. Everyone, including me, was surprised by the focus of Gingrich's assault. The Deputy Chief Counsel stammered to explain. Gingrich waved her off, returning to his demands. After an hour the meeting dissolved. Gingrich had made himself clear, he needed to get on to other items.

Shaken by the encounter the Deputy Chief Counsel collected her dumbstruck staffers and headed for the door. As they entered the hall one staffer mumbled something. "Oh, don't worry about him," the Deputy Chief Counsel said in a stage whisper, "Gingrich is only a Republican. Republicans don't matter."

Three weeks later America elected Ronald Reagan president of the United States. The Republican revolution had began.

22 ACT

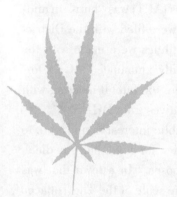

AS THE MEDICAL marijuana issue continued to grow we realized public demands
and state laws alone could not crack the
prohibition. The drug warriors were too
strong, entrenched and arrogant. Increasingly it seemed the only way
to escape the prohibition's power was through Congress. After all,
Congress had passed the laws that prohibited marijuana and, later,
the laws that would grant federal agencies the authority to impede
research and block access.

It seemed to us that Congress could, like Alexander the Great,
slice through the Gordian knot of federal drug regulation and free
marijuana for medical access.

Or, to put it in a more American way: If at first you don't succeed
get a bigger hammer. The States had tried, and failed, to loosen the
federal stranglehold on medical access to marijuana. Congress, we
reasoned, was a bigger hammer that could resolve the problem for
everyone.

There were, of course, those councils of wisdom who said "impossible." In the still lingering wake of the Bourne Affair, the drug
war was escalating. There was a growing backlash against the "coun-

terculture." Congress would never consider a medical marijuana bill, the wags would say, never.

We understood the odds. In a Washington landscape dominated by huge lobbying firms staffed by skilled people on lush payrolls it seemed unlikely that two political neophytes could make a difference but there was, from our perspective, little choice. Besides, the two "neophytes" had already accomplished a great deal.

The Alliance for Cannabis Therapeutics (ACT) was "born" in mid-1980 when the Articles of Incorporation were filed with the District of Columbia government and additional filings were made with the IRS to obtain tax-free status. We officially announced ACT's formation in September, just one week before the fateful meeting with Newt Gingrich, Mona, and the representatives from DHHS.

ACT's purpose was "to promote the public interest in and work to ensure the adequacy of cannabis supplies for legitimate medical, therapeutic, scientific and research purposes." In a town that was packed with nonprofit organizations on the scale of the The Tobacco Institute or the American Association of Retired Persons, ACT was an institutional microdot: an organizational illusion.

Financially, ACT was a disaster. While medical marijuana enjoyed broad public support, it was not a mass movement and its strongest supporters—the seriously ill—were often desperately poor. Such people would give themselves body and soul to fight the good fight. But they had no cash. Direct mail appeals elicited few contributions. Hundreds of grant requests to major and minor philanthropies also came up empty. Medical marijuana was too controversial for many, not controversial enough for some. We did obtain a "seed grant" of $5,000 from The Playboy Foundation but we were unable to parlay it into anything meaningful. Christie Hefner made good on her promise to provide ACT with free ad space in the slick, widely read magazine. The *Playboy* ad featured a handsome, eye-catching map outlining the states with medical marijuana laws. *Playboy* was mass media. Eight million Americans read it every month. The ads increased public awareness, resulted in hundreds of requests for information but failed to increase contributions to ACT.

Yet, for all it did not have, ACT did enjoy certain advantages. By design it was nonmembership; lean, easily directed, without internal strife. A very closed system nearly immune from external distraction. We had seen what internal strife could do to an organization. We had watched as NORML slowly descended into chaos after the Bourne debacle and Keith's departure. We purposefully established a small Board of Directors: President, Vice President, and Secretary-Treasurer. We occupied two of the three slots. Mae Nutt later agreed to serve as our Vice President.

To that core we added a battle-proven board of advisors that included some old friends: Mona Taft, the Ripples, Anson Chong from Hawaii, Ara Cron from Kansas, and Vince Mustachio from West Virginia.

There were many others who agreed to join the Advisory Board of our new group: Dr. Andrew Weil, professor of medicine at Arizona State University and budding author; Dr. Norman Zinberg, coauthor of the first modern study on marijuana's medicinal use by cancer patients; Dr. Dorothy Whipple, a noted pediatrician who helped secure the rights of women in the medical profession when she became the first married woman admitted to Johns Hopkins Medical School in the 1920s; Antonio G. Olivieri, City Council member from New York City, who helped spearhead passage of the New York State marijuana-as-medicine bill and would later die of cancer; Rep. Virlyn Smith of Georgia, mentor to Rep. Newt Gingrich; Rep. Miller Hudson of Colorado; Senator Jerome Hart of Michigan, and others. We were tremendously exhilarated by the willingness of others to help our cause.

Even the absence of funds, while unfortunate, was not debilitating but liberating. Operating on anger, hope and the adventure of discovery, we were not obsessed with making money. All we needed was enough to pay the rent. Ah, youth!

ACT had the advantage of a compelling argument and the benefit of broad public and press support. ACT also had the *pro bono* assistance of Steptoe and Johnson.

Our old friend at Steptoe, Tom Collier, had moved on, becoming a deputy assistant secretary at the Department of Housing and Urban Development (HUD). Prior to his departure from Steptoe, Tom had encouraged us to break away from NORML and establish our own group. But we resisted, wary of the obvious problems which accompany running an organization. Finally, however, the chaos and disintegration at NORML left us little choice.

Tom referred us to several attorneys in Steptoe & Johnson who had assisted on my case in May 1978. As we outlined our plans to approach Congress there was an excitement from the lawyers about expanding on the precedent established in my case and extending it to others via codified law. Once again the issue of medical marijuana was brought before Steptoe's *pro bono* committee and, to our great delight, the firm agreed to help us. Steptoe's considerable skills, vast resources and well-seasoned reputation could help give credibility to our congressional enterprise.

Was this a recipe for success? Combine two dedicated people with one highly credible law firm, a score of state laws, appealing allies, broad public backing and a cogent message. Mix in massive doses of media amplified by local human interest and perhaps it was possible for Congress to enact federal marijuana-as-medicine legislation.

Stranger things had happened, especially in Washington.

23 Government Is the Problem

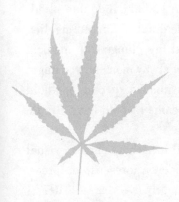

THE REAGAN REVOLUTION rode to Washington in a limo. For the first time since Herbert Hoover, Republicans took off their cloth coats and put on mink. The opening act in an age of excess.

The moralizing Carter of wide smiles and Plains conceit was washed away by a flood of newly rich Hollywood glitz. Plutocrats parked their private jets in neat rows. Luxury hotels were booked. Expensive perfume filled the air. There were grand fireworks, lavish parties. American hostages were released from Iran. The USA beat the USSR for Olympic gold in hockey. A new beginning.

Our drug reform friends greeted Reagan's arrival with foreboding. But Bourne's elitist coke snorting had already consigned drug reform to the ash heap of history. Reagan could not harm them any more than they had harmed themselves.

We were not alarmed. The campaign to enact state laws was fueled by conservative anger and my initial encounter with Newt Gingrich— a new breed—was encouraging. We believed medical marijuana could survive, might even thrive under Ronald Reagan. Anything's possible.

Anything.

For example: I was not blind. From 1972 on I had been repeatedly assured I would be blind before turning thirty in the year 1978. The experiences at UCLA, John Hopkins, Howard and Duke Universities keenly reinforced this bleak prognosis. When I first secured legal marijuana in 1976 there were limited expectations. It was assumed that marijuana, like conventional drugs, might work for awhile then fail to provide relief. When that happened I would slide into blindness. No one expected marijuana to provide durable, long-term relief.

This expectation—blindness—enabled my plunge into medical marijuana. Why bother with a career when, at any moment, you might go blind? I threw myself into medical marijuana expecting it would be a short avocation. When the darkness came I would learn Braille and find new pursuits.

This Scarlett O'Hara logic worked until it became obvious visual annihilation was not in my immediate, or even foreseeable, future. My sight was stable, had been stable for nearly five years. In 1977 I had marveled at the Voyager project and envied those who would be able to see the photographs from deep in space. Already I had seen the pictures from Jupiter with its distinctive moon Io and had sat spellbound as the rings of Saturn beamed into my living room in 1980. Marijuana had saved my sight and my future prospects.

As the stress of impending blindness receded and time offered reflection on my options I could think of no alternative employment. What job would permit me to practice mass rhetoric, write press releases, do interviews, alter public opinion, enact laws, engage in national politics and smoke ten joints a day? An expectation of blindness and an odd convergence of events had thrust me into an illuminating universe peopled by interesting actors asking ancient questions on the nature of power and the character of humankind. Jobs like this aren't advertized in the classifieds.

I would cope with blindness when and if it came. In the interim it seemed wise to have an interesting life. Medical marijuana, at the intersection of law and medicine and prohibition and power, was interesting. Why stop?

At the dawn of the Reagan Era another dozen states moved to enact medical marijuana laws. But the bureaucratic strategy of synthetic substitution was beginning to take hold. States promised federal marijuana were given an ultimatum: THC or nothing.

THC was a deal most states could not refuse. California illustrates this point. After a year of wrangling with the FDA the California Research Advisory Panel (CRAP) requested 1 million NIDA marijuana cigarettes. When the feds just said "no," CRAP confronted a dilemma. It could demand the marijuana California was promised, go to the state legislature, and appeal to the state's huge congressional delegation to pound the drug warriors into compliance. That would have been the right and noble thing to do.

The officials at CRAP, however, are appointed not elected. They were not particularly concerned with battling for the rights of Californians to receive legal marijuana. More than anything else they were bureaucrats. From their perspective the officials at the FDA and NIDA were not adversaries, they were colleagues. Surely state and federal drug officials could come to an accommodation. Bit by bit, day by day, California's legislative intent was sacrificed on an altar of bureaucratic schmoozing. The state IND, which once demanded enough marijuana cigarettes for 7,500 patients per month, was dramatically altered. Under the revised CRAP/FDA plan, eligibility requirements were established that severely limited the number of cancer patients who could participate. Soon it was estimated that only 3,000 patients a month would "benefit" from the program. Expecting marijuana, the patients who did meet the stringent eligibility criteria received THC.

In fact, only a handful of hospitalized patients on the three most infrequently used anti-cancer drugs were allowed to smoke marijuana. One oncologist noted, "I had used only one of these drugs in the course of my decade-long practice. The other two were so rarely used that the marijuana portion of the California program was essentially a dead end."

These deals gutted California's medical marijuana program. In the five years that the program would operate, fewer than 2,500 patients would receive THC and barely more than 100 would get federal marijuana cigarettes.

Nevertheless, CRAP proclaimed victory. In its 1986 report it would proudly claim, "[T]he Panel has met the "compassionate access" aspect of its legislative mandate." The feds were also victorious. In coming years they would point to California and claim "no physicians asked for marijuana" and "the claimed advantage . . . through smoking is only a hypothesis and has not been scientifically proven."

But cancer patients knew better. They continued to obtain marijuana illegally, often with the full knowledge of their frustrated physicians.

In other states, like Washington, locals trusted "the experts back East" and swallowed THC substitution hook, line and sinker. Washington officials scoffed at the delays New Mexico encountered, and publicly vowed it would not happen to them. When the FDA shoved THC down their throats state officials tried to make it look delicious.

By flooding NCI-related centers around the country with THC, the FDA gave local bureaucrats a way to undo the state medical marijuana laws. THC was free, the state was relieved of monitoring results, and the NCI and FDA would collect the data. In the end the government's strategy of synthetic substitution prevented most states from receiving any marijuana. By 1983, 34 states had medical marijuana laws. But only six states—New Mexico, Georgia, Michigan, New York, California and Tennessee—actually established therapeutic treatment programs that employed marijuana.

Even in this handful of states supply irregularities were frequent. In some cases bureaucratic attempts to conceal the supply shortage led to outright fraud. In Illinois, health officials held a press conference to celebrate the arrival of the state's first shipment of federal marijuana. Then, when the press conference ended, state officials dutifully shipped the photogenic tin of NIDA marijuana back to North Carolina. Show 'n tell for the benefit of bureaucrats and the press. No cancer patient in Illinois ever received marijuana, yet when THC failed the federal government attempted to blame marijuana and headlines across the country read "One in five cancer patients prefers nausea to marijuana." Careful reading of the article revealed that only THC had been used. Whoosh goes the memory hole.

States that strongly resisted THC substitution were able to break through these bureaucratic barriers. In Georgia, the determination of Mona Taft together with the editorial punch of *The Atlanta Constitution* and threats from Rep. Gingrich, compelled the FDA to meet that state's marijuana supply needs. But, even here federal red tape minimized the number of patients receiving marijuana.

In Michigan, press and political pressure forced federal agencies to deliver the goods. But the marijuana sent to Michigan by NIDA was old, dirty, and of only .88% THC potency. Medical marijuana is 2% THC or higher. Many Michigan cancer patients fled the state study saying they could buy better marijuana off the street. Unable to resolve these supply problems, Michigan health officials surreptitiously referred cancer patients to Arnold and Mae Nutt who continued to operate their "Green Cross" service well into the 1980s.

Deprived of legal access to marijuana, some cancer patients pliantly accepted THC. But the results were predictable. In San Francisco, oncologist Ivan Silverberg signed up for the CRAP program expecting to prescribe marijuana. Instead he was forced to dispense THC. Dr. Silverberg provided four cancer patients with THC. All four returned the synthetic complaining of erratic benefits and adverse effects. One patient actually threw her bottle of THC across the room screaming, "What are you trying to do, poison me?"

These federal/state frictions and alarming patient reports, amplified by the media, validated our strident attack on THC. Newspapers editorialized against the pot pill and ran features personalizing the plight of patients. Physicians, like Silverberg, publicly complained. Many cancer patients tried THC, then turned to the streets for marijuana. Others took THC, had panic attacks, found it ineffective, stopped chemotherapy, and died.

By the time Ronald Reagan came to Washington few Americans were fooled by the government's synthetic bait 'n switch. In the dawning Reagan years I was able to crystallize this public discontent by asking over and over again, "Who, but a bureaucrat, would be dumb enough to give a vomiting patient a pill?"

While America understood medical marijuana, Congress was less aware. How do you introduce an idea to 535 people, attract their attention, and get their support? Using ACT as our vehicle we settled on a strategy of "info-osmosis."

As the FDA's synthetic storm raged through the states, ACT recycled the flood of newsprint into Congress. Pure information with no appeal for action. I believed information delivered at high velocity would elicit interest and act as its own persuasion. Then Congress, like the state legislatures, would respond.

ACT's information saturation campaign was made possible by technology. When nearly no one had a computer, we struggled to master DOS, CP/M, eight inch floppies—which actually flopped—and the agonizingly intricate instructions needed to merge letters with addresses.

By November 1980, ACT was directing a constant flow of information into Congress. Good timing. Congress was in recess, its members home in their districts. It would be the staffers who read our letters, then slowly spread the news: info-osmosis.

By the time Congress returned in January 1981, ACT had blanketed Capitol Hill with information. Congressmen from states with medical marijuana laws received multiple letters. Every pertinent newspaper article was reproduced and forwarded to the appropriate Senators and Representatives. Pure information. No plea for help.

We began to wonder if a computer could expand media generation and spent several weeks in the Library of Congress consulting reference books on radio and television, newspapers and other outlets. By Spring, ACT had compiled 2,500 media outlets accessible by city, state, region, format, market, and megawatts. ACT used these lists to generate media in the states, then recycled that media into Congress. The result was a dynamic dialogue between us, the states, media outlets and Congress.

This info loop, while very overt, fell below the bureaucratic horizon that relies on *The Washington Post* and little more. We made no effort to excite *The Post* or *The New York Times*. Our goal was to inform the nation and Congress, not the elite liberal press. This reliance on regional press and radio talk sustained a national media bubble, maintained public support and rapidly enhanced Congressional awareness. It was, we reasoned, just a matter of time.

April 10, 1981
Cannon House Office Building,
Capitol Hill

After months of information saturation, I finally received the call I had been trying so hard to provoke. "Could you meet with Rep. McKinney regarding this medical marijuana problem?"

Stewart McKinney was a middle-aged, middle class, middle-of-the-road Connecticut Republican, married, Catholic, with a large family. His private office was modest and modern. The Congressman sat at the head of a long conference table, within easy reach of a Mickey Mouse phone, surrounded by eager young staffers. No pretense. Very human. Stewart began by mentioning that his friend, Governor Ella Grasso, was battling cancer. He had also been told about a bill in Connecticut that was making its way through the legislature. His interest was piqued. "What's this about medical marijuana?" he asked.

The meeting was brief. Rep. McKinney was sponsoring a bipartisan bill to allow the Amerasian children of G.I.'s into America. But, that bill was "in the hopper" and about to become law. Stewart was looking for another issue. "If you develop a medical marijuana bill, I'd like to look it over," McKinney said, ending the meeting. I was delighted. A moderate Republican interested in medical marijuana.

Doug Herbert, my newest Steptoe attorney, was an Alabama native with an interest in drafting legislation. Doug enlisted several Associates and after a few weeks they produced a federal medical marijuana bill. The draft was very straightforward. Congress would recognize marijuana's medical uses, reschedule marijuana to Schedule II so it could be prescribed, and establish a reliable system of supply and distribution. Under the bill marijuana was handled like any prescription and any licensed physician could call on the federal government for supplies.

The bill, couched in conservative concerns—State rights, doctor/patient control over medical care—was radical in intent. To provide background I worked with Doug to develop a detailed supporting memo. The end result, a handsome product, was given to Reps. McKinney, Gingrich, and Neal on June 24, 1981.

Two weeks later, on July 9th, Rep. McKinney agreed to sponsor the bill. "I like the scope and style of this bill and I'm happy to sponsor it." McKinney said, "But we need a few cosponsors."

The next day Newt Gingrich called and expressed his support for the bill and agreed to cosponsor. He had sent the bill to his mentor Virlyn Smith, and the ailing Georgia legislator lost no time in making his opinions known. He called Gingrich's office on the 9 and followed up with a letter.

> I know Bob Randall and ACT have put a lot of time and thought into this proposal, and I think they have a good bill. I would personally appreciate your support of it.
>
> Even though we have a workable program in Georgia *NOW*, thanks only to *your interest and support*, most of the other 32 states that have tried to help in this most humane cause have not been so fortunate. It is not reasonable to think that under the limitations of research as viewed by the FDA, NCI, and DEA, that any more than just a few of these states will ever have an effective program.
>
> This denies access to a great majority of the suffering patients, or worse yet, involves them or someone trying to help them, in the criminal process of buying and using street marijuana.
>
> Again, I ask your support of this. I think you will *feel great satisfaction* in helping a segment of our society that is doomed to much suffering. Any relief that can be given seems almost a miracle.

On September 16, 1981, Representatives McKinney and Gingrich publicly introduced ACT's federal medical marijuana bill. Two other Republicans, the moderate Millicent Fenwick of New Jersey and conservative blue blood Hamilton Fish of New York, joined as co-sponsors. McKinney and Gingrich held a press conference that sparked favorable editorials in their states. Wire services carried the news across America.

• • •

We were playing political jujitsu: A "pro-marijuana" bill backed by four Republicans. While very different, Stewart and Newt worked well together. Stew McKinney was a secure, mature, go-along/get along politician who moved quietly through the House, was well-regarded by his peers and had few enemies. Stewart promoted "his" bill with soft persuasion. He sent out "Dear Colleague" letters—written by me—and inserted favorable press clippings into the Congressional Record. Using this approach Stewart reached out to other Representatives and encouraged their support.

Newt Gingrich was an Alpha pup, scrappy, less secure, but far more aggressive. Newt's "Dear Colleague" letters targeted lean young conservatives looking to fight the feds. Newt was tenacious in promoting "his" bill and secured considerable Republican support. While McKinney was without pretense, Gingrich fancied himself an intellectual: an historian. He was much more verbal than Stewart and anxious to succeed. I frankly enjoyed listening to Gingrich practice the formative outlines of his "Opportunity Society." He was a man of ideas and action.

The combined efforts of these very different men propelled congressional support for medical marijuana. Press clippings, editorials, and notices of new cosponsors poured into the Congressional Record. After a year of info-osmosis Representatives on both sides of the aisle were quick to respond. By the end of September House Resolution 4498 had more than twenty cosponsors.

More begets more. As new cosponsors signed on ACT made certain they received favorable press coverage "back home." These clippings were then inserted into the Congressional Record or used to launch another volley of "Dear Colleague" letters. The number of cosponsors continued to climb.

All previous marijuana reform measures had the spotty support of ten or fewer left-wing liberals. By ignoring the left and coming from a conservative base, the federal marijuana-as-medicine bill gained bipartisan support. Medical marijuana, driven by Republican sponsors and conservative aspirations, had appeal across the political spectrum. By the end of 1981, 90 Members of Congress—from Barney Frank on the far left to William Dannymeyer on the farthest right—were backing medical marijuana. H.R. 4498 was a roaring success. Gingrich and I looked forward to hearings and a successful floor vote. Stewart, more seasoned, cautioned against excessive optimism.

With hindsight we can now see Stewart was right.

But in the waning days of 1981 there was no hindsight. Our sights were set on the future which, like Reagan's shining city, seemed bright and promising. These were halcyon days. Our faith in the American system seemed overwhelmingly validated. In 1976 we had placed our faith in the courts and it was rewarded. From 1978 to 1981 we trusted in the people and were rewarded by 34 state laws that legislatively recognized marijuana's medical use. A constitutional amendment requires just 33 states to be enacted! The support was clear-cut and the issue had passed the nation's toughest standard—a two-thirds majority of the states.

Now, it seemed, Congress was equally supportive of marijuana-as-medicine. As we moved into 1982 there were more than 100 cosponsors on the bill and more good news was on the way. In February, the National Academy of Science released a report on marijuana's medical uses. The Dept. of Health and Human Services (DHSS) had been ordered by the Court of Appeals to review "scientific and medical findings" on all of marijuana's substances. It was yet another legal round in NORML's long-standing suit to reschedule marijuana, first filed in 1972.

The Court order came at an inopportune time for the agencies. They were just beginning the Group C distribution of THC and an agency review of marijuana's medical utility could be politically inconvenient. So, the DHHS, in an effort to stall the legal proceedings, asked the National Academy of Science, Institute of Medicine (IOM) to review the question of marijuana's medical uses.

At a lavish dinner held in the NAS building near the White House, the report was released to a select group of attendees. There were, in the classic Claude Rains line from the movie *Casablanca*, "all the usual suspects" from the FDA, NIDA, and DEA. I was invited, no doubt the token "citizen" and legal marijuana user. Also in the hall that night was Rep. Millicent Fenwick, Republican Congresswoman from New Jersey and one of the four original sponsors of H.R. 4498.

Millicent Fenwick was a Washington legend. A strikingly handsome woman, she was wealthy and looked it. She had briefly been a Vogue model in her youth, which was not surprising. She possessed enough quirks to get her noticed and cement her "legend" status. She smoked a corn cob pipe and was reputed to eat spaghetti for dinner nearly every night. She liked the pasta, she noted, and found the process of deciding what to eat "boring." So, when she ate at home, she ate spaghetti.

These numerous quirks, coupled with her bold style and frank talk won many admirers. Many claim she was the model for Lacey Davenport in Gary Trudeau's "Doonesbury" cartoon strip.

I had never met Mrs. Fenwick and, aside from my info-osmosis campaign, had never dealt directly with her office. Her support for H.R. 4498, like that of Rep. Hamilton Fish, came out of the blue. I accepted the support and concentrated my energies elsewhere.

As I sat through the NAS dinner I listened to various speakers discuss marijuana's medical uses not in terms of "maybe" but in absolute terms. The NAS/IOM report went far beyond any previous discussion of marijuana's medical use in treatment to stress the drug's important medical potential in the treatment of numerous life- and sense-threatening diseases. While it stopped short of any policy recommendations it was critical of the federal approach to marijuana's use in medicine.

It was a glad-handing evening for sure. Everyone seemed to warm to the occasion and I listened, in astonishment, as officials from

NIDA and the FDA spoke in glowing terms of how they had "helped pave the way" with their compassion towards Robert Randall.

I could not be still and, when finally recognized, told the gathering that compassion towards one man was not enough. Whole states were seeking relief and where was it?

There was some tsk-tsking from the crowd. Murmurs raced through the room. There was a sense of isolation as I realized I was alone in a mass of bureaucrats who wanted to hear none of my moaning and groaning. "There's that Randall, again," they would say. "He's never content." It was a scene all too familiar.

But on that night I would have a champion, and a beautiful one at that. In her clear yet gravely voice, Millicent Fenwick spoke directly. "Depriving glaucoma and cancer patients of medical access to marijuana is inhumane." The room became very quiet. "My office recently received a letter from a 74-year-old man who had to purchase marijuana illegally for his wife who is undergoing chemotherapy treatments. I think that is wrong."

Federal officials rushed to assure the Congresswoman that marijuana "can be obtained legally." Fenwick listened and then leveled both barrels at the bureaucrats. "I contacted health officials in New Jersey and was bluntly told it is easier for patients to get marijuana off the streets than from their doctors because of all the federal red tape involved in getting it legally." The bureaucrats studied their coffee more carefully under the wilting gaze of the New Jersey representative. "That," she concluded "is an outrage."

There were no spontaneous bursts of applause to greet the good Representative's common sense observations. To say I was bolstered by this event is putting it mildly. For six years Alice and I had worked hard to instill the basic message. On February 25, 1982, like the echoes through a canyon wall, the message came back, delivered by the lovely Lady from New Jersey.

The dinner concluded and I sought out Mrs. Fenwick to thank her.

She was intrigued with my case and peppered me with questions as we shared a cab back to our Capitol Hill homes—hers closer to the brilliantly lit dome than mine. We said goodbye. I would never speak to her again. Rep. Fenwick retired at the end of 1982. She would live another ten years, dying on September 16, 1992, eleven years to the day after H.R. 4498 was introduced.

24 Profiles in Pathetic

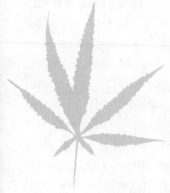

1982 BEGAN WITH promise but storm clouds were gathering. As *The Washington Drug Review* had noted three years before, "Marijuana . . . has enjoyed for a short time a small amount of breathing room as a public policy issue. No more."

The changing tide was subtle at first. The Carter Administration had continued to publicly back decriminalization (while doing nothing for the medical use issue) but behind the scenes there was a quiet transfer of emphasis and money. Government funds were quietly diverted to "parent groups," organizations throughout the country that were concerned about growing drug use by adolescents. These groups had already targeted the medical marijuana issue, echoing the public bulletins of the DEA, calling medical marijuana "a stalking horse for legalization" and printing broadsides under the banner of Families in Action. These were reinforced by a vociferous publication called "War on Drugs" purportedly funded by the rightist of wingers, Lyndon LaRouche.

By the time Reagan arrived in Washington the giant bureaucratic machinery of the drug agencies was poised to engage in a radical shift of direction and in Nancy Reagan the agencies found their engineer.

In the latter part of 1981, Mrs. Reagan met with representatives of the National Federation of Parents for Drug-Free Youth, an organization chaired by the wife of the Republican party chairman. The Federation was a new offshoot of the Georgia-based PRIDE (Parent Resources and Information for Drug Education) which had been receiving government grants for a number of years, some of it funneled through the anti-poverty agency ACTION. The folks at PRIDE were delighted when their new friends from the Republican party took an interest in their cause. They knew it could mean increased funding, both private and public. But they were reluctant to relinquish their own power so the Federation was born. PRIDE was right about the fund-raising. The Federation would see *lots* of money pour in, including a $500,000 contribution from the Sultan of Brunei. Another group was later formed, the Nancy Reagan Drug Abuse Fund. It received $1 million from King Fayed of Saudi Arabia. Ironically less than 10% of these funds would help the battle against drug abuse. The remainder was used for "administrative" costs and funneled to appropriate antidrug, i.e. Republican, political candidates.

All of this was in the future. That first meeting at the White House in November 1981 was a trial balloon and it floated very well indeed. The First Lady had been severely criticized for her spendthrift ways at the White House and the Administration was anxious to find a "cause" in which she could engage. Staffers wanted something less political than drugs but Mrs. Reagan insisted that this was the area in which she wanted to concentrate her energies.

In April 1982, the First Lady spoke to the Ad Council—a private, nonprofit organization, founded in 1942 to rally support for the war effort—at a wine-soaked luncheon at the State Department. The Council was famous for its public service announcement campaigns that raised billions in War Bonds, encouraged the planting of Victory

Gardens and recruited 2 million women into the work force through the powerful symbol, "Rosie the Riveter." After the War, the Ad Council continued its work through such notable campaigns as Smokey The Bear and the United Negro College Fund's "A Mind Is a Terrible Thing to Waste."

Mrs. Reagan encouraged the group to take up the campaign against the use of drugs by children. She derided the numerous subtle ways in which "drug acceptance is everywhere" in the culture. She criticized music, movies, television, advertising, and, obliquely, the news media. At one point Mrs. Reagan said, "I wonder if anyone stops to think what perceptions kids are picking up from some of the stories about the therapeutic effects of a chemical found in pot." She went on to tell the story of a fifth grader in Atlanta who believed, "if you smoke pot you won't get cancer or have to wear glasses. Now how do you suppose a fifth grader gets ideas like these?" The inference was clear. The media was expected to censor such stories, to save the kids, of course.

From this lunch was born the "Say No to Drugs" advertising campaign. A short while later Mrs. Reagan would modify the slogan into the battle cry of the 1980s—"Just Say No!"

Initially we were not particularly worried by these efforts. Concern about drug use among kids was not inappropriate and besides, the medical issue was separate. We naïvely thought that 34 state laws and close to 100 cosponsors on a federal marijuana-as-medicine bill in Congress would delineate the two issues—drug abuse v. controlled medical use. It seemed simple and clear cut to us. As different as black and white.

But as more and more money was pumped into so-called "parents groups" the bureaucrats used these mercenary parents to counter patient demands for care. Rather than spend their federal grants to prevent kiddie drug use, these parent groups targeted medical marijuana. The broadsides issued by Families in Action specifically took aim at H.R. 4498, filling half a dozen pages with misinformation and outright lies about the bill, marijuana's effects, research, and the struggling state programs such as the one in Georgia.

"It sends the wrong message," blared the party line from a dozen newsletters. As Nancy Reagan's "Just Say No" crusade gained momentum, attacks on medical marijuana became routine. DeKalb Families in Action—a coven of the concerned in Georgia—sent an attack memo to Gingrich.

The press in Georgia picked up on the brewing feud, but backed Gingrich and his federal medical marijuana bill. Enraged "parents" then started disrupting Newt's District meetings. The anti-med/anti-pot parents were loud, mildly abusive. Having won reelection by a slender margin, Newt began to sweat.

Curiously, Gingrich's reaction was unique. Stone-age conservatives like Hamilton Fish and William Dannemeyer were unshakably committed to ending federal controls over medical marijuana. Liberal lefties like Barney Frank were committed to meeting human needs. But Newt was committed to Newt. And Newt was concerned medical marijuana might injure his budding career as a conservative revolutionary. Could he offend the First Lady, the federal drug control establishment, and a few crazed constituents, and ever hope to succeed in the Republican Party of tomorrow?

While government-funded "parent groups" mauled Newt, Washington drug warriors found a liberal ally. There was an odd alarm among senior Democrats who feared medical marijuana might make Republicans look compassionate. Representative Henry Waxman of California was chairman of the Subcommittee on Health, part of the Energy & Commerce Committee. It was this committee that would eventually forward H.R. 4498 to the House floor for a vote and it was Waxman's subcommittee that had to start the ball rolling.

A liberal reformer from a big state overwhelmingly in favor of medical marijuana, Waxman seemed a likely med/pot supporter. But Mr. Waxman was deeply addicted to pharmaceutical PAC money and intellectually in hock to the FDA. If conservatives love bureaucrats with badges, liberals love bureaucrats in lab coats.

I met several times with Waxman aides trying to understand why the Congressman would not support McKinney's bill. But, by summer it was clear Waxman would block medical marijuana hearings until after the 1982 election.

With the prospect of prompt hearings and a rapid floor vote receding, Gingrich realized medical marijuana would not be quickly resolved. He grew increasingly nervous as 1982 slid along and the Just-Say-No crowd increased the pressure on him. His old mentor, Virlyn Smith, had died of cancer in March 1982. Without Virlyn's common sense approach and courageous articulation of "the right thing," Newt abandoned H.R. 4498 at the start of 1983.

In an inartful letter to me he withdrew his support for H.R. 4498. "The factual case [for marijuana's use in medicine] is sustainable, but the cultural case is not," Newt wrote. In a similar letter to Rep. McKinney, Gingrich elaborated. "The medical case for the use of marijuana is sustainable, but the cultural case isn't. There are millions in this country who are terrified of the drug problem. . . . At a time when our efforts should be toward crushing the illegal drug culture, and destroying the illegal dealers, it's simply unwise to confuse the message with a bill which is not understandable to our own allies—people who are with us on the effort to destroy the illegal drug culture."

I had observed Gingrich's wilting enthusiasm and anticipated his departure. I could accept, if not respect, Gingrich's gutless decision, but was enraged by Newt's pathetic, revealing rationalization. What culture was Newt defending? Certainly not the mass culture. Polls indicated 80% of the American people believed marijuana should be available by prescription. Courts had ruled marijuana to be a drug of "medical necessity." Scientific studies confirmed marijuana's medical usefulness. The political culture, reflected in the votes of elected state legislators, overwhelmingly favored ending the medical prohibition.

So, what culture was Newt defending? Like so many conservatives, Gingrich got trapped in a political paradox. While deeply fearful over the aggregation of centralized power, conservatives are suckers for authoritarian coercion. Newt abandoned medical marijuana and the facts to defend an odious bureaucratic culture built on institutionalized lies. In less than a year drug warriors neutered the frisky Newt. Exploiting Gingrich's lust for power, bureaucrats turned a conservative bomb-throwing revolutionary into a cringing sycophant of a fraudulent system.

I told a friend on Gingrich's staff, "It's dumb statements like Newt's that put Jews into ovens and Blacks into slavery." They were brutal remarks and overtly threatening. "If Newt withdraws his support, fine. But no press and no effort to drag other conservatives off the bill. If Newt does not go quietly I'll release his letter, my line about Jews and Blacks, and let Newt publicly explain why facts— the fact that sick people are suffering—don't matter."

Newt went quietly.

The twin profiles in pathetic—Gingrich and Waxman—condemned Americans to needless suffering for decades to come. The pendulum had shifted. Through the release of THC and by skillful use of the parents' groups, the government had regained its footing.

The seriously ill could no longer count on the facts to win the day, at least not in Congress.

Newt Gingrich's ignoble departure had little effect: no other Republican jumped ship. While Newt's absence was barely missed, Representative Waxman's refusal to hold congressional hearings effectively retarded progress: a super-liberal, gushing compassion, blocked reform.

In 1983 and 1985 Stewart McKinney's federal marijuana-as-medicine bill was reintroduced into the 98th and 99th Congresses with broad bipartisan support. At the peak of its support McKinney's marijuana-as-medicine legislation had 110 cosponsors. In each subsequent Congress the number of cosponsors was greater than 100.

The proposed legislation also gained powerful endorsements. Nearly every major legal organization in the country including the American Bar Association (ABA), American Civil Liberties Union, National Association of Criminal Defense Lawyers (NACDL) and the National Association of Attorneys General (NAAG) passed resolutions supporting McKinney's bill. But without the necessary hearings in Congress all this support was for naught.

The bill languished but not Stewart's support. In March 1987, the Connecticut representative phoned to ask about reintroduction of the medical marijuana bill in the 100th Congress. The last several times I met with him the Congressman seemed fatigued and even in this last phone call there was a weariness to his voice. There had been bouts of illness and it was clear something was wrong with Stewart McKinney.

There was no indication Rep. Waxman would permit Congressional hearings on medical marijuana and ACT had shifted focus to a new project—hearings before the DEA on medical marijuana. I explained to Stewart that ACT could not simultaneously cope with federal legislation while preparing for DEA hearings. I suggested we return to Congress in 1989, after the DEA hearings. Stewart accepted the decision with some sadness.

Two months later, Representative Stewart McKinney became the first member of Congress to die from AIDS. The bill would resurface seven years later, this time introduced by a liberal. When it finally reemerged it would demonstrate all too well how medical marijuana had become fodder for the drug warriors.

25 Changing Gears

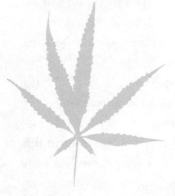

ACROSS THE NATION the political enthusiasm which had fueled the enactment of
34 state laws in five years began to cool,
partly because of THC's release and
partly because our focus shifted to Congress. Mostly the point had
been made, and for the first time since our arrest the river of energy
which carried us forward slackened.

Six states managed to apply enough political pressure to receive
federal supplies of marijuana: California, Georgia, Michigan, New
Mexico, New York, and Tennessee.

The criteria for inclusion in the marijuana studies varied from
state to state but, in the final analysis, hundreds of cancer patients
legally received medical supplies of marijuana under the aegis of
these short-lived, state-sponsored marijuana research programs.
Every state study found marijuana safe and highly effective in reducing chemotherapy-induced vomiting. In the first half of the 1980s
the states routinely reported these favorable findings to the FDA
which routinely ignored the data.

Federal drug agencies continued to consolidate the gains they had secured through the Group C release of THC and sought to "privatize" the distribution of the drug. The FDA offered a sweet deal—an absolute marketing monopoly for a ready-to-go drug. No expensive research needed. No reason to fear those pesky FDA committees. Here was a drug, developed entirely at the taxpayers' expense, that would absolutely clear the hurdles of the New Drug Application process. 100% guaranteed. Every major pharmaceutical company in America reviewed the data and rejected the deal. It was clear THC was not a remarkable drug and the pharmaceutical companies had serious doubts about its formulation. An erratic drug with little profit margin is hardly what major pharmaceutical companies are looking for in the cutthroat world of drug marketing.

The FDA finally convinced a small New Jersey company to take THC. Unimed was developing anti-cancer drugs but had never reached the final approval stage nor marketed a drug in the United States. (Ironically, the chief executive officer of Unimed, Paul V. Bollenbacher, was a neighbor to the late Anne Guttentag.) The small firm undoubtedly felt that THC would swiftly clear the barriers of approval and, by comparison, it did. Nevertheless it required four years for Unimed to negotiate the final hurdles of FDA-regulatory procedure. In an Orwellian twist, THC was renamed dronabinol and would be marketed under the trade name Marinol. It was officially approved in June 1985.

The Compassionate IND model developed in response to *Randall v. U.S.* expanded, although not necessarily for patients needing marijuana. In 1984, responding to the pressure of the expanding AIDS crisis, the FDA created "treatment INDs" which permitted people with AIDS to legally obtain medical products before they received full FDA marketing approval. The Treatment IND approach was modeled on the Compassionate IND and it pleased me to see that Steptoe & Johnson's *pro bono* work really was extended for the "public good."

My access to marijuana had been, for the most part, secure since

1978. There were occasional minor glitches in supply deliveries. But, all in all, my prescriptive access to marijuana was locked in by the artful work of Tom Collier and Steptoe & Johnson.

A handful of others had used the Compassionate IND program to secure federal marijuana, Jim Ripple had successfully used marijuana for a couple years but then his doctor grew weary of federal intrusion and withdrew from the program. The Ripples were unable to locate another doctor and Jim Ripple would lose his sight. Alice and I became reluctant to put desperately ill people through such a cumbersome and bruising regulatory process. I candidly told cancer patients "By the time the FDA responds to your request you'll be dead or cured." Many of the other patients we dealt with were unable to convince their doctors to cooperate in the IND process.

In mid-1983, Alice and I moved from our huge old apartment on Capitol Hill into a modern minimalist condo on Willard St. N.W. between DuPont and Adams-Morgan. The move, in part, was occasioned by Alice's job as administrative officer for the Society for Scholarly Publishing (SSP). She greatly enjoyed SSP, gave the fledgling organization a distinct style, and became absorbed in the rapid advance of new publishing technologies.

During this time I continued to lobby for Rep. McKinney's marijuana-as-medicine bill but there was no funding for ACT which severely curtailed activities. In 1985, I received a $25,000 grant from New Jersey to develop IND protocols for cancer and glaucoma programs, as authorized by that state's 1981 law. I was happy to have an income and completed the work, but New Jersey never submitted the proposal to the FDA.

Weeks, then months passed without urgent calls to Steptoe or meetings with Rep. McKinney. There were no supply problems. My access to marijuana was secure, my sight stable. I continued to send out press releases, travel and do radio talk. The media sporadically reported on medical marijuana, but political stalemate sapped drama from the story.

The mighty steam engine of the medical marijuana issue had run out of fuel. The American myth—the lone citizen fighting evils, changing the course of the nation—had not let us down but Congress had.

This much needed respite came to an end in 1985 when federal agencies, anxious to complete the regulatory procedures necessary to market the newly dubbed "dronabinol," offered NORML a deal. If NORML did not oppose the rescheduling of dronabinol/THC, the DEA would hold hearings on marijuana's medical utility.

An interesting offer, if slightly disingenuous. The DEA had been ordered by the U.S. Court of Appeals, on several occasions, to conduct public hearings on marijuana's proper classification. The delays had been infuriating to NORML, which had initially filed the legal suit in 1972. Now, years later, DEA was trying to cut a deal in order to secure the final piece of regulatory paper before Marinol could hit the market.

ACT had no objections to THC's release if the DEA guaranteed public hearings on natural marijuana. While inferior to marijuana, we could see no reason to block Marinol; it might help someone. Some drug reformers, however, wanted to delay the synthetic's "for profit" marketing, arguing the drug had been developed at taxpayer expense and should not be handed over to a private pharmaceutical company. Others just objected to "giving in" to the DEA. The prospect of "sticking it" to the agencies was appealing. Hearings would take several years and could gum up the works royally. Besides, these reformers argued, the U.S. Court of Appeals had already ordered the DEA to hold hearings on marijuana.

Eventually, less ideologically inclined minds prevailed. NORML agreed to permit THC's prescriptive use and, in April 1986, the DEA ordered public hearings on marijuana's medical value.

We would have another chance to present the facts.

26 In the Matter of...

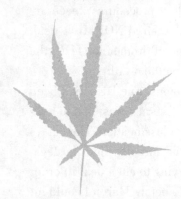

Summer 1986
Steptoe & Johnson
Washington, D.C.

"Can you see anything at all?"

"No."

"No shapes. No color."

"No."

"How long you been blind?"

"Since I was seven."

"So. Can you remember colors or shapes?"

Several Steptoe Associates squirmed in their seats as I asked Frank Stilwell what it was like to be blind.

Frank was a large, round man—no edges. I wondered if being blind made Frank so round. Frank sat at the head of a conference table, his blinded eyes hidden behind super-black wraparound sunglasses. Frank's suit was half a size too large, his shirt cuffs spotted by stains he could not see. Not your typical, scrubbed-for-success Steptoe Associate.

But Frank *was* a Steptoe Associate. Which meant, despite the lack of vision, he had graduated at the top of his law school class. Good minds are hard enough to find, but I reasoned Frank must also have a great will and strong spirit. Without hesitation I welcomed Frank as ACT's new lead attorney.

It was a curious pairing—the man who would be blind but for marijuana and an attorney blinded so young. We would be an instruction to one another.

Frank was young—under 30. He had never handled a major legal case, had little political experience, was naïve to a courtroom. An Ohio boy, big as a farmhand, with a full moon face and formal manner, Frank dressed like a Blues Brother—dark suit, starched white shirt, thin tie and ultra-black shades. He was comfortable in his blindness; rode the subway to work, walked D.C. streets guided by a cane. His office was less cluttered, more organized than most. He took Braille dictation at a furious rate and had a computer programmed to scan printed text into memory so he could retrieve the words in Braille on paper, by synthesized voice playback, or displayed on a Braille reader. I marveled at the high tech gadgetry that gave Frank access to the world of words.

Frank reflected his upbringing in a conservative Republican family steeped in Christian values. A close relation to World War II General "Vinegar Joe" Stilwell, Frank was deeply patriotic with a solid sense of morality and no evident prejudices. Frank loved his ham radio, often listened to police scanners, went to movies with friends, swam almost every day. Round, yet square.

"Have you ever smoked marijuana?" I asked.

"Heavens no," Frank replied, with mock horror. Then, more seriously, "Absolutely not. I'd like to be a judge some day."

The legal trail that led to the proposed hearings had been long and arduous. To recapitulate briefly, in 1972, NORML, together with the American Public Health Association, petitioned the Bureau of Narcotics and Dangerous Drugs (soon to become the Drug Enforcement Administration) to recognize marijuana's medical value and remove the drug from Schedule I of the Controlled Substances Act. Five years later, in 1977, Alice and I delivered a similar petition to the DEA, this one signed by thirteen seriously ill patients. In both instances the petitions were summarily dismissed by the agency without a hearing—a violation of the law. These petitions—ours and NORML's— were eventually merged. Several trips to the U.S. Court of Appeals reinforced the petitioners' right to be heard but the DEA, and later the Dept. of Health, Education and Welfare, imposed severe delays on the proceedings. In October 1980 the agencies were again ordered to hold public hearings but, as the previous chapter notes, the DEA continued to delay the process until 1986 when it traded THC's medical release for hearings which would formally be known as *In The Matter Of Marijuana Rescheduling*.

We felt the DEA hearings offered ACT an opportunity to create the most complete record of marijuana's medical use in the 20th century. Steptoe's *pro bono* committee agreed and authorized resources for the effort. It would be a monumental, and expensive, task. Our new lead attorney was hesitant.

"I'm not certain we should spend a lot of money," Frank cautioned.

My response was politic. "This is history, Frank. If we spend too little and lose everyone will notice. There will be lots of second-guessing. But if we spend what we need to win no one will care how much we spent, just that we won. After all, Frank, this is Steptoe & Johnson. They like to make history."

The DEA hearings revolved around one elemental question: does marijuana have a "currently accepted medical use in treatment in the United States?" The law, embodied in the Controlled Substances Act, contended marijuana had "no accepted medical use in treatment." ACT and NORML argued it did. This single point, accepted medical use, was the difference between Schedule I drugs—totally prohibited, like marijuana—and Schedule II drugs—tightly restricted but available by prescription, such as morphine.

The hearings were conducted by the DEA's chief administrative law judge, Francis L. Young, a kindly looking 60-year-old man who spoke with a light Louisiana lilt, had wispy gray hair and exercised firm control over his courtroom. Initial planning sessions began in the autumn of 1986. There were three principle parties—ACT, NORML and the DEA.

As always, Steptoe was uneasy about working with NORML. Frank seemed especially reluctant to become entangled with a "pro-drug" organization. I appreciated, even shared these concerns, but felt they could be overcome. Better to know what NORML was doing then be blindsided.

Kevin Zeese, a young lawyer, was now in charge of NORML. We had known Kevin for almost a decade. He arrived at NORML as an intern, played a role in the litigation involving Paraquat spraying of marijuana and knew the legal issues. By the time Kevin became NORML's director the once proud organization was struggling to pay the rent. Kevin was working to put things back on track.

A New Yorker, Kevin talked fast, smiled easily, was playfully cynical and easy to like. He was less overtly complicated, more grounded than most reformers. Kevin was practical as a Dutchman.

After several meetings it was decided ACT and NORML would develop independent, but parallel cases. By default the burden of case development fell on ACT.

To facilitate such a large case, Judge Young decided legal testimony would be taken by affidavit. Frank and I settled on a division of labor. I would collect testimony, write affidavits and, with Alice's help, coordinate the accumulation of research reports, medical studies, political facts and supporting materials. Frank would edit the affidavits, but his primary concentration would be on legal arguments and the development of briefs and motions.

For more than a month I conducted detailed interviews with witnesses via speakerphone in a windowless conference room at Steptoe. I would then prepare affidavits for each individual.

A few witnesses were new, their names culled from newspaper articles and public statements. Many were physicians and pharmacists who approached their testimony with clinical detachment. Others were dear friends, veterans of the struggle to enact state laws. My goal was to blend each separate account into a larger story.

Dr. George Goldstein, New Mexico's Secretary of Health, outlined bureaucratic problems. Dr. Daniel Dansak clarified the results of New Mexico's landmark medical research on cancer and marijuana. Katy Brazis, an oncologic nurse, spoke in human terms of how cancer patients in New Mexico benefited from the state's medical marijuana program.

Other witnesses spoke to broader concerns. Andrew Weil, M.D., an ethnopharmacologist trained at Harvard, and John Morgan, M.D., Director of Pharmacology at the City College of New York, helped define marijuana's pharmacologic profile, medical benefits and potential harms.

Robert Stephan, the conservative Attorney General of Kansas—and a cancer patient—testified to the need for prescriptive marijuana. Stephan explained his own situation, then outlined the reasoning behind the National Association of Attorneys General support for marijuana's medical availability. Several other politicians spoke to the intent of their state laws recognizing marijuana's medical value.

The pivotal point of the hearings was whether marijuana was medically "accepted." By whom? The law said "in treatment" so we sought out oncologists, ophthalmologists and neurologists with vast treatment experience to testify on behalf of marijuana's use as a therapeutic agent. These physicians from throughout the United States described how smoking marijuana eased the suffering of their patients and favorably altered medical outcomes without adverse effects. Many of these physicians, including my doctor, Richard North, had never publicly discussed their opinions and findings.

Interviews conducted with patients or, in many cases, the surviving relations of patients were emotionally taxing. Over the speakerphone, Mae Nutt painstakingly described her son Keith's battle with cancer and, as I scribbled furiously, I was astonished to see tears falling on the yellow legal pad. With trembling voice Mona Taft, so strong and controlled throughout the passage of Georgia's marijuana-as-medicine law, sadly recounted her husband Harrison's protracted death and wistfully recalled her efforts to help Georgia cancer patients.

There were new patients including John Dunsmore and his son, John Jr. The Dunsmores lived in Durango, Colorado. Mr. Dunsmore had contacted the Alliance (ACT) because his son, afflicted with bone cancer, had been threatening to quit chemotherapy. Then they discovered marijuana. John Jr., a teenaged amputee fighting for his life, eloquently spoke of how marijuana eased the devastating effects of his anti-cancer treatments. His father reflected on his daily struggle to find—and afford—the marijuana his son needed to continue chemotherapy. Kind people in sad circumstances.

Not all outcomes were sad. Janet Andrews, an Idaho mother, testified about giving her five-year-old son marijuana cookies to get him through chemo. Josh, a cancer survivor then turning ten, had won his battle with cancer. What difference did marijuana make? "Josh would eat a marijuana cookie, get chemo and ride his tricycle down the hall while other kids were bedridden and vomiting," Janet said with bracing honesty. "We still have Josh. Most of those other children are dead. Marijuana cookies saved Josh's life."

Day after day I listened to the many voices of medical marijuana. Each witness offered personal insights, but told the same story. It was like passing through many rooms and looking out the windows onto the same landscape, each window affording a particular point of view, but the scene was always the same. In the quiet after mid-

night, I tried to capture these voices with their different cadences
and tonalities intact—to turn each witness' private journey into cogent testimony which, when combined with other voices, would tell
the larger story.

ACT presented testimony from 37 witnesses. NORML produced
less detailed testimony from 5 witnesses. The DEA responded with
nearly 30 affidavits. Many DEA witnesses were federal bureaucrats
who parroted the party line. Lacking factual evidence they advanced
a looping argument: marijuana has no medical value because the law
says marijuana has no medical value.

One DEA witness was surprising, Dr. Robert Hepler. Representing the American Academy of Ophthalmology (AAO), Hepler's affidavit had an odd flavor about it. It noted the obvious—marijuana's
ability to reduce intraocular pressure. But the AAO had developed
a peculiar side step to the question of marijuana's effectiveness in
the treatment of glaucoma. Their official statement read:

> Effective treatment of glaucoma involves the use of pharma-
> ceutical agents or surgical procedures that prevent progressive
> nerve damage. To date, the only clinically effective method of
> accomplishing this is by lowering intraocular pressure. How-
> ever, merely reducing intraocular pressure is not necessarily
> beneficial to the eye, and pressure reduction does not neces-
> sarily prevent glaucomatous optic nerve pressure.

The AAO stressed the need for a drug or surgical procedure to be
safe and not cause "unacceptable damage to the eye or to other parts
of the body and reduce the pressure sufficiently to prevent optic nerve
damage."

Marijuana, the ophthalmologists concluded, had not been proven
safe to "other parts of the body" so it could not be accepted as safe
for medical use in treatment. There was, of course, no mention of the

side effects of currently available glaucoma medications. Ironically it was at about this same time that the press began to report some disturbing side effects from Timolol, primarily an adverse impact on cardiac rhythms. And, of course, all the existing medications that were available had some adverse systemic impact: cataracts, kidney stones, itchy eyes, blurred vision.

In short, marijuana was being held to a higher standard. Of course the AAO generously acknowledged that marijuana should be investigated further.

Hepler, it seemed, was caught in a squeeze play. The AAO had asked him to join the Ad Hoc Committee on Marijuana Legislation to draft a response to McKinney's bill. No doubt he was pleased just to have the AAO endorse further research and acknowledge the drug's ability to reduce IOP. But then the DEA hearings came along and the AAO tapped him to be the spokesperson.

I was mentioned in his DEA affidavit. "Several years ago . . . Robert Randall was one of my first test patients. As a result of some of the earlier testing, I concluded that marijuana was effective in lowering his intraocular pressure when combined with traditional glaucoma medications. With the subsequently developed information about glaucoma and marijuana, I fully support the Academy's position on this issue."

Whoosh! Without realizing it Hepler was caught in the vortex of the memory hole. It was a tightrope he was walking.

Hepler would have the odd distinction of being a witness for both sides. His 1978 affidavit for *Randall v. U.S.*, standing in stark contrast to his now "official" view, was included as an appendix in ACT's testimony.

ACT and NORML challenged the relevance of testimony from nearly a dozen DEA witnesses. Largely law enforcement officers with no medical knowledge, these witnesses offered boilerplate prattle of marijuana's link to lurid violence, insanity and other fictions. Judge

Young struck the testimony of a third of DEA's witnesses. This was to be a case about marijuana's medical use, not a platform for drug war hysteria.

Once the witness list was finalized any party could require any other party to physically produce a witness for cross-examination. Frank, Kevin, and I had differing views. The ACT/NORML testimony was richer, more varied and much stronger than DEA's stale case. I argued there was no need to call any DEA witness. Kevin disagreed. Frank was uncertain. Eventually, only one DEA witness, Dr. Keith Green, the clinical researcher who developed the failed THC eye-drop, would be cross-examined.

DEA attorneys took a precisely different tact, demanding to cross-examine nearly every witness who testified in favor of ending the medical prohibition. I was delighted by the DEA's decision. The resulting record would give oral weight to the written testimony. To accommodate the DEA's demand to cross-examine nearly all ACT and NORML witnesses, Judge Young scheduled multiple hearings to be held in New Orleans, San Francisco and Washington, D.C.

After a year of preparation Judge Young opened the first public DEA hearing on medical marijuana in New Orleans on November 18, 1987. There were two days of hearings in New Orleans. Frank, distracted by the commotion of travel, the sounds of a new city, his role in a courtroom, the two female DEA attorneys, and my incessant instruction had difficulty focusing on questions for witnesses. At one point he seemed utterly lost. Judge Young became impatient and Kevin quickly intervened, redirecting the questioning. It was deeply disturbing and I wondered if Frank could handle the challenge. Kevin thought Frank should get a second chance. "I was really nervous my first time in court," he said. "I think Frank will work it out."

After returning to Washington, Judge Young's office informed all parties something had gone wrong during the first day of testimony.

The taped transcript of the hearing could not be retrieved. Attempts to find an alternative tape also proved useless. An NBC radio reporter who taped much of the testimony, discovered his tape had also been wiped clean.

Coincidence? Conspiracy? Perhaps the DEA was playing games and goofed. Who else would have the technical wherewithal to accomplish such a feat? Rather than place blame, however, everyone pretended the destruction of evidence was a mysterious mechanical occurrence beyond human understanding.

The second series of hearings was in San Francisco three weeks later. This time we planned a more leisurely travel schedule. Frank and I flew out several days early to do final interviews with several witnesses and to give Frank a chance to "settle in" before the next court date. On our first day we "saw" some of the city together. We rode on cable cars and I would describe the buildings and streets as they glided past. Then we settled down to work.

December 7, 1987
Dr. Ivan Silverberg's Office
San Francisco, California

I had some early afternoon appointments and arranged to meet Frank around 4 p.m. We wanted to review Dr. Silverberg's testimony and make certain the doctor was comfortable with the upcoming court appearance.

When I arrived, Frank was already sitting in Silverberg's private office. He did not look well. The young lawyer was pale and clearly uncomfortable.

"Is something wrong, Frank?"

Frank slowly nodded. "I got here early and Dr. Silverberg put me in here while he finished treating a few patients in the next room." Frank moved his head in the direction of the wall and stopped to collect his thoughts. "I heard him come down the hall with a patient and could hear Dr. Silverberg give the chemotherapy. The first man complained a lot, then I heard him throw up. It was awful. He just couldn't stop vomiting. And it was so violent."

Frank stopped for a moment and wiped his brow. "There's a second patient in there now. Dr. Silverberg brought him in a little while ago. I heard them talking. The guy is getting the same chemo. I've been sort of waiting for . . . but he hasn't vomited."

"See what a difference marijuana makes, Mr. Stilwell?" Silverberg was in the doorway, watching Frank recount the tale to me.

The physician and I watched as the realization of what had happened swept across Frank's face. "I had no idea," Frank exclaimed. "No idea. I've been reading about this for over a year. But I had no idea. I guess hearing is believing, huh?"

The three of us chuckled at Frank's "blind" humor and Frank began to relax. But I could see that Frank was transformed, just as Merritt had been when he measured my eye pressures after the first marijuana cigarette. All the abstract testimony and stale statistical studies made rational sense which Frank could verbally defend. But the physical realities of the cancer patients in the next room—one vomiting violently, the other not—made medical marijuana graphically real to Frank. For the first time the young lawyer understood medical marijuana was not a technical legal matter, but a desperately real question of basic human care. On that day in Ivan Silverberg's office, Frank Stilwell found the soul of the issue.

After reviewing testimony I asked Dr. Silverberg why the patients in his waiting room seemed so young. "AIDS," Silverberg replied. "AIDS-related lymphoma. It's ironic, really. Initially, I specialized in pediatric oncology, but couldn't bear writing out death certificates for children. So I shifted into lymphoma—mainly a disease of older people. But now," Silverberg said with choking sadness, "I spend one day a week writing out death certificates for young men who have died from AIDS-related lymphoma."

"Mention this in your testimony," I urged. "So far all the focus is on marijuana's medical use in cancer and glaucoma, with a few references to multiple sclerosis. Until now no one's mentioned AIDS."

On December 8, Ivan Silverberg testified before Judge Young. He was a superb witness. His credentials were impeccable. In practice since 1972, Silverberg also taught at the University of California, San Francisco; a practitioner and an academic. He commanded attention from the witness chair.

When asked to recount some patient experiences he told of a young man with AIDS who found marijuana the only drug that allowed him to eat. "Without marijuana," Silverberg said, "that young man would have died much sooner. For him, marijuana made a critical difference."

When Silverberg completed his testimony a young, obviously gay court reporter walked over to the oncologist. "I'd like to shake your hand, doc. My friends are dying from AIDS. I'm glad you were here to support their needs."

Silverberg took the young man's hand. "Anything less would be wrong."

The hearings in New Orleans and San Francisco lasted a total of four days. The Washington hearings, held in a federal courtroom on Lafayette Park by the White House, stretched over a month with almost eleven days of testimony.

By the time the hearings began in Washington, Frank and Kevin worked well together. Kevin was still more skillful in examining witnesses, but Frank proved a fast learner.

After six or more hours in court, Frank and I would have dinner with one or more of the next day's witnesses. Frank would then go home, reread the witness's affidavit and prepare for the next morning's first witness. It was a grueling work load, but Frank just got better and better.

Most witnesses testified to a nearly deserted courtroom with just the judge, the attorneys, and myself in attendance. Occasionally reporters wandered in. Media interest was not intense, but it was constant. Witnesses would often be interviewed by D.C. reporters representing hometown papers.

Mae Nutt and her husband, Arnold, rode the train from Michigan to testify. Mae was a riveting witness and Herb Kaplow was so taken by her story he did a piece for "CBS News" which highlighted the hearings.

The DEA attorneys, both women, proved dogged advocates. But their questions often provoked detailed answers that only underscored marijuana's medical effectiveness. Unable to attack the treatment decisions of practicing physicians they began assaulting the credibility of witnesses. But how can one attack the credibility of a mother who has watched a son die?

I was the last witness to testify. The courtroom was filled to capacity. Alice, who had testified earlier, was unable to bear the strain. "It's easier to walk on hot coals then watch you testify," she explained. Having agonized through her testimony I understood. Still, there were many familiar faces in the room. Many more unfamiliar. Some reporters. More than a few DEA types. Looking for payback.

It was contentious. And very, very long. For eight hours—far longer than any other witness—I answered questions. There were nearly no surprises, but the experience was exhausting.

By the end of the hearings the record included 15 volumes of oral testimony, 60 lengthy affidavits and more than 5,000 pages of exhibits, evidence and other supporting materials. Now it was time to write the briefs.

Unlike Tom Collier, whose great talent was in reaching out to tap the talent of others—building a team and fully exploiting Steptoe's vast resources—Frank relied primarily on himself. He did recruit one Associate, Roberto Laver—an Argentine attorney working at Steptoe. I was the third member of the team. We divided the case into chunks. Frank and Roberto researched legal questions. I began pulling the factual case together.

It was, in the end, an immense case. Thousands of pages of testimony and evidence, with mountains of supporting materials that were footnoted, referenced and cross-referenced. All was neatly bundled and delivered to the Office of the Chief Administrative Law Judge.

The case was now in Judge Young's hands. It would be five months before the decision was delivered.

On September 6, 1988, DEA chief administrative law judge Francis L. Young ruled marijuana had "an accepted medical use in treatment in the United States." Young called the medical prohibition "unreasonable, arbitrary and capricious," and recommended marijuana be reclassified to permit its prescriptive medical use.

It was a smashing victory, all the sweeter because so many doubted the possibility of winning. Judge Young was "their guy," the top DEA law judge. No one expected him to rule in our favor. We knew the facts supported our cause but we had learned, from Newt Gingrich, that facts did not always prevail. This time would be different. Judge Young would not ignore the facts. It was a courageous decision.

The DEA still had the upper hand. Young's decision could be accepted or rejected by the DEA administrator. Two weeks after Judge Young's decision *Time* Magazine reported that a cable was sent from DEA headquarters to all field offices. "DEA counsel will be filing vigorous exception to the findings." Administrative law decisions are not ordinarily overturned but this was not your ordinary decision. We began the waiting game again, this time waiting for the DEA administrator, John Lawn. Realistically we did not expect an embracing of Young's decision.

In the meanwhile, the press coverage of Young's "unprecedented" decision was overwhelming. Once again the medical marijuana issue reclaimed the public's imagination. Headlines screamed the news. "Judge OKs Medicinal Use of Pot" was the banner in *USA Today*.

Ironically Judge Young's decision did not extend to glaucoma. He determined there was accepted medical use for marijuana in treatment for cancer, multiple sclerosis, and a variety of rare disorders but not glaucoma. It was a disappointment but the overall decision was so monumental that the glaucoma exclusion was lost in the merrymaking. I can't be certain why Young ruled in this way. From my perspective the evidence was solid. Perhaps it was Hepler's defection that swayed the Judge's thinking. Perhaps it was an attempt to placate the hard-liners at DEA. "Well, at least he stuck it to Randall," they could say. Who knows?

An even greater irony was the date of the decision—September 6, 1988, precisely sixteen years to the day I had been diagnosed with glaucoma. On that day in 1972, Dr. Fine had looked across his desk and, with some sadness, predicted I had "3 to 5 years of remaining sight." Marijuana had undeniably altered that dire prognosis. I could still see. Well enough to read Judge Young's decision, well enough to enjoy the beauty of Washington as I walked back to our apartment from Steptoe and Johnson on that historic day.

In the Matter Of Marijuana Rescheduling created the most extensive record of marijuana's medical use in the 20th century. It was a monumental collection of materials standing more than five feet high. It was a trove of information and we knew others would benefit from the data and insights it provided. But how would anyone ever gain access to such a massive record? Eventually, the DEA would ship the entire record off to long-term storage. Where it would end up only the gods knew. The memory hole, no doubt, would suck away great portions of the record. "Sorry," the persistent researcher would be told, "we don't seem to be able to locate those records." It was essential to preserve the information and, after some fretting, the answer presented itself in that most subversive of all enterprises— publishing.

Franklin Roosevelt once said, "books are weapons" and in the evidence of *In the Matter of . . .* we had a vast arsenal with which to battle the memory hole.

Through her job at SSP, Alice had the opportunity to learn about the emerging field of desktop publishing. Why not translate critical portions of the factual record into accessible print via this new technology? We realized we could do the work ourselves, with minimal financial investment. And so we decided to become publishers.

The goal was to create a viable reference work that reflected the views of all parties. After reviewing the case we decided to create two volumes. The first would include the written testimony of all the witnesses. *Marijuana, Medicine & the Law*, Vol. I was published in November 1988. A second volume published a year later contained the complete legal briefs submitted by ACT, NORML and DEA, and the complete text of Judge Young's historic ruling.

Once again we became an arsenal of information. *Marijuana, Medicine & the Law* was distributed to hundreds of legal libraries, medical and law schools, universities and local libraries. These books, still available from Galen Press, remain the most complete record of our society's encounter with medical marijuana.

IV

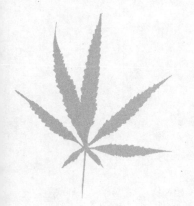

New Allies

27 The Necessity of Necessity

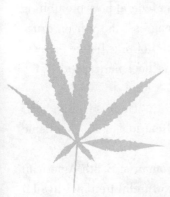

THE DEA HEARINGS had consumed my attention for two years. But as the final testimony was heard before Judge Young in Washington, I realized the case would come to an end and I began to wonder what path I should be taking. I didn't have to wait long for the answer.

The medical use of marijuana was widespread and well-known but legal access to the drug was virtually impossible. Of the thirty-four states that had enacted laws acknowledging marijuana's medical utility only six managed to implement programs of legal access and, by 1988, most of those had closed. Federal drug agencies would point to this fact and offer it as "proof" that no one really wanted medical marijuana except the "pro-drug groups." But the truth was far less sinister—it was simply easier to obtain marijuana illegally.

But illegal marijuana carried considerable danger, mainly arrest.

My own case in 1976 had given medical marijuana users a defense—medical necessity. Judge Washington's ruling was tightly drawn and could not be used carte blanche. A patient must have exhausted all legally available medications and the illness had to pose a great danger to the patient. In other words, medical marijuana use for hangnails would not pass the test.

Since Judge Washington's ruling there had been only one additional successful argument of medical necessity. It involved a multiple sclerosis patient in Washington state, Sam Diana, who successfully raised the medical necessity defense on appeal after he was convicted of marijuana possession in 1977.

But in the late 1980s, as efforts to reform federal laws prohibiting medical access to marijuana stalled in Congress, the war on drugs simultaneously heated up. It was just a matter of time before patients who were medically using illegal marijuana became trapped in the cross fire.

On March 6, 1988, I received a phone call. "Hello, Mr. Randall," said a middle-aged woman with a Ricky Ricardo accent. "My name is Elvy. Elvy Musikka—with two K's."

Elvy Musikka, in her late 40s, was a woman of South American and Norwegian extraction. She had two grown children and lived a quiet life under the palms in Hollywood, Florida. Elvy needed help. Nearly blinded by glaucoma and more than twenty surgical procedures, Elvy had been arrested for growing six marijuana plants in her backyard. Sound familiar?

Elvy Musikka's medical history was an ophthalmologic horror story. Elvy was born with congenital cataracts and developed secondary glaucoma. Efforts to control her glaucoma with drugs failed. She had undergone surgery—for both cataracts and glaucoma— many times. These surgeries failed to control her ocular tensions and repeated operations had weakened and mutilated the shape of her eyes. During her last operation a blood vessel ruptured, immediately blinding that eye. Her remaining eye was badly damaged by unrelieved pressure and surgery. There seemed to be no hope. Then, Elvy found marijuana.

That was in 1976, the year Judge Washington established the

medical necessity defense. "I read everything about your case," Elvy said. "Funny. I knew one day we would meet."

In addition to reading about my case Elvy also learned about marijuana's use in glaucoma treatment from one of her doctors. He encouraged her to try marijuana brownies. They worked. For more than a decade Elvy Musikka had quietly smoked or consumed marijuana, kept her ocular pressures under control and avoided additional surgery. While legally blind, her condition was stable and she was still able to get around with modest help. Things were going well until policemen raided her home, seized her small marijuana crop and hauled Elvy off to jail.

It was the next morning, after being released on bail, that she called me. I was just getting accustomed to Elvy's unique accent and detailed story when she said, "Oh, I have to go. The television reporters have arrived."

Later that day we would talk again. "All the reporters gone?" I asked.

"Oh, yes. But they were all here. And so nice."

"If we're going to work together, no more press," I said.

"But how will people know?" Elvy sounded crestfallen. Having just been arrested she was angry and wanted to get her story out.

"First, we develop a legal case. If that works we go to trial. Once you are in court everything is public and there will be plenty of press."

With considerable reluctance, Elvy agreed.

The case came together with surprising ease. Elvy's current doctor, Paul Palmberg of the Bascom-Palmer Eye Institute at the University of Miami, had treated her for many years. He was aware of her marijuana use and, while not overtly approving, encouraged her to keep doing "whatever works." I spoke with Dr. Palmberg and he was frank. "She's my only patient where it's quite clear-cut this is the only thing that will help her." After some consideration he agreed to testify on

Elvy's behalf. More importantly he agreed to help Elvy apply for
Compassionate IND access to marijuana.

Elvy's attorney, Norman Kent, agreed to represent her on a *pro
bono* basis. I guided him in developing the legal case and wrote
detailed affidavits for Elvy and her physician. At the same time I
provided Dr. Palmberg with a draft IND. Palmberg submitted the
IND application without hesitation.

In August, after months of telephone chatter, I flew to Florida for
the trial. Elvy was a handsome woman, lively and loving. Unlike my
blind lawyer Frank, she wore clear glasses, her surgery-damaged
eyes magnified by cataract lenses.

Elvy had befriended Irvin Rosenfeld, who received FDA-approved
marijuana under a Compassionate IND for a rare disease that caused
painful bone spurs and tumors. I had started assisting Irvin in the
late 1970s. After nearly five years of effort, Irvin's IND was approved
in September 1982 and he began receiving supplies of government
marijuana two months later. For several years, following the closure
of the state marijuana-as-medicine programs, Irvin and I were the
only two individuals receiving legal supplies of marijuana in the U.S.
Irvin, who lived in North Lauderdale and worked as a stockbroker,
liked to remain in the background, but he agreed to testify in Elvy's
case, if necessary.

The August 15th trial was a carbon copy of my own case. A po-
liceman testified regarding Elvy's arrest. A chemist declared she was
growing marijuana. The state rested, case closed.

Elvy's attorney admitted the crime and raised a defense of "medical necessity." I was the first to testify on Elvy's behalf—a glaucoma
patient legally smoking U.S. government marijuana to save his sight.
I was followed by Dr. Palmberg who reviewed Elvy's extensive medical history. Palmberg concluded, as Robert Hepler had a dozen years
before, that, if legal, "he would prescribe marijuana for this patient
for her medical use." He was a convincing witness who acknowledged

his discomfort in the role. "I'm a Presbyterian elder, and I've had to be dragged kicking and screaming to say this."

Elvy's testimony was heartfelt and oddly dramatic. "Marijuana," she said, "saved my sight. I don't think the law has the right to demand blindness from a citizen."

As I predicted, the press was there and they were wowed by the story. So was the judge. Unlike my own case, Elvy's decision came on the spot. Judge Mark E. Polen ruled from the bench that Elvy was not guilty by reason of medical necessity. "I don't see where a better case could ever be made for medical necessity. In this case, Miss Musikka is trying to preserve herself from serious bodily injury."

Promising a full written decision in short order, Judge Polen warned against others thinking this decision "was a green light" for widespread marijuana use in South Florida. "That's not the message that I want to convey," he said. "The ruling of this court is limited to the precise facts of this case."

Elvy would win the first part of her battle with a speedy trial and rapid justice. Waiting for her Compassionate IND would take longer.

There were two other medical necessity cases that summer but the results were not as happy. Ironically both took place in Kentucky.

James Burton was a 39-year-old glaucoma patient living on a ninety-acre farm near Bowling Green. He made no secret of his use of marijuana to treat his glaucoma nor did he particularly try to hide the marijuana he was growing to treat his illness. But he was growing a lot of marijuana, more than 100 plants.

Kentucky was not one of the 34 states recognizing marijuana's medical utility but Burton, foolishly, was certain he was safe. When the Kentucky State Police raided his farm Burton told them of his medical use. They didn't care.

Jim Burton found himself in a dirty little skirmish that would have a brutal ending. Because of the large number of plants involved he was tried on federal rather than state charges. The jury believed his claim of medical necessity enough to mitigate the charges against him—manufacturing and intent to sell. But it found him guilty of simple possession and he was sentenced to one year in prison without parole. Worse yet, a new weapon in the war on drugs had been hatched by the U.S. Congress. It was called forfeiture and, simply put, it meant the government could seize the property of individuals charged with drug possession. Jim and Linda Burton would lose their home of eighteen years and be given ten days to vacate the 90-acre property. The seized "drug property" would then be auctioned to the highest bidder. When Burton was finally released from jail he and his wife would flee the U.S. and settle in Holland, which was more sympathetic to his medical needs.

Rick Morris was a 31-year-old cancer patient in Paintsville, Kentucky. He was arrested in November 1987 with more than seven ounces of marijuana. He could have plead guilty to a misdemeanor charge and paid a $250 fine but Morris decided to fight on medical necessity grounds. In late July I flew to Kentucky to testify on Morris' behalf.

Morris' case had fewer complications than Burton's, not the least of which was his being charged by the state rather than the feds. There was no question of forfeiture. Rick Morris had little in the way of possessions. His cancer, ostensibly, was cured but he continued to experience severe nausea and vomiting. At one point his weight dropped from 200 pounds to 130.

Dr. Daniel Dansak, a psychiatrist who worked with New Mexico's Lynn Pierson Therapeutic Research Program, testified that this was not unusual for cancer patients. The lingering effects of radiation and chemotherapeutic treatments could last for years.

The prosecutor, clearly swayed by Morris' predicament, urged the jury to convict the Kentuckian but also asked for leniency. The jury convicted Rick Morris and sentenced him to a $1 fine.

The prosecutors in both cases would argue that medical necessity should not be considered because "the court was not the place for this argument." Instead, they contended, "proponents should take their case to the legislature." Elvy Musikka lived in a state that had enacted legislation and she successfully argued her case of medical necessity. Perhaps, if Kentucky had enacted a marijuana-as-medicine bill Jim Burton and Rick Morris would have been found not guilty. We'll never know.

Necessity was becoming a necessity. Congress ignored the needs of the seriously ill and let stand a situation that forced these three individuals, and countless others, into criminality to meet their medical needs.

After nearly six months of waiting Elvy would finally receive legal supplies of marijuana. In October 1988 she became the third individual in the U.S. receiving legal supplies. She would be the second woman to acquire such a unique status—Anne Guttentag had been the first.

Elvy's case began to rekindle interest in the Compassionate IND process. In the coming year I would assist another individual into our exclusive lifeboat. Corrine Millet, a 60-something Nebraska grandmother with glaucoma, doggedly pursued legal access and began receiving federal marijuana in October 1989.

There would be one more Compassionate IND approved in that year. It would go to an AIDS patient in Texas and it would spark a firestorm of interest that would force the issue of medical marijuana back into the public spotlight. This time the light would shine bright enough to strip away the mask of "compassion" and reveal the federal government's absolute denial of marijuana's medical utility.

28 Prizes, Pawns and Patrons

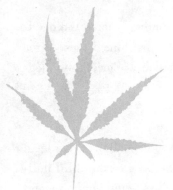

"I HAVE AIDS," Steve said, choking on the stigma.

At the dawn of the Reagan era a mysterious affliction came to America. Gay men in the prime of life were dying of rare cancers and pneumonia. A small ripple of death moved through an outcast community. There was silence. Then, with stunning rapidity, the unnamed disease leapfrogged from homos to Haitians to hemophiliacs then to heterosexuals. Near-panic gripped epidemiologists as outbreaks of this demon disease doubled and redoubled. Scientific alarm slammed into political indifference.

AIDS. By 1983, the mystery disease had a name—Acquired Immune Deficiency Syndrome—and a profile. A virus carried in blood-based body fluids destroyed the immune system. Once the immune system collapsed infected individuals were prey to all manner of microbes. Death was inevitable.

"Marijuana helps with my AIDS," an unidentified caller told me in 1983. I pressed for details. "It just helps me eat," the man said.

As the incidents of AIDS multiplied, calls to ACT became more frequent. "Would you like to apply to get marijuana legally?" I would ask. Every man—all the callers were men—declined. With frail voices they would say, "I'm dying. I don't have time for cops and courts and bureaucrats. I just want you to know pot helps." ·

In retrospect it is hard to fathom the political silence and bloated hatreds which welcomed AIDS into the 1980s. There was good reason for fear. A society suckled on medical marvels could find no defense. Science was stymied. There was no cure, no effective treatment. AIDS was 100% fatal: a fearsome epidemic loose on the land. Uncertainty over how AIDS spread intensified social anxieties. Christian fanatics attributed the accelerating slaughter to divine retribution. Sinners were dying. Who cares? Then, sinless children infected by transfusion were cast from schools. Mobs formed. Homes burned. Plague and political silence. Shame.

In 1986, AIDS touched us personally for the first time when we learned our college friend, Bobby Evans and his lover, Walter, had AIDS. Walter died the following year. "Horrible," Bobby said, his voice conveying a concern for his own future. "Just horrible." Not yet 40, Bobby moved to San Francisco to prepare for his own demise.

In 1988, the AIDS Quilt came to Washington. We walked among the brilliantly colored panels spread on the Ellipse, just across the street from the White House. We wept over the deaths of so many so young. Among the panels there we would find a tribute to Rep. Stewart McKinney. Another marked the death of our neighbor Rusty. It was an awesome display that called out for acknowledgment but in an act of supreme neglect President Reagan did not bother to visit the Quilt.

Despite escalating death rates, AIDS, enveloped in bigotry and fear, was not yet part of the national dialogue. This disconnect was even reflected in the massive record *In The Matter Of Marijuana Rescheduling*. Buried within thousands of pages of testimony on marijuana's medical value in cancer care, glaucoma therapy and spasm control was but one fleeting mention of AIDS. One sentence of concern lost in a million words of testimony.

"I have AIDS," Steve said choking on the stigma. "And I want your help." In early October 1989, Steve L. called for help from his bed at the Audie. L. Murphy Memorial Veterans Hospital in San Antonio, Texas. He was dying.

"I told 'em if I kept looking I'd find you," Steve said, sad as a sick puppy. "I told 'em I'd find you."

Steve L. was a backwoods Texas boy. Reared in poverty he quit school in the seventh grade and worked odd jobs doing lawn care, chopping firewood, etc. By the time he reached thirty Steve was just another aimless, angry alcoholic, addicted to methamphetamine and selling blood to make ends meet. A dark bedeviled life of hard scrabble and hard luck.

Steve's life got much harder when, unable to breathe, he ended up at Audie Murphy diagnosed with AIDS from a dirty needle. He lapsed into coma, then awoke to slow recovery and transformation.

"What happened in your coma?" I wanted to know.

"I remember walking down this path," Steve began. "Trees, like a tent overhead. Dark, but there was people, shadow people, standing off to both sides. But I paid 'em no mind, just kept walking 'til I come over a rise and saw this wide, black river, flat as glass. So I walked on by the river awhile 'til I come upon this small boat. I was getting in to go to the other side when a man with no face stopped me. 'Not yet,' he said. 'Not yet.' Then I woke up. And now I've found you."

"Were you looking for me?" I asked, trapped by the imagery.

"Oh, yeah. Looking hard," Steve said with gravity. "Looking a year or more."

Steve's pneumonia-induced coma was followed by ineffective, highly toxic medical treatments and rapid weight loss. Constantly nauseated by disease and drugs, his weight collapsed. "I'm not a big man," Steve explained, "but I lost half my weight; down to 80 lbs. Skin and bones. Then I discovered marijuana."

Following his comatose journey to the River Styx, Steve emerged spiritually transfigured. "No booze. No drugs. No anger. No fear. Like I woke from a bad dream. Happy," he said.

Happy, but terribly thin. A friend, alarmed by Steve's bone-bruising thinness, urged Steve to take a toke of marijuana. "He said it might help me eat. I thought, 'What the hell?' And it worked."

"How?"

"Well. I could eat. Once pot took my nausea away I couldn't stop eating. Gained back my weight, mostly, started chopping firewood again. It's like I come back to life. My doctors, everyone are real amazed. I'm telling you true; without pot I'd have died last year. That's when I started looking for you."

"How did you find me?"

"Weren't easy. I knew you existed 'cause I saw you on TV. So I started looking, making calls. I asked my doctors, the people at V.A., local police, the Texas Rangers, FDA, even the DEA. I kept telling people there was this man who legally smokes pot. But they all told me you didn't exist. That got me real confused so as I didn't know what to do. Then I got arrested."

"You've been arrested?"

"Yep. Six months ago: March 1989. The police they come storming in 'n took my pot. That was real bad. Without pot I ended up back in the hospital. That's when I started looking for you again."

"So how did you find me." I needed to know who guided this messenger from the edge of death to my door.

"Well, I called all over again. And everybody kept saying no one gets legal pot. Then I called the DEA and this real nice guy, he listens to what I'm saying. Then he told me all about you. Even gave me your phone number. That's how I found you," Steve said with the pride of a hunter who has finally cornered his quarry.

"So. You've found me. How can I help you?"

"I want you to get me legal pot," Steve said.

"Why?" I probed for motive.

"Because people with AIDS are dying—starving to death. That's not right. They should know marijuana helps. So I want you to get me legal pot. Then people with AIDS will know, right? That's what I want you to do."

Steve L., returned from death, was on a mission. He had, after a long, frustrating search, delivered his message inviting me to be his guide. "It's why I came back," Steve said with sweet certainty. "So you could help me."

Steve spoke with fate's voice and issued a summons I could not— dared not—refuse. He approached me with a certainty that I would somehow lead him to a new place, a new level. But it was Steve who would be the guide and he would lead me to a new universe.

Until Steve L. medical marijuana was about cancer and glaucoma and, ever so slightly, spasms and chronic pain. Could Steve's case stretch the Compassionate IND to include the use of marijuana in treating AIDS? Steve L. was eager to try. I could not deny him the chance.

Steve L. had good friends, chief among them Papa Bear (a.k.a. Robert C. Edwards), a big, burly, bearded man in his mid-fifties. Papa Bear founded and ran the San Antonio AIDS Foundation (SAAF), a charity that cared for AIDS patients in southeastern Texas. The SAAF, fueled by Papa Bear's energy, provided dying men medical care, operated food pantries, prepared a hot potluck dinner every night and delivered meals to men too weak to leave home. A human response to the spreading plague. Edwards—the father of a gay son—could not deny Steve's plea for help. "A lot of my guys smoke pot and say it helps," Bear told me. "Steve kept telling us you existed but we thought he was imagining things. Maybe he's on to something. How can I help?"

Papa Bear helped a great deal. He encouraged the SAAF doctor to apply for a Compassionate IND. I altered a cancer protocol and wondered how the FDA would react to a marijuana IND for AIDS. "Then there's Steve's arrest," Bear reminded me.

Steve was set up; busted after buying 13 ounces of marijuana from a vice cop. "I was getting enough marijuana to last me the rest of my life," Steve explained. Instead, Steve ended up several thousand dollars poorer, out on bail, dying of AIDS while facing criminal charges and prison.

"We told the court about Steve's condition," Bear said. "So the judge just keeps postponing the trial. No reason to drag a dying man to court."

But Steve L. wanted his day in court. "Hell, I wanna fight 'em. They oughtn't be doing this to sick people," Steve said.

I contacted Kevin Zeese for help. Within days Gerry Goldstein, a San Antonio attorney and one of the nation's finest criminal defense lawyers, agreed to represent Steve L. *pro bono*.

Within a week of calling, Steve L. had a doctor willing to apply to the FDA, and his criminal case was in capable hands. Within two weeks I had drafted the nation's first Compassionate IND for marijuana/AIDS. Steve's doctor submitted the IND and we began tracking its progress through the FDA. Time was short. Steve was sick.

Aware of the stress that comes from waiting, I made a point of speaking with Steve nearly every night. Despite his lack of formal education Steve was an intelligent, articulate fellow who wrote hauntingly beautiful poetry. Steve often spoke of his dog, Cool Breeze— C.B.—and frequently reflected on his return from death; the path and the ferryman. I listened for hours as Steve pondered the meaning of the mythic imagery he was living.

"Why wouldn't the ferryman let you in the boat?" I asked.

"Unfinished business," Steve replied with simple certainty.

As I listened to Steve night after night I found myself far removed from congresses and courtrooms, plunged into a more ethereal, less material realm governed by only vaguely apprehended energies. Ghosts of fallen allies would manifest themselves in Steve's simply articulated goals. I hoped I could faithfully discharge the commission he presented.

In 1988, when Mae Nutt came to Washington, D.C. to testify before Judge Young, she encountered Alice in the hallway and the two women shared an emotional moment as each complimented the other on their testimony. Wondering together at the final outcome of the long battle in which they had engaged, Mae looked the younger woman square in the eye and said, "There's no need to worry, Alice. We've got angels on our shoulders."

In the Fall of 1989, as Steve L.'s IND bounced around FDA, those angels manifested themselves with a dramatic, unanticipated event.

Our friend Kevin Zeese had left NORML and, together with American University professor Arnold Trebach, established a new group called the Drug Policy Foundation (DPF), a Washington "think-tank" established to develop alternative public policies in the war on drugs. Among the activities of the DPF was the annual presentation of awards named for various individuals who had made significant contributions to the reform of drug laws. I was honored when Kevin and Arnold informed me that in 1989 DPF would establish the Robert C. Randall Award for Achievement in the Field of Citizen Activism. I would be the first recipient of the award. Along with a nice plaque, the DPF award came with a check for $10,000.

The award and prize would be presented during DPF's annual banquet in early November, part of a three-day conference. I arrived at DPF's welcoming reception before Alice. Being near-blind and not much good at mingling I found a corner of the room and settled.

People came by, extended congratulations, made small talk and moved on. Kevin asked if I'd like a drink and then vanished in the direction of the bar.

"Didn't I see you smoking marijuana on Larry King?" someone asked.

My eyes moved in the direction of the voice and worked hard to focus on the large, friendly man smiling down at me. "That was me, all right."

"Good job," the large man said. "Good job," he repeated, then shyly retreated as Kevin returned with my drink.

"You know who that was?" Kevin asked.

"Haven't a clue," I replied.

"Rich Dennis," Kevin said with pride.

Richard J. Dennis. I had first encountered the name in a newspaper several years earlier. Richard J. Dennis, the article read, made a cool $80 million in 1986 to become the fourth highest earner on Wall Street. Not much more than 40 years of age, Richard J. Dennis was a very wealthy man who helped bankroll DPF's start and the awards that would be presented later that night. As we chatted about the interesting Mr. Dennis, Kevin revealed the philanthropist was looking for other good works to support.

As an imminent recipient of Rich's obvious generosity I was grateful to have met him but thought little of the encounter. I had given up chasing after rich men in hopes of phantom philanthropy. Money, I feared, was the ultimate addiction: tedious to pursue, difficult to sustain, enslaving in the extreme. I could either write unrequited grant requests to wealthy men or draft IND protocols for people like Irvin, Elvy, Corrine, Steve and others. No contest.

The next evening the banquet and award presentation was held. For fifteen years I had held press conferences, handled reporters, given thousands of interviews. But only rarely did I give a formal speech. I found the process intriguing. Rhetoric is more than mere words.

The speech was well-received and I was much relieved. I shook hands, made small talk without really connecting to any of the individuals. On autopilot I reached for the next extended paw. "That was a very fine speech," Richard J. Dennis said. "Give me a call. Maybe I can help."

"Seriously?"

"Seriously," Richard J. replied with a smile.

Days later someone from Chicago phoned. "Could you outline what you would like? That will give Rich a chance to review things before you talk." Seriously.

With zero expectations I wrote Richard J. a long, sometimes clever, sometimes rambling overview of drug reform and medical marijuana. I made it painfully clear we had no interest in empire building. There would be no organization to support, no fund-raising effort, no direct mail campaign, no outreach to activists nor seminars nor membership drives nor bake sales. I didn't give a damn about such frivolous distractions. Given a choice between creating a big organization or a vital issue I would build an issue. All I really wanted was to pursue medical marijuana. No strings.

It was a brutally honest, utterly unorthodox "non-proposal": heartfelt, but hardly politic. Without pausing to consider the consequences, I dropped the missive in the overnight mail bin. Chicago called the next day to give me Richard J.'s L.A. number. "Call any time," Chicago said.

Shortly after sunset on Sunday, December 7, I left Alice on the sofa watching TV and wandered to our small office upstairs. I dialed L.A. and Richard J. answered, a football game blaring in the background. "I could call back," I suggested. "No need," Richard J. replied. "And call me Rich. So, how would you win medical marijuana?"

"That's an unfair question; a bit like me asking you how to win in the stock market. There's no easy answer. The point is I know how to win."

"What's important to you?" Rich asked.

"Aesthetics," it tumbled out. "Ethics, style and an ability to communicate. That's the problem with drug reform—all argument, no aesthetics."

"So, what are you working on now?"

"I'm working with some people in Texas. We're trying to make medical marijuana available to people with AIDS . . ."

It became a long, elliptical conversation. Rich asked unusual questions. I responded with unusual answers. "Would you like me to support ACT or you?" Rich asked.

"ACT is an illusion," I replied. "I'm very real."

"In your proposal—I guess that was a proposal—you mention $100,000?"

"Yes. But I've decided it will take more," an honest, too-candid response.

"How much more?"

"$150,000 total."

"Would you like that in a lump sum or installments?"

I made my way downstairs and found Alice in the kitchen. "So, how'd it go?" she asked with casual interest.

"Swell," I replied in a daze, "just swell."

In the span of a phone call, football blaring in the background, we found a patron and gained economic freedom.

There was some additional back and forth with Rich's aides. Formalities. After that Rich's checks arrived in quarterly allotments, the first appearing in the mail on my 42nd birthday. "That's more than I make in a year," Alice said, staring at the numbers. "And we get three more just like it this year," I happily noted.

With angels on our shoulders we faced a new beginning for medical marijuana. Fate was arming us for the struggle ahead.

• • •

On December 13, a week after Rich's fateful phone call, the FDA approved Steve L.'s Compassionate IND request for medical marijuana. Steve's goal was to let others know about marijuana's medical use so I lost little time in preparing a press release. Wire services around the world carried the news: "FDA approves marijuana in AIDS care." Rich saw the story in the *L.A. Times* and told Kevin, "That's what I call a fast return on an investment."

In our rambling calls throughout that autumn, Steve had often told me he wanted to inform the world about marijuana's usefulness to people battling AIDS. Fax machines had arrived on the scene and we embraced this new technology to spread the word about Steve. I pushed the buttons and Steve's story circled the globe. Several weeks later I obtained a copy of the UPI story from a Tokyo newspaper and forwarded it to Steve with a note, "You wanted everyone to know, Steve. Now, even the Japanese know marijuana can help people with AIDS."

The FDA's approval of Steve's IND, under anxious prompting from myself, Papa Bear, and Steve's doctor, was unexpectedly fast; less than six weeks. But when would Steve L. actually receive his promised supplies of legal pot? We had seen how long this could take. The decade-old memory of Lynn Pierson was still fresh in our minds.

Christmas came and went. Our great good fortune—the promised funding from Richard Dennis—was celebrated with close friends but like anxious poker players we held the good news close to our chests. I issued no press release nor did I announce my new benefactor's generous support in any way. "I'd like to keep this discreet," I told Rich. It was a very uncharacteristic approach. Rich thought the desire for discretion a bit curious, but readily accepted the decision without complaint.

Steve L. had a far less happy Christmas. Even though his IND was approved the DEA was delaying the first shipment of medical marijuana. It was not unusual for the DEA to drag its feet in approving shipments but this particular delay seemed especially cruel and premeditated.

These delays made no sense until Friday, December 29, 1989. On the last business day of the decade, with reporters rushing home for New Year's Eve weekend, DEA Administrator John Lawn formally rejected Judge Francis Young's recommendation that marijuana be rescheduled for medical use. In Administrator Lawn's skewed view marijuana had no accepted medical use in the United States.

A group of glorified gumshoes rejected the testimony of ACT's witnesses as "pro-drug." Ignoring the factual record DEA argued that ending the medical prohibition would unleash sin upon the land and, of course, "send the wrong message." It was a deeply stupid statement. ACT and NORML would appeal.

But the timing of the release made it easy to understand why Steve had not received his promised supplies of marijuana. How very awkward it was for our zealous federal bureaucrats. Two weeks before the DEA planned to assert the fiction that marijuana has no medical use, the FDA moved to expand marijuana's medical use to include AIDS. Clearly, communication between federal agencies had broken down.

Officials at the DEA knew such hypocrisy would not go unnoticed by the press. So they simply ignored the approved IND until after the Administrator's decision was released. To hell with Steve. A national policy was at stake. The AIDS patient would have to wait.

Steve L. was a pawn, caught in the dreadful cross fire of the war on drugs.

For several weeks, as Steve's condition worsened, I tried to find a remedy. Instead, I got the red tape run around. DEA Washington blamed DEA San Antonio. DEA San Antonio blamed the Audie L. Murphy V.A. pharmacy. Steve, the subject of all this finger pointing, remained moot.

From the beginning of our association Steve had insisted on remaining anonymous. Ashamed of his illness, Steve was adamant about staying out of the public spotlight. I respected this and in press releases designed to build public pressure on the DEA I referred to him only as a "Texas AIDS patient named Steve."

"If you don't become real I'm not sure I can help you," I warned. This was not a minor matter. It was time for Steve to escape his sense of stigma or shut up.

"I told you I don't want no one to know about my AIDS," Steve and his stigma said.

"Look. We're headed for criminal court. That's public. Everyone will know who you are and what disease you have. But without your help right now I won't be able to force the DEA into action."

"Alright. What should I do?" Steve said, the will to complete his mission finally overtaking his fear of exposure.

As soon as Steve relented, I arranged for a San Antonio television station to carry the story. It was the second week in January. Steve, still in the hospital, appeared in the report wearing a surgical smock and mask—still anxious to conceal his identity. I was interviewed by an affiliate station in Washington, smoking my legal joints, demanding to know why the DEA was depriving Steve of FDA-approved access to similar care.

The separate video clips were merged into a single report. At the conclusion the reporter explained that the DEA had, that very day, decided to comply with Steve's request. Problem solved? Hardly. Having deflected a minor media hit, the DEA returned to delaying tactics and refused to release Steve's shipments. It was New Mexico all over again. Apply a little public pressure and the agencies would say what the public wanted to hear. Once the video lights turned off the feds returned to the trenches.

And, like New Mexico, the federal bureaucrats were hoping Steve would die before they were compelled to make good on their promise of legal access to marijuana. The stakes were just as high. Lynn Pierson spoke to thousands of cancer patients and unleashed a tremendous demand for medical marijuana. Steve L. could do the same for AIDS. Why set a precedent?

Flush with cash thanks to our new patron, I flew to San Antonio the next week, walked into the Audie L. Murphy Memorial Veterans Hospital and asked to see the director. Working my way through the hierarchy I tried to ascertain if there were any remaining problems that could prevent DEA from releasing supplies. A gaggle of doctors swore the V.A. was not to blame. I met the hospital pharmacist who told me, "We're ready to go; just waiting for supplies."

After these brief encounters, I finally met Steve. Gaunt and tired-looking, Steve had the look of a man near death. On his arm were medication patches. His hair was thin and wispy. Only 34 years old, he had the slow mannerisms of an elderly man.

"I'm sure glad you came. I get no straight answers. Do you think I'll ever get my pot?"

"Yes," I said without promise. "I think so."

The next day I increased the media pressure, working the phone and speaking to several local reporters who then called the DEA. Struggling to not look purely evil, the DEA relented, assuring reporters that Steve would receive his first shipment of marijuana the following day. The news blanketed Texas and moved out into America.

The following day Steve L. smoked his first legal joint. The logjam had finally been broken. The phone rang in my hotel room and the soft twang of Steve's voice immediately conveyed the good news. "Guess what I'm doing, Robert?" he asked from his hospital bed. "I'm smoking a fat, juicy joint, and eating lunch." The joy was unmistakable as was the renewed resolve. "So, when can we talk to more reporters?" he asked.

The next morning Steve L., released from Audie Murphy, arrived at the AIDS foundation as reporters from San Antonio and Dallas were setting up their equipment. "Don't worry," I told Steve. "You've won. Now it's time to get the news out."

Steve L. was a touch scruffy; thin moustache, old baseball cap, heavy flannel shirt, dark sunglasses: just another Texas good ole boy. Now "legal" Steve's fear of exposure quickly faded as we sat under quartz lights, answering questions. "I think we should smoke a joint," Steve suggested. Matches flared: Cameras rolled.

"Half the state of Texas is drooling right about now," Steve told me through a haze of smoke.

"And the other half wants to arrest us."

An odd pairing. The nearly blind Washington man in a blue wool suit and a thin, scruffy Texas redneck dying from AIDS. Steve got his legal pot, made news. But, after so much excitement, he was anxious to retreat deep into his piney woods, get home and see C.B. "I'm making my coffin," Steve explained without sadness. "But I'll be here if you need me."

In his battered pick-up truck Steve drove me to the airport and we said our good-byes. "Thanks for everything, Mr. Randall," he said, giving me an unexpected hug. Beneath his thick work shirt, Steve was bone thin.

A few days after smoking his first legal joint Steve was back in the hospital. Doctors said his spleen was failing. No one knew why. When I phoned the hospital a kindly woman answered.

"Are you the nice man who came to Texas to help my baby?" Ollie, Steve's mother, asked. "Steve's asleep right now."

"How is he?"

"It's bad, real bad. Mind, they don't tell me much. But a mother knows. He's in a lot of pain."

"Your son is a remarkable man."

"Thanks. Maybe I shouldn't say this. But AIDS gave me back my baby," Ollie confessed. "Before Steve got AIDS he was just plain mean. Don't know why. Always was. But then, after he near died, he came back so kind. I just wish my baby had longer to live."

I phoned often. Ollie always answered. Together we shared Steve's rocky decline. "When he's awake we write his will," Ollie said. "His pain's worse."

On a few occasions Steve and I spoke briefly and in these micro-conversations I heard Steve's crushing pain. His spleen was threatening to rupture.

"Don't they give him morphine?" I asked Ollie.

"No," Ollie said with exhaustion. "The V.A. doctors say he might get addicted." I phoned the hospital director and soon Steve was given a morphine drip. "Is he better now?" I later asked.

"Ever so better," Ollie said with relief.

On February 12, 1990, Steve L. died. He was buried several days later at a military cemetery in a pauper's pressboard coffin. His mother was not told of Steve's handmade oak coffin hidden deep in the piney woods.

Steve's death came less than a month after he received his legal marijuana and was oddly devastating. Steve L. had enticed and guided me into a new universe, then abandoned me to fate. I was richer, true, but I wasn't certain I was any wiser. Steve had been so certain that he was returned from death's door to find me. There was a burden that had been conveyed.

I sought refuge in travel, attending a silly psychedelics conference in Oakland where cartoon activists and no-account joyloaders pretended to be relevant. Their "concerns"—legal LSD and a drug called Ecstasy—seemed ridiculously petty.

I crossed the Bay to San Francisco and spent time with our dear friend Bobby Evans, who, despite his AIDS, still looked healthy and fit. Bobby helped me accept Steve's abrupt departure. "Why be sad? You helped him achieve what he needed to achieve. Put your hurt to work." Sage advice from a dying friend.

I returned to Washington, still reeling. Out of the blue an editor at *High Times* Magazine called. "We got this press release about the

Texas AIDS patient," the editor explained. "We were thinking maybe you'd like to write his obit?"

"I think I'd like that very much."

It was mid-February and *High Times* wanted to include the obit in their next issue, scheduled to hit the stands in mid-March. I'd have to write fast.

Steve proved a person with AIDS could get legal pot from the government. A new, publicly acknowledged use of the drug was born. But all was not rosy. At least one person we had worked with for years expressed alarm. "Why do we have to be associated with the kind of people who get AIDS?"

An insensitive, but honest question. I considered what AIDS might mean to medical marijuana—a meditation on medicine and medical care.

Glaucoma is a disease of the self. Painless, invisible to others, glaucoma was a very private, almost unshareable thing. There were no glaucoma support groups. A glaucoma patient in a doctor's waiting room was not surrounded by other glaucoma patients, but by people who needed an eye exam or new contact lenses or cataract surgery.

Cancer, by contrast, seems a disease of the family. Cancer patients communally receive chemotherapy. They and their close relations attend support groups, speak among themselves, share the sorrow and sickness of a malignant disease.

AIDS was altogether different. Unlike cancer patients often diagnosed at death's door, HIV-infected people, like my good friend Bobby, could live normal, active lives for months, even years. But, unlike cancer, AIDS in America began as a disease within a community—gay, white, middle-class men. While the rate of AIDS infection for gay males was waning, the gay community—talented, comparatively wealthy, educated—was an emerging cultural force. Articulate. Increasingly aggressive. Demanding. It did not take a prophet to know the gay AIDS community would rapidly rally to medical marijuana. The resulting release of energy would be far more intense than anything generated by lone glaucoma patients or scattered, near-death cancer patients.

As I wrote Steve's obit and ruminated on these ideas I began to realize the potential energy of this emerging therapeutic use. There would need to be new torch carriers to complete the job Steve had begun. Were those angels still on our shoulders or had they fled with Steve's spirit?

29 Two American Kids

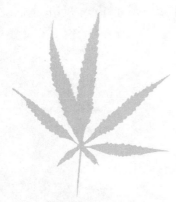

April 2, 1990
My Office
Washington, D.C.

"Hello? This is Kenny. Kenny Jenks. Hello? Is this . . . Is anyone? Hey, Hop, it's a answer machine."

"So? Tell 'em why we're calling."

I listened with some amusement. These two were young, very young. Probably just another request for information.

"Oh. Yeah . . . Hello," the voice continued. "This is Kenny Jenks. Me and my wife—Barb and me—we just been arrested—eh, 2 plants—that's all. We just got out of jail 'n . . ."

"Tell 'em about Steve, Kenny. Tell 'em about Steve . . ." It was a woman's voice in the background.

"Oh, yeah. We got this *High Times* and there's this story—about Steve. Steve L. It says here you helped Steve. Well, Barb 'n me, we're like Steve. Ah . . . we got what Steve has—had. My wife and me, we . . . Barb and me we . . . we're just like Steve. . . ."

"Can he help us Kenny? Can he . . . ?"

"Shush, Hop. I done told you it's just a mach . . ." click.

• • •

You never know where fate will take you. Steve wanted to send a message. So we helped Steve send his message. Message sent: Steve died. In that first call from Kenny and Barbra there was the fading echo of a dead man's desire to be heard.

Here we have a story which smiles at its own sadness. This is not long ago, far away fiction; no once-upon-a-never-was. Fate has summoned us here to tell a tale of how cruel circumstance can conspire to open a door to Life's better side.

Young, in love, so very alive, so utterly alone, Kenny and Barbra Jenks were dying of AIDS. Blood crimes had mortally wounded a man and his mate; disease condemned them to terrible afflictions and death. Into this sea of sorrow a pitiless state was now seeking to convict this dying young couple for the crime of growing medicinal weeds.

Kenny and Barbra were people of little consequence. A K-Mart couple wearing hand-me-down clothes, easily overlooked. Exceedingly ordinary people about to engage in an extraordinary experience. Fate sent me to guide them and, before we were done everything would change—everything but the outcome.

May 7, 1990
Regional Airport
Pensacola, Florida

Dazed by sunlight, disoriented in the crowded terminal, I felt lost. I was entering an America I did not know. "Mr. Randall? You Mr. Randall, sir?"

"You're Kenny?"

"Yes sir," said the tanned young man wearing dark glasses, a pink baseball cap and dirty white T-shirt. "And this here's my wife, Barb," he said, squeezing her small shoulders. "I call her Hop."

"It's Barbra," Kenny's short wife said. "Barbra. Like in Streisand."

I followed the young couple into an illegally parked gold-flecked Pontiac. As Kenny popped the clutch I was thrown back into the seat. There was a slight squeal that left a little rubber and a small puff of blue smoke in front of the terminal. "Good pickup, huh?" Kenny shouted as he drove the aging car into a blazing Florida day.

"How's about some music, Hop?" Before I could protest the radio was blaring.

It was a long, hot ride from Pensacola to Panama City Beach. Kenny—I would quickly learn—abhorred silence. A motormouth, he talked incessantly, repeating cliches of the day. Barbra occasionally interrupted his gab to point out a cool Chevy passing on the far side of Interstate 10.

"Local folks call this the Redneck Riviera," Kenny said proudly while pointing out the sites. Panama City Beach is a very bubba-on-the-beach place. A cluttered collection of cheap motels and kiddy attractions, goofy golf courses, high-rise condos and a few good hotels.

Since Kenny's first disjointed call in early April I had, with Kevin's help, found a local attorney, John Daniel, to represent the young couple *pro bono*. Working with an AIDS group in Pensacola, I had located a doctor willing to explore marijuana as an AIDS treatment. Having gained these commitments, I flew to Florida to meet the principal players and prepare for the upcoming criminal trial.

The morning after my arrival Kenny and Barbra were scheduled to meet their new attorney. I was surprised to find the young couple still wearing the same clothes from the day before. I was struck by how vulnerable they seemed. "Nervous?"

"Yes, sir, Mr. Randall. A little." Kenny admitted. "We ain't never seen no lawyer before."

"No need," Barbra interjects in anxious protest. "No need."

John Daniel's office overlooked a small river and possessed a pleasant feeling that matched its occupant. Daniel was around 50. Tall and wiry, with glasses, a ruddy face, thinning hair, red-gray moustache, toothy smile and down home charm. A small town criminal lawyer, he was well-respected in the Florida legal community. John had taken this difficult case out of love for the law. "You gotta believe in justice," he says. "What's happening to these young just ain't right."

Initially shy, Kenny soon realized he was expected to speak and chattered out his story. Barbra was mostly silent—letting the men talk. Occasionally she would interrupt Kenny's rambling to condense his paragraphs of misdirected words into a surprisingly sharp, stunningly simple sentence. It was an unexpected talent.

After a while Kenny and Barbra were asked to wait in the reception area while Daniel and I conferred. "I cannot believe the D.A. will prosecute these kids," Daniel exclaimed. "They're dying. My God! Who cares if they smoke a little pot? If this case goes to trial I'll do my best to defend these poor, young children."

"If there is a trial," I asked, "how will Panama City react to a young couple with AIDS who smoke marijuana?"

"Not sure," Daniel said. "Depends how they're told. There are a lot of fine, caring people in this community. But this is North Florida. There are some real bigots. How will people react? We'll only know that when we get to court."

The three of us left the lawyer's office, looking for lunch. At a greasy spoon down on the docks I watched Kenny and Barbra wolf down burgers and fries—"I love fries," Barbra smiled—and considered the young people before me.

Barbra, 23, was transiting between eighteen and infinity. Once plump, she had a large, English face framed by raven black hair. She was born in Enid, Oklahoma into an abusive family where loutish parents raised criminal sons and paid no mind to "the girl." Her smile was generous, her laugh warm. But Barbra was deeply suspicious of a world that had seldom been kind. She occasionally flared with anger.

Kenny was five years older, but hardly more mature. Tall, thin, with angular features, bony arms and knobby knees. His sharp tan face was shielded by badly scratched photosensitive lenses. A baseball cap covered brown, close-cropped hair. He was often loud, always opinionated. A military brat, the kid of a low-ranking NCO, he grew up in pain and modest poverty. He read the local paper every day, but had nearly no connection to what he read.

As they ate their lunch I learned the story of their "courtship." They met in Tucson when Barbra was 15. "Love at first sight," she sighed. "Kenny'd sneak over 'n spend the night. 'Til we near got caught," Barbra relished relating the tale of her seduction.

"One night I told Barb's parent we was going to eat at the Red Lobster," Kenny continued the story. "But we didn't go to no Red Lobster. Not in Tucson anyway. I just kept driving 'til we got all the way to here."

They reminded me of the Dorothea Lange photographs of the Great Depression—stark, compelling and very real. They had only the most basic education. Kenny does not know where New York is. Barbra does not care. Most Americans would simply dismiss Kenny and Barbra as poor white trash. Kenny would bristle at such a suggestion. He and Barbra held a mortgage, paid their bills. But they have never not been poor. They have few skills, but work very hard. As a song lyric once said, "They were two American kids doing the best they can."

After lunch that day we went to Kenny and Barbra's home—a small trailer set on a wooded lot—and I began to collect the facts about Kenny and Barbra's life. I started with Kenny.

Kenny was a hemophiliac—a bleeder. At 30, he was an old hemophiliac: a product of miracle medicine and wonder science. Paradoxically he was both surviving and dying because of Factor VIII—an infused clotting factor refined from the blood of thousands of donors. Kenny got AIDS from HIV-tainted blood products.

"Them blood companies and Hemophilia people just plain decided to kill us," Kenny said with bitterness. "They didn't give a damn about people, just profits."

A harsh indictment: mass murder for money. But, of course, true. The philanthropic fellows at the Hemophilia Foundation, a creature of the companies that trade in blood, made the fiendish decision to sell HIV-infected blood to hemophiliacs. The FDA did nothing. Nor was this a uniquely American decision. The same logic dominated blood boardrooms in Paris, Tokyo and elsewhere. Now those craven decisions made by powerful men were killing Kenny. He was not alone. Nearly every hemophiliac in the industrial world was dying.

"Them men decided to kill me," Kenny repeats. "And kill my wife, too."

Kenny got AIDS from a tainted Factor VIII injection. Barbra was infected by love. Alone and together they were doomed beings pursuing inevitable outcomes.

Hemophilia is a lifelong affliction. Kenny had been in and out of hospitals all his life. He bled nearly every week. A major bleed could send him to the hospital for weeks, even months. If the hemorrhage was severe, blood collected under his skin. The resulting pressure on joints and nerves could cause temporary or even permanent paralysis. Like most hemophiliacs, Kenny walked with a slight limp.

"Things got a lot better when Factor VIII came along," Kenny would tell me. "It's real expensive; $800 an injection. But it's better than weeks in the hospital or being a cripple."

When Kenny first asked his doctors about AIDS in the mid-1980s they laughed at his concerns. "One chance in a million," they assured him. "One in a million," Kenny scoffed. "Hell, Mr. Randall, every hemophiliac I know has AIDS."

It was Barbra who became sick first. Unable to breathe, hospitalized, and tested, she lapsed into a coma just before Christmas, 1988. While watching Barbra struggle for life, Kenny learned they both had AIDS. "Like getting a death sentence."

After Barbra's hospitalization she was too weak to work. But Kenny, despite his diagnosis, continued to work 8-hour days. "It was the only way we could make ends meet."

Barbra and Kenny began intensive AIDS treatments: massive doses of highly toxic AZT to slow the virus and megadoses of antibiotics to stop infections. "Just look at all them drugs," Kenny would say, pointing to nearly 50 brown bottles containing dozens of potions and hundreds of pills.

"It's kinda hard just remembering what to take when," Barbra interjected.

"Them pills, they was killing Barb," Kenny noted. "We was taking all these drugs and we just couldn't eat. Barb couldn't stand the smell of food. She really started losing weight, nearly 50 lbs. Ain't that right, Hop?"

"At least 50," Barbra affirmed, dryly.

"She was wasting away. Dying in front of me. Then we started going to this AIDS group at County Health." One young man in the group approached Kenny after a meeting. "Your wife," he said, "needs to gain some weight. Why don't you smoke some pot?" The young man handed Kenny two joints.

Barbra—a Reagan baby—Just Said No. She had never smoked marijuana and was terrified to try, unwilling to break the law. Kenny, slightly older, was less reluctant. When they got home, and over Barbra's stern objections, he took a couple of hits.

"It was amazing, Mr. Randall. Amazing. First, my nausea just vanished. And I got real talkative. Me and Barb, we had kinda stopped talking. But that night I told Hop how sorry I was she got infected cause of me."

"That was real nice," Barbra added. "AIDS was pushing us apart.

We couldn't even say the word, AIDS. But talking brought us back together."

"And then I got hungry. Real hungry." Kenny continued. "I started going through the kitchen, eating anything I could find. Amazing."

"I hadn't seen him eat nothing for 6 weeks. But he just ate the rest of that night. Eating and talking."

The next evening Barbra asked Kenny if she could smoke some marijuana with him. Together, they smoked half a joint, talked some more, fell into a laughing fit, then sat down to eat together for the first time since Barbra had gone to the hospital three months before.

"It was like we was husband and wife again," Kenny said. "And Barb, she really started gaining weight." When the couple discovered marijuana Barbra weighed 102 lbs. With marijuana's help she regained over 25 lbs.

Over the next year Kenny and Barbra hid their AIDS, smoked pot and stayed out of the hospital. Kenny went to work. Barbra stayed home and fixed dinner. Their only problem was finding and affording enough marijuana. "My wife would die without pot," Kenny said with certainty. "That's why we decided to grow some."

They grew two small marijuana plants in their bedroom. Then, an informant turned them in. On March 29, 1990, they were sitting down to dinner when nearly a dozen heavily armed policemen stormed their small trailer in the piney woods. They were taken away in cuffs and chains, charged with felony cultivation.

May 9, 1990
Holiday Inn
Panama City Beach, Florida

Kenny and Barbra arrived at my hotel shortly after noon for more discussion about their lives and the circumstances leading up to their arrest.

Barbra was not certain she had anything to add to what Kenny had said. Nor was she accustomed to being asked her views. While Kenny lounged on the bed, Barbra haltingly began to tell her story.

She began to get ill in July 1988, just before her 21st birthday, when she developed a massive yeast infection.

"My tongue got all white. I brushed 'n brushed, but it wouldn't go away. It got so bad I went 'n seen the doctor. He gave me some pills and told me to get tested." She paused. "But I didn't."

Kenny interrupted to explain. "It's like we told you yesterday, Robert. We was scared. There was these stories on TV. People find you got AIDS they go crazy; run you outta town, set fire to your home."

Barbra nodded her agreement and continued her story.

"The yeast cleared up . . . sorta. Then I got a bad cold that wouldn't go away. By Thanksgiving I was real tired. Then one day I couldn't barely breathe. So I went to the doctor and told 'em it was an emergency. But them nurses made me wait 'n wait. So I come home. I was gonna go back, but I barely made it inside the trailer before I passed out."

"Flat out," Kenny energetically picked up the story. "I come home 'n Barb's on the floor. Burning up, Robert. Just on fire! So I took her to the hospital." He paused and became more subdued. Looking at his wife he continued, "By the time I got Hop to the hospital she was hardly breathing. So the docs put her on oxygen 'n IVs 'n all. But we was too late. Barb went into this coma . . ."

I immediately thought of Steve's pneumonia-induced coma. "You remember any of this?" I asked the suddenly quiet woman.

"Naw, I was good as gone." It was almost a whisper.

"Yeah, Robert. Hop stayed in that coma three weeks. The docs told me she was done for. Wouldn't make it."

"Did you have a near death experience?"

Barbra, visibly jolted by my question, was slow and awkward in reply. "Maybe . . . yeah."

We had come upon a deep and secret memory. Kenny, with a trace of hurt, said, "Hey, Hop. You never told me."

"Course not, silly. Cause I didn't want you thinking I'd gone nuts or something."

Barbra was reticent but I sensed she wanted, very much wanted, to tell us about her experience. I gently probed. "Would you like to talk about it? What did you see?"

"A light." The response was without hesitation. "A bright, white light." She was bolder now, remembering something she could not forget. Kenny, uneasy, hummed the "Twilight Zone" theme. "Quit that, Kenny." Her tone was abrupt and she slapped him hard on the leg. To Barbra this was very serious stuff.

"Did you know you were dying?" I prompted, trying to regain the moment.

"Oh yea! I was a gonner." Barbra gratefully returned to the dialogue. "But it didn't upset me none. The light was so nice, really beautiful. I was in this dark place and I was moving, floating, to this wonderful light. I was trying to get to that light, floating closer 'n closer."

"Did you know if you went into the light you would die?"

"Uh huh. But that didn't matter none. It was so peaceful 'n all. I'd have been happy to die."

"So, why didn't you go?"

She hesitated, unsure again, but continued on, "You'll think I'm crazy. . . . Well, I was being surrounded, swallowed up like by this light, getting sucked right into it . . . but I suddenly wondered who was gonna fix Kenny's dinner. As soon as I thought about Kenny things changed. The light got further away so's I couldn't reach it no more. And then it just disappeared 'n everything got dark 'n suddenly I was in all this pain. That's when I woke up 'n come out of my coma."

"So it wasn't your time?"

"Yeah. Cause Kenny needed me 'n . . ." she paused. "Oh, I dunno, Robert. It's like I wasn't done; like there's something I still need to do—gotta do—before I can go."

"That's what Steve said," I remembered.

"That man in the magazine story?" she asked.

"Uh huh."

"So, why didn't Steve go, Robert?" It was more of a demand than a question. Barbra was beginning to sense something.

"Same reason. Steve says—said—he came to a river, but couldn't go across because he still had things to do."

"Yeah! We're all here to do something. We're supposed to help each other. That's what I think." Barbra was beginning to see a different light. "You liked Steve, didn't you Robert?"

"Yes I did. Steve wanted to help people; people like you and Kenny. He thought people with AIDS should know marijuana helps. So I helped Steve do that. He was the first person with AIDS to speak out. That took guts."

Kenny had been listening intently and begun to realize where the conversation was heading. "That was so strange, Robert. After Barb 'n me got out of jail, that same morning, I got this magazine 'n opened it up and there's this whole big story all about Steve 'n AIDS 'n marijuana. It was like I was reading about Barb 'n me."

"You write that story, Robert?" Barbra wanted answers.

"Yes, I wrote that . . ."

"So me 'n Kenny, we found you because of Steve. That's what I think. That story you wrote 'n all. It's like Steve was reaching to us. Like a message in a bottle. You know, Robert?"

"Yes, Barbra. I know."

I had known since the previous day when I entered the pine filled lot that held their trailer, saw the pound pups lazing under a rusting pick-up truck on blocks in the front yard. Kenny and Barbra Jenks were people Steve L. would have known and liked. Simple folk.

"Spooky, huh?" Barbra suddenly shivered with a chill.

"Yeah. Spooky," Kenny admitted. Once again he hummed the "Twilight Zone" theme.

"Quit that, Kenny," Barbra reached across the bed to give Kenny a slap but this time it was more playful and relaxed.

For the rest of the afternoon we would talk about Steve, AIDS, and marijuana. Barbra's recollections of her near-death experience had led us to an unexpected understanding of our purpose together. After a room-service dinner Barbra decided it was her turn to find out about me.

"So, can me 'n Kenny ask you questions, Robert?"

"Sure. Only seems fair. What do you want to know?"

"You get pot from the government, right? Legal pot?" Kenny wanted to know how that worked.

I patiently explained about my glaucoma and the long road that led to my legal access.

"So was you the first American to get medical marijuana?"

"Uh huh. Nearly fifteen years ago." As I spoke I realized Barbra was only six when I smoked my first legal joint.

"Are you famous, Robert?" Barbra's question was so unawaredly paradoxical I began to laugh.

"Some people probably think I'm famous. But I'm not famous. Being famous takes too much work."

Kenny, wondering about his future, asked "How many people get legal marijuana, Robert?"

"Five."

"Five people! In the whole United States?" Kenny wasn't sure those were good odds.

"And Steve," Barbra was trying to keep things straight, "he was the first AIDS patient to get legal marijuana?" I nodded. "So, me 'n Kenny, we'd be the second and third people with AIDS to get legal marijuana?" The words trailed off. Barbra was putting the pieces together.

"So you just fly around 'n help people?" Kenny was trying to figure out who I was and what I did. Before I could answer Barbra spoke up again. "So, Robert, you think me 'n Kenny can really get legal pot?"

"Uh huh. I think we can do that. It won't be easy. There are no guarantees."

"But do we have to go to court?" Kenny feared exposure.

"Yes. Unless you admit you're guilty and hope the judge gives you a reduced sentence. In your case—first arrest—they'd give you probation and send you home." The easy way out.

Kenny, looking for an easy out, says, "So then we wouldn't have to tell nobody we got AIDS?" I nodded.

"But we'd be guilty? Me 'n Kenny we'd have criminal records 'n stuff?" Barbra was wary of easy outs.

"Yes. You'd have a criminal record," I replied.

"So we'd be criminals," Barbra concluded, "and them policemen, they could come arrest us again?" She was coming to grips with her jeopardy.

"If you're out on probation and keep smoking pot the police can arrest you anytime they want."

Barbra had heard enough. "No way! I ain't no criminal. I ain't gonna let anyone make me no criminal. I ain't gonna die with no criminal record."

"Then, you've got to go to court and convince the judge you're innocent. We will argue there's no crime in growing marijuana to save your life." I outlined the defense.

"So, would this all be in the newspapers 'n stuff?"

"If we do it right your story will be in every newspaper in America. TV, too." I paused and considered the two silent individuals before me. "Scared?" I asked.

"Yeah. It's real scary," Kenny said. Barbra amended his fear, "Kinda. Sorta."

"Good," I advised. "It's good to be scared. Life's scary."

"What if crazy people, nuts 'n stuff start calling us on the phone?"

Kenny remained unconvinced. Barbra, bored with being frightened, had a different question, "Robert, you think me 'n Kenny going to court 'n all would help other people? Other people with AIDS?"

"Barbra, I'm here because you and Kenny got Steve's message. Now, you and Kenny need to decide if you want to send that message to others. Win or lose in court, if you speak out other people with AIDS will learn marijuana can help."

"But we could lose?" Barbra wanted assurances. I declined her hope. "You could lose, go to jail, die in prison. I don't think that will happen. But there are no guarantees."

It was a dialogue of destiny. Fear was the barrier. I knew things I could not say. I had been summoned to assist, not to play a tempting serpent. I could provide insight, allies, instruction. But alone together Kenny and Barbra had to elect the path. If they clung to fear there was little that could be done. The state would condemn them as criminals; their fast-ebbing lives would be consumed in isolation and despair, grim beyond bearing.

Arrest, paradoxically, had opened an alternative path. If Kenny and Barbra ignored their fears to accept the path fate now offered they would enter a universe beyond their imaginings. I knew these things but dared not speak them. After all, there were no guarantees. And the decision was not mine to make.

It was Barbra who made the decision. "I ain't no criminal 'n I ain't gonna die with no criminal record."

Fate smiled.

30 Hearts and Minds

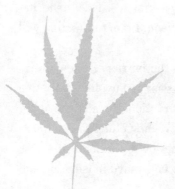

WE WERE ENTERING a vortex of events which would irrevocably alter the dialogue. It was the night before the trial. For Kenny and Barbra these were the last isolated moments of their lives. And the most terrifying.

I arrived in Panama City two days earlier to meet a CNN crew. None of the broadcast networks or wire services were alerted. I approached CNN with an exclusive. It was a calculated decision. Network news had degenerated into "info-tainment." Kenny and Barbra were not "info-tainment." What Kenny and Barbra were about to say had global implications and CNN had global reach.

The day before trial had been spent with the CNN crew in Kenny and Barbra's front yard. Sitting shaded among the pines they prepared for their first interview. Kenny maniacally chatted with the crew while I huddled with Jeff Levine, the CNN medical reporter handling the story. Barbra was silent; dazzled by the men, mikes, tripods, lights and muttered instructions. Levine conducted the interview with great skill and, after some early fidgets, Kenny and Barbra settled into easy conversation.

Earlier in the day CNN had dropped in on the arresting vice

cops—a blond Don Johnson clone and his rugged partner—then visited the prosecutor. With CNN's arrival alarm bells began to ring in the Bay County Courthouse. What was up?

As Kenny and Barbra began their interview with CNN, Alice, in Washington, began faxing a news release to major and local media outlets. In Panama City reporters received the notice early enough to allow a mention on the evening news and in the morning paper but too late to do more than confirm essential facts. Just enough to ensure their presence at the trial. A little after six o'clock the phone in my hotel room rang. It was Kenny, breathless with excitement and sounding a little scared. "We was on the TV news!"

Two Panama City stations had run with "Local AIDS Couple Says Marijuana a Medicine." One station even flashed mug shots of the allegedly criminal couple.

The hermetic news seals were beginning to rupture. Right on schedule.

July 26, 1990
Bay County Courthouse
Panama City Beach, Florida

The Bay County courthouse sits in the center of a sea of hardy grasses: virtually treeless, it shimmers in the July heat. The case of *Florida v. Jenks* was to be argued in the second floor courtroom. Judge Clinton Foster, a grandfatherly fellow who looked as if he lost an election for sheriff, presided. There was no jury.

The courtroom was white: without adornment or grandeur. Usually, marijuana cases are quickly, quietly dispatched absent public notice. Attorneys wheel and deal: clients pay a fine, go to jail or get paroled. Panama City is a law and order town. Unless there is violence—a murder, say—the local press is blasé about pot cases down at the courthouse.

Today was different. An historic case had come to town. By design, Florida had TV-friendly courtrooms. CNN and the local stations were already set up: their harsh quartz lights further flattening an already stark scene. Kenny and Barbra, wearing second-hand clothes, were captured on video as they entered the arena of their fears. Poor, dying, they evoked sympathy and compassion in the brittle light.

I considered wardrobe and suppressed the impulse to buy an alternate image for them; Kenny and Barbra *are* poor and, deep down, I believed the world should see how America treats her children.

The prosecutor, having been confronted with CNN the day before, had fled town, leaving execution of the law to his assistant prosecutor. In the glare of watching lenses the barbarity of the state's assault was evident to all.

The state's case was basic. Police raided a trailer, seized two pot plants. A vice cop testified regarding the arrests. A chemist verified "Cannabis." Case closed. For me it was all too reminiscent of a Washington, D.C. courtroom fourteen years before.

John Daniel informed the Court he would argue Kenny and Barbra Jenks broke the law to save their lives; that any sane person would make the same decision. He would prove that marijuana's ability to enhance the appetite of people with AIDS created a "medical necessity."

The prosecutor objected, claiming there was no precedent. The Musikka case was mentioned and citations intoned for the record. Judge Foster, aware of the watching lenses, agreed to take testimony on "necessity" before ruling on the merits of such a novel defense. John Daniel called his first witness—me.

I provided background, explained my unusual status, and reviewed the FDA's approval of Steve L.'s marijuana/AIDS IND. I concluded by telling the court Kenny and Barbra's doctor had asked the FDA for legal permission to provide them with medical marijuana.

Kenny and Barbra's doctor was a no-show but he provided a written statement for the judge, stipulating that he had been unable to effectively treat their nausea with legal drugs and if he could legally prescribe marijuana he would.

Kenny, then Barbra entered the dock. These were gripping minutes of testimony as each explained their sad circumstances.

Kenny's testimony was reasoned and steady. "We were growing the plants because we couldn't get the marijuana we needed and if it was available we didn't have the money to buy it." No one doubted the young man's story. "I really didn't have a choice," he continued, "Anybody in my position would do anything they could to have a decent life. I fully believe without marijuana my quality of life will deteriorate and I will die. And my wife will die too. Your honor, my wife would not be alive without marijuana."

As I listened to Kenny testify I realized how quickly he had absorbed the concepts of medical necessity and the righteousness of his action. Despite his "motormouth," Kenny did listen.

Barbra's testimony, while similar, was more pointed and dramatic. "I don't feel I was doing any harm at all. I was doing it to survive, so that I could eat. I've got to smoke marijuana. I've got to or I'm gonna die. I'm gonna die anyway but I would like to have my life a little better."

It was an electric moment. Throughout the courtroom the simple words invoked a heartache of understanding. It was a sad madness that people so already wretched would be called to trial for growing weeds.

The final witness was Dr. Daniel Dansak, the former director of New Mexico's pioneering marijuana/cancer study. As Dansak approached the witness chair I couldn't help but think of Lynn Pierson. Dansak was Lynn's contribution to the case as ripples of his long ago acts washed across the years.

Now at the University of Alabama in Mobile, Dr. Dansak continued to work with terminal patients and was aware of marijuana's spreading use among people with AIDS. He was a superb witness;

engaging and friendly. Judge Foster, skeptical throughout, listened as the good doctor carefully outlined how marijuana helps people with AIDS survive.

Closing arguments were spirited. The state argued crime is crime. John Daniel argued it is not a crime to save your life. Staring into the quartz lights Judge Foster promised a decision "next week."

Jeff Levine's CNN package played and replayed on Headline News for nearly 18 hours. An excellent piece. While earth orbiting satellites beamed the news worldwide, the local impact was of more immediate concern. Kenny and Barbra's case was all over the local newspapers. Clips of their haunting testimony were featured on local news shows. In a day they had catapulted out of anonymity and into the hearts and minds of 40 million people.

The morning after the trial, Kenny and Barbra were walking out of a drugstore when an excited middle-aged woman stopped them. "Ain't you that nice young couple in the newspapers?" Reflexively they began to recoil as the woman rushed on, "I sure hope you win your case. I'll be praying for you."

Kenny's greatest fears were phantoms. The people of Panama City Beach did not assault them with pitchforks and torches. Three days after the trial, before the decision was rendered, the local *News Herald* editorially declared "Trial Unwarranted in Marijuana Case" and instructed the local citizenry on tolerance and the need for compassion. It was a thoughtful, but unnecessary sentiment. In the space of a few days Kenny and Barbra had become something I have always avoided: "recognized." Kind people approached them, wished them well, promised to mention them in their prayers.

So far so good.

• • •

The judge had promised a decision in a few days but it was more than two weeks before the good judge rendered his verdict. Alice and I were in Juneau, Alaska when CNN reported Judge Clinton Foster had found Kenny and Barbra Jenks "guilty." To temper his verdict the judge sentenced them to "500 hours of community service to be defined as loving and caring for one another."

A cream puff conviction that left them guilty of a crime but extracted no punishment. In the short CNN clip Kenny and Barbra appeared agitated. "I ain't no criminal," Barbra protested. John Daniel also appeared. "This isn't justice. We will appeal."

Later in the day CNN expanded the clip slightly, borrowing from footage shot two weeks before. Once again the story would replay for hours, assuring maximum, global coverage.

Morley Safer, correspondent for "60 Minutes," saw the story while on assignment in France. The story piqued his interest and he made a note to speak with the show's producers about it. Perhaps it would make a good segment.

We were stepping through the looking glass.

August 26, 1990
Newark, N.J.

Kenny and Barbra emerged from the crowd looking flush from their flight. "Welcome to Newark," I said leading them into a waiting limo. Barbra balked at the door. "Get in," I prodded.

"Is this your car, Robert?" Kenny was impressed.

"Sorry Kenny. This is the TV station's limo."

As Manhattan slid by on the far side of the Hudson Kenny marveled at the sights. "Them are tall buildings."

Barbra, uneasy with big, dared to glance at the passing skyline. "Is it always this busy, Robert?"

Delivered at the hotel we all spent a restful evening. The next day was important.

Early the next morning the limo delivered us to WWOR, located in a Jersey marsh. "9 in the Morning" is broadcast in New York and fed to scores of cable systems throughout the U.S. The producer took us into a cold, cavernous studio with bleacher seating for 400. The audience was filing in. The stage—little more than cheap flats, carpets and chairs—looked tiny.

In the Green Room Kenny and Barbra were taken away for makeup. "Never been through a thing like that," Kenny sputtered, brushing powder from his upper lip. Barbra appeared with lipstick and rouge. The producer came to collect them. "Ain't you coming, Robert?"

"No. The first segment is you and Kenny."

Watching in the Green Room, I was apprehensive as the stage manager counted away the seconds. The couple was dazzled by the lights, distracted by the commotion of camera crews, aware of the raucous studio audience in the dark beyond their sight. They were ON AIR: unedited, live.

The host introduced them and asked his first question. Kenny, after briefest hesitation, settled into conversation. Barbra, nervous answering direct questions, was shining as she interrupted Kenny to finish his thoughts. They were a likable, familiar couple. As the camera panned the crowd I watched women in the audience identify with Barbra. For many it was the first time they had seen a woman with AIDS. The effect was riveting.

A New Jersey trooper and I were introduced into the second segment. The trooper was "the balance," there to present the other side. He was law and order: lock 'em up. He quickly offended the studio audience which rushed to Kenny and Barbra's defense. "What," one angry audience member demanded of the trooper, "would you do if Barbra was your daughter and had AIDS and marijuana helped?"

Looking Barbra in the eyes the trooper honestly replied, "I'd probably go buy her some marijuana." Cheers. "But it's still against the law." Boos.

It was a rout. At the end of the show the studio audience was polled. For medical marijuana—sustained, standing applause. Against medical marijuana—four hands, from two people who arrived with the trooper, clapping into a vast silence.

"We do all right, Robert?" Barbra wonders.

"You heard the applause. We won," I replied. "Now, let's go see New York."

Through prior arrangement with the very pleased producer we piled into the WWOR limo and headed for Manhattan. Passing through the Lincoln Tunnel made Kenny queasy. "Gosh, I wish I'd smoked before we got going."

"Smoke now," I advised as the long black limo glided down 8th Avenue. "I don't think the driver will mind." The chauffeur chuckled.

The limo left us in Battery Park. We rode the ferry to Staten Island, ate lunch and returned to the Battery where we watched a violent thunderstorm from the safety of the Ferry Building. As the rain stopped we started walking towards Wall Street.

It was one of the sweetest days I can remember. Everything was new to them. The flight, the limo, the TV studio, the ferryboat, the huge buildings and crowded streets. "What's that smell?" Barbra asked as we descended into the subway. "New York," I replied.

After dinner and a hot fudge sundae, Kenny was anxious to discover more of New York. But Barbra was deeply fatigued. "I wanna go to the motel," she said.

In the incandescent glare of Times Square—Kenny and Barbra in tow—I approached three cops to ask directions. "Excuse me, officer? Could you tell me where . . ."

"It's you guys," the large cop in the middle shouted. I was thrown. Kenny looked as if he was about to bolt. "You three," the cop repeated, wagging his thick finger.

"I was just telling my buddies here about this couple with AIDS who was smoking marijuana. That was you guys, right?"

"Yeah," Kenny nodded with uncertain relief. "That was us. Sir."

"Well, let me shake your hand," the cop said extending his big paw. "You kids like New York?"

"Oh, it's excellent, sir. Excellent," Kenny gushed. Handshakes all round. I got directions. "Best of luck," the big cop said, retreating with his buddies into the Manhattan night.

"How'd he know us?" Kenny worried.

"Well, they may be following us," I teased, "or maybe he was just one of the four or five million people who saw you on television this morning."

"That many?" Barbra marveled. "Millions?"

Marvelous it was. The kind prayers of the people of Panama City, a firm handshake and "best of luck" from a New York City cop, and the lopsided embrace of a studio audience's applause fell like rain on dry earth.

Without effort offers of additional news coverage developed. In September I met Kenny and Barbra in Philadelphia and did more media, then traveled by train to Washington. The travel was new, the cities were new, the train was new. There was a constant acceleration in available energies.

Even as they were dying, Barbra and Kenny's universe expanded with each trip. In Washington they met Alice. She was, like nearly everyone who met them, stunned by how vulnerable they seemed. Contrarily, I sensed how rapidly they were maturing.

In October, Kenny and Barbra asked Florida Governor Bob Martinez for a pardon. It was my idea and could be easily executed with John Daniel's help. It was just before the election and I felt there was a chance of succeeding. But the Governor responded with silence. No matter. The gesture generated news throughout Florida where the

Jenks' story was fast becoming an unfolding drama. Martinez would lose the election. President Bush would appoint him Drug Czar.

The pardon story attracted "Florida Spotlight," a statewide TV magazine show. In November I returned to Panama City to guide Kenny and Barbra through the interview. The resulting network-quality piece was nearly 14 minutes long and immensely powerful. In one telling moment the camera captured the amazed look of Barbra's former doctor as she entered the room. He told the reporter, with evident wonder, "Every AIDS patient I was treating when Barbra got sick is now dead. Barbra looks marvelous." His obvious joy and astonishment spoke volumes.

We have won the battle for hearts and minds. Steve's message has been sent. I was pleased to be the messenger, happy to serve these two young people whose courage was inspiring to me just as it was to millions of others. But as 1990 was drawing to a close I began to see the greater role I had in this drama. I had helped Steve get his marijuana. I was helping Kenny and Barbra. But others also needed help. There were vast energies, already in play, that had to be coalesced into coherent action. That was my role.

Behind the escalating media screen much was happening that was hidden from public view. Calls to ACT were up dramatically, and many patients were willing to invest the time and effort needed to secure legal marijuana from the federal government. We were preparing dozens of requests for a variety of disorders—glaucoma, cancer, multiple sclerosis, and paralysis. But AIDS altered the dynamic. Alice was quick to recognize the danger. If ACT attempted to craft patient-specific Compassionate INDs for each new AIDS request we would be swamped; our energies sapped. It was a trap of paper that could easily bury us.

It was time to reconceptualize the Compassionate IND—that little known and seldom employed means of penetrating the medical prohibition. Since 1978, we had prepared about half a dozen marijuana INDs for individual patients.

Each IND contained volumes of personal medical data. If the FDA refused to respond the resulting document was designed to function as a basis for legal action. Constructing one of these iron-clad and cumbersome applications could take weeks. Draft INDs were then mailed to the sponsoring physician who had to absorb the information, fill out the final application forms and haggle with the FDA over inane details. In 1979, Anne Guttentag suffered need-lessly while the FDA insisted on miniscule changes to her IND request. In 1988, Elvy Musikka's physician, Dr. Paul Palmberg, estimated he spent more than 50 hours responding to often frivolous FDA demands. It was not unusual for doctors to withdraw from the process after initially agreeing to help. It was an intensely intimi-dating regulatory procedure. It was never meant for the private in-dividual.

This unresponsive, paper-heavy system, if wrongly engaged, could consume us utterly without seriously threatening any aspect of the medical prohibition. It was time to define an alternative approach that shifted the stress from patients and physicians back into federal agencies. Feedback.

We began reviewing the IND, seeking ways to simplify the process as much as possible. We soon realized that with AIDS there was a uniformity of disease progression that offered a means of accomplish-ing our goal. Our objective was to translate the abstract, highly skilled craft of IND construction into a simple formulation any pa-tient or physician could follow.

Our goal was mass production.

Even before Kenny and Barbra appeared, I faxed an outline of this strategy to our patron Rich Dennis. No response. No matter. Rich seldom responded. We continued to refine new IND models.

In the early Fall I met Rich at the Four Seasons Hotel in Wash-ington for drinks. Rich was impressed by media reaction to the Jenks case and listened with interest as I outlined the emerging plan. "Sounds good," Rich said. "Send a budget."

We met again before the Drug Policy Foundation conference in November. The Robert Randall Award for Citizen Achievement was being presented to old allies, Mae and Arnold Nutt. The presence of the Nutts, coupled with the media coverage of the Jenks case, was creating a buzz in the drug reform community that would begin to manifest itself in the coming months.

At that moment, however, my focus was on momentum. Without funding it was foolish to continue. Rich agreed, increasing our base funding to $200,000. An additional $30,000 was targeted to support two ACT projects. One would generate Compassionate INDs for people with AIDS. A second, less advanced project, would do the same for people with spinal cord injuries resulting in paralysis.

"What are we going to call these projects?" Rich wanted to know.

"Don't know about the spinal cord project," I replied. "For the other I'm thinking of Marijuana/AIDS Research Service or MARS."

A small smile eased from the friendly face. I took it as approval. We seemed to have a solid, easy, odd relationship. There was no formal agreement. No requirements. No demands. I faxed reports to Rich every week or so. Rich never responded: was never expected to respond. His checks arrived on time and did not bounce. A commodities broker, Rich placed his bet and did not intrude. A wise man, Mr. Dennis weighed results and enjoyed winning.

In November 1990 we were definitely winning.

December 18, 1990
Pawklawn Building
Rockville, Maryland

Once again Alice and I stared at the looming mass of the Parklawn Building. It had been years since we were last here. The memories of endless committee meetings from the late 70s and early 80s were still fresh in our minds. On the drive out from Washington Alice had begun to feel queasy at the thought of entering this sterile edifice again.

The FDA had summoned me to Parklawn for a meeting. The agency had noticed an increase in Compassionate IND applications and wanted to discuss matters. It was the first time in 15 years the FDA had indicated a desire to talk. Suspicions were raised.

Sensing danger, I brought along Alice and an attorney from Steptoe & Johnson. My arrival—with two witnesses—caused a commotion. The agency had planned a very intimidating and conspiratorial meeting; just me and one or two FDA staffers.

With witnesses present the small, private meeting became a major production. Government attorneys were called, the entire New Drug Therapies Unit staff assembled. More than a dozen anxious bureaucrats crammed into an airless room, glanced at one another. With witnesses present—with everyone present—how to deliver the message?

Curtis Wright, M.D., an oafishly rumpled man with unkempt hair and dirty fingernails spoke as the voice of the State. An unfortunate choice. Wright was not in charge of the Unit, merely an IND review officer recently imported into the FDA from the DEA. A man of mingled motives and no authority.

With so many eyes watching, Dr. Wright was slow getting to his point. The FDA wanted to turn Compassionate INDs into "N-of-1 studies." A bureaucratic desire to adjust semantics. "N-of-1" is virtually the same model as a "single patient Compassionate IND," but by eliminating the word "compassion," the FDA hoped to escape the trap of public condemnation that was sure to accompany refusal of some requests.

"If you accept our N-of-1 approach," Wright suggested, "you might be able to claim a proprietary interest in medical marijuana."

"Are you saying I could own medical marijuana?" That was precisely what FDA IND Review Officer Curtis Wright, M.D., was suggesting. A dozen bureaucrats leaned forward for the answer. "We could be of great help," another voice said.

"I'm not interested in owning medical marijuana," I busted their balloon. "I want to solve this problem."

"With Compassionate INDs?" Wright scoffed.

"If necessary," I replied. "That's for the FDA to decide."

"Compassionate INDs are a lot of work," Dr. Wright responded. "What if the FDA decides to stop Compassionate INDs? Where would you be then?"

Threat delivered—fail to cooperate and we will shut everything down . . . including you. I had been here before. At least Wright was smart enough not to put it in writing.

I realized the enticement I rejected would be offered to others. The threat, however, was for me alone.

I also realized that "proprietary interest" in marijuana would render me mute. New drug developers, i.e. pharmaceutical companies, are prohibited from publicly "advancing" a drug not yet approved for marketing. Such "minor" regulatory concerns could be overlooked in some cases. I doubted I would qualify for such an oversight.

It was an odd, inconclusive meeting fraught with sinister overtones. The Steptoe attorney was virtually speechless upon our exit. "They were threatening you," she exclaimed. That much I already knew.

Perhaps in a vain attempt to seduce me into acceptance the FDA demonstrated "good faith." On December 20, 1990, the FDA signed off on seven Compassionate INDs, including the Jenks'. In a relatively short period of time we had tripled the number of approved INDs. As 1990 drew to a close there were approximately fifteen approved INDS with five patients, including me, receiving supplies.

• • •

After months of retooling and prototype testing we were poised to engage the drug control system in a way bureaucrats could not imagine. MARS, the poetically potent acronym that invoked the mythical god of war, was coming together piece by piece. This time the battle was not for the heavens, it was a battle for hearts and minds.

Kenny and Barbra were the key. Before we could advance they had to get legal marijuana. Approval of their Compassionate IND triggered another round of media. "Marijuana Approved for Couple with AIDS" headlined the local paper on December 23rd and wire stories carried the announcement across the country.

Kenny and Barbra briefly celebrated. But the DEA, as usual, snarled the marijuana shipment in red tape. Christmas came and went. No marijuana. The regional DEA office refused to authorize a shipment without first printing up formal, official, special DEA marijuana order forms. It was all too reminiscent of Steve's experience. I strafed the regional DEA office with media volleys but the bureaucrats refused to budge.

January became February. More salvos fired. Despite a terrible pounding in the Florida media, the DEA continued to obstruct the shipment. It looked as if the DEA would let Kenny and Barbra Jenks die before allowing marijuana to flow into the hands of another AIDS patient. Then, against a backdrop of growing public antagonism the DEA finally relented.

"We got our pot today," Kenny happily shouted into the phone. It was February 19, 1991, nearly nine months after their application was filed and two months after it was approved.

Three days later I joined them in Panama City, along with John Daniel, to publicly celebrate the arrival of their legal, FDA-approved pot. Cameras rolled. Shutters snapped. "AIDS Couple Receives Govt Pot." The story managed to poke through the media haze of the imminent Gulf War.

The Marijuana AIDS Research Service (MARS) was slated to be launched in less than a week in Rich's home town, Chicago. Kenny and Barbra were the Honorary Cochairpersons of MARS and would be a part of the official announcement on February 28. The final countdown had begun.

On Monday, February 25, John Daniel drove the couple to Tallahassee where he argued for the reversal of their conviction before the Florida Court of Appeals. The argument before the Court hinged on the defense of medical necessity and with the recent arrival of FDA-approved marijuana the Court couldn't help but draw the obvious conclusion: If the FDA was giving them legal marijuana perhaps marijuana was a "medical necessity." The DEA's idiot delays afforded a sweet conjunction.

The next morning Kenny and Barbra were on a plane to Chicago. The window to MARS was opening.

31 MARS

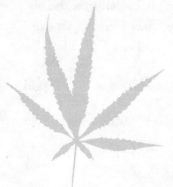

"ONLY SEEN SNOW but once before." Barbra was shivering in the Chicago cold at Midway Airport.

The launching of MARS was upon us and, after weeks of collaboration, the mechanics were now in the hands of Rich's Chicago staff. Rooms had been rented; certain groups informed; select members of the press primed.

We arrived on February 26th and a driver from Rich's office collected us at the airport and then showed us the sights. He took us around the Loop and up the Sears Tower. Kenny was wowed by the City of Big Shoulders. Barbra was less taken with urban delights, but thought Chicago was cleaner than New York. She seemed poorly.

The second day was spent in Rich's office where a small staff worked the final details of tomorrow's announcement. I was absorbed. Kenny and Barbra were bored. Rich briefly said hello, invited us to dine with him that evening, then vanished into a trading room of video screens flashing commodity prices.

One of the women on Rich's staff, Noma, took me aside and delicately tried to explain there was a problem. "They cannot go to dinner dressed like that." I tried to explain that Barbra seemed dead set against shopping. "Let me take care of it," smiled the lovely Noma.

From across the room I heard her engage Kenny and Barbra, speaking softly about "Mr. Dennis' media consultant, Mike, thinks you should get some new clothing for the upcoming events. He's going to take you to a store and will take care of everything. Okay?" Barbra would not be able to escape this shopping trip. Hours passed and they did not return.

"You're going to be late for dinner with Rich," Noma warned me. "You go ahead. I'll send them on to the hotel."

Returning to the hotel I met Jim Barnes and Gil Hansen, a gay couple who have driven in from the cold woods of Michigan. Jim has AIDS and contacted ACT in the summer of 1990. In November 1990 he applied for a Compassionate IND using the prototype of the MARS IND. It was approved in the same week that Barbra and Kenny received their supplies. Now he would wait for his supplies. He was our first Man from MARS.

We waited for our ride to dinner and, forty-five minutes late, Rich's "media consultant" Mike finally arrived. "Sorry we took so long. Kenny and Barbra are in the car. You ready?" It was a dash across Chicago to the Four Seasons. The trip was filled with introductions and chatter. We were rushing inside the hotel when I realized Kenny and Barbra had been transformed.

"Nice suit," I tell Kenny.

"Thanks Robert. It's a Armani," Kenny read the label. "Fits real good."

Barbra was in a blue dress with matching earrings and shoes, even a bit of rouge. I had never seen her in a dress. She was stunning, but awkward as a child playing dress up.

The shopping trip was a great success. Kenny and Barbra looked grand. Rich was waiting at his table. We were more than an hour late. His close friend Mary Ann Snyder wondered what took so long.

What took so long? Months later Rich would confide the shopping spree became extended when Kenny and Barbra did not know their sizes. "How," Rich asked, "can that be?"

"No one ever bought them new clothes before," I replied.

The change from rags to fine threads was appropriate. Everything was about to change. The curtain was going up.

February 28, 1991
Morton Hotel
Chicago, Illinois

"We are here to announce the formation of MARS—the Marijuana/AIDS Research Service," Rich told the packed room. The press was out in force. In Chicago, Richard J. Dennis is a draw.

"Kenny and Barbra Jenks legally smoke marijuana. Jim Barnes, our first man from MARS, won FDA approval using the MARS model IND," Rich explained. "These individuals are living proof that people with AIDS can apply to the FDA and legally obtain marijuana. MARS allows any AIDS patient in America to petition the FDA for legal access to medical marijuana. I'm honored to back such a worthy enterprise."

The MARS launch was flawless. Wire services carried the news out of Chicago. WGN satellited MARS news across the continent. NBC transmitted the story for optional play on local news screens. In Washington, Alice added to the density of coverage by faxing MARS announcements to New York, D.C. and San Francisco media plugs.

Initial telemetry was excellent. Before the Chicago press conference was over people with AIDS were phoning ACT for MARS packets.

• • •

MARS was an act of faith and aggression: a double-edged sword designed to pierce the prohibition to its heart or unmask the menace at its core.

For more than a decade federal agencies had evaded medical marijuana by mumbling a trite mantra: Marijuana has no medical value, and anyone who medically needs marijuana can legally obtain it. A doctor need only ask.

The first contention, the DEA's official line, was a widely recognized lie. Americans know marijuana has medical value. The public mind was very clear on this point.

The second contention, the FDA's "compassion posture," emphasized the fraud of the first. If the FDA provided marijuana to people with legitimate medical needs then obviously marijuana has medical value. The FDA conveniently deflected this logic by calling such access "research."

This distorted good-cop/bad-cop routine confused the public mind and, by 1991, confusion was deep. Medical marijuana had been news for fifteen years. Everyone had read the headlines. The courts and thirty-five states recognized marijuana's medical value. A DEA judge had ruled that marijuana has important medical uses. Some people, like Kenny and Barbra, legally received marijuana.

"So," the public asked, "what's the problem?"

If federal agencies kept their promise—anyone who medically needed marijuana could legally obtain it—there was no problem. But, as this narrative suggests, legal access to marijuana was altogether rare.

MARS was designed to clarify the public mind and, like a touchstone, test the value of the government's tender.

MARS embraced the government's promise of care by providing AIDS patients with what they needed to apply for legal access to marijuana. By bundling IND forms with clear instructions, MARS altered the dynamics of the Compassionate IND system. Prior to MARS, physicians who requested IND forms from the FDA could wait for weeks, even months for the forms. When the papers did arrive there was often no explanation about how to complete the 31 questions. Some were relatively routine but others were head-scratchers. For example:

List numbers of all investigational new drug applications (21 CFR Part 312), new drug or antibiotic applications (21 CFR Part 314), drug master files (21 CFR 314.420), and product license applications (21 CFR part 601) referred to in this application.

This intimidating question can be answered simply with "Reference NIDA master files 1631 and 366." But no one in FDA would ever tell a doctor that little bit of information. Private physicians were forced to play the same shell games as New Mexico and the other states, stabbing in the dark to find the right answer, trying to find the little bit of correctness that would inspire an FDA official to say, "you're getting warmer."

Our MARS IND forms were approximately 90% completed. Only personal information about the doctor and patient was required and we developed a series of checklists to simplify this aspect of the form's completion. Physicians who once struggled for hours to answer arcane FDA questions, could sit with an AIDS patient, open a MARS packet, go through a checklist and put an application in the mail in under an hour.

MARS made applying for a Compassionate IND easy and accessible. We theorized, correctly, that such a MARS-induced collapse of application time would trigger intense interest in the AIDS community. Even before Kenny and Barbra, word was already spreading in the AIDS community that marijuana seemed to help people with AIDS live longer. Kenny and Barbra coalesced the thought and MARS harnessed energy behind it.

MARS unlocked a landscape of intentions. Positively engaged,

MARS would rapidly increase the number of AIDS patients receiving marijuana. This, in turn, would cause an explosion of knowledge as treating physicians evaluated marijuana's medical utility. MARS was an extremely robust, highly accelerated research model. If the government wanted to know if marijuana could help people with AIDS, MARS could quickly and inexpensively provide the answer.

A happy ending? Perhaps. But there was a darker, alternative path.

It is possible our federal government does not want to know if marijuana can help people with AIDS—or any disease for that matter. It is possible the prohibition is more important than people. In which case bureaucratic efforts to maintain the medical prohibition— to resist MARS—would put federal agencies on a collision course with public opinion.

In the starkest of terms MARS was a game of cosmic chicken played with human lives. There are only two possible outcomes.

If the FDA responded to MARS with optimism the needs of many sorely afflicted people would be eased and the medical prohibition would melt into antiquity. This would happen only if the government could be trusted to keep a publicly made promise to provide medical care to dying people.

If federal agencies failed to deliver on their promise "that anyone with a legitimate medical need can legally obtain marijuana," and if bureaucrats blocked MARS, the feedback would disrupt the control system and irrevocably tear up the institutional illusion of compassion.

Two possible outcomes: Fusion or fission. MARS favored the former, but either would serve our interests.

We were approaching critical mass.

MARS was barely off the launch pad when there was a disruption in my access to marijuana. On March 4, 1991, just five days after the Chicago announcement of MARS, my pharmacy in the Washington

Hospital Center couldn't fill Dr. North's script. A shot across the bow? A tug on the leash? Just a coincidence?

Explanations are requested. NIDA reported the FDA failed to process the pharmacy's supply request in a timely fashion. The order arrived at the FDA shortly after the December 1990 meeting at which Curtis Wright asked me, "What if the FDA decides to stop Compassionate INDs? Where would you be then?"

The order sat in the FDA for so long—more than six weeks—that it became invalid. A glitch. Just a glitch they say. NIDA cooperated fully and the pharmacy received supplies within 48 hours but the low tearing sound of fission was unmistakable.

On that same day, March 4, a hearing was held in the U.S. Court of Appeals, Washington, D.C. ACT appealed the DEA's refusal to accept Judge Young's decision *In The Matter Of Marijuana Rescheduling*.

Our old friend Tom Collier, now a senior partner at Steptoe & Johnson, returned in a cameo appearance to argue ACT's case. He strongly stated ACT's basic argument: Marijuana clearly has an "accepted medical use in treatment in the United States." Any other conclusion is, as Judge Young said, "unreasonable, arbitrary and capricious."

Department of Justice [DoJ] attorneys argued that only the DEA Administrator can decide if marijuana is medically useful and they cited regulations which allowed the administrator to ignore the recommendations of the agency's chief judge.

The three-judge panel asked several inconsequential questions. Then one judge wondered why a law enforcement agency like DEA should decide if a drug is medically useful. Shouldn't doctors, patients and health care professionals make such a decision?

Another judge wondered what "accepted" might mean. "Accepted" by whom, under what conditions? For example, if FDA was approving marijuana for medical uses like cancer, glaucoma and

AIDS then how can DEA claim marijuana is medically useless? Seemed like a contradiction.

The DoJ attorneys stammered. The judges called for additional briefs. The once slight divide between the FDA and DEA's publicly uttered mantras was suddenly a legal chasm. Each approved IND for marijuana eroded the DEA's legal argument before the U.S. Court of Appeals.

Two weeks after the Court of Appeals hearings "60 Minutes" came to call on Kenny and Barbra Jenks. Every newspaper and television station in Florida covered "60 Minutes" covering Kenny and Barbra. The biggest of big media had arrived.

Kenny and Barbra were only vaguely familiar with the show. I resisted the urge to fly to Florida and monitor the taping. When I started giving instructions Barbra told me "We can handle it, don't worry."

It had been less than a year since their arrest. Eight months previously, they had agonized about friends in Panama City Beach learning about their AIDS. Now they were about to meet Morley Safer and appear on America's most popular news show. Barbra's nonchalance was charming and wonderful.

Morley Safer had followed through with his interest in the Jenks story after seeing the CNN report on their trial and asked "60 Minutes" producer Gail Isen to look into it. Gail had found her way to ACT. We had worked through the story for several months. It would be many more months before the segment aired.

"Mrs. Isen? Oh, Gail. She was real nice," Kenny reported. "Smart, too. And that Morley—Morley Safer?—he was real good."

Gail was "delighted" with the Jenks, John Daniel, even the vice cops. A colorful collection of improbable characters living through unusual circumstances with national implications. A great story.

"What those poor kids are living through," Gail said of Kenny and Barbra, "is so very moving."

While America celebrated victory in the Gulf War, news of MARS flashed through the AIDS community, ricocheted into the gay community, and then slowly settled into the national mind. The response was stunning.

In December 1990, just before the meeting with the FDA, I had written to the Steptoe lawyers and explained the MARS strategy. "The target," I wrote, "is to get 1,500 IND application forms in the hands of AIDS patients/physicians, with 200 completions into formal IND applications from physicians to FDA for access by the end of 1991. It is difficult to know if these targets are wildly off the mark."

By the end of March 1991 we realized these estimates were, in fact, far too low. AIDS groups in San Francisco and Miami requested permission to copy the MARS packet. Soon AIDS groups in New York, Los Angeles, Atlanta, Dallas, Minneapolis and Chicago were also photocopying MARS. We quickly began to lose track of how many MARS IND applications were "out there." In many ways it wasn't important. Our goal had been to enable others to apply on their own behalf. Goal accomplished.

On March 15, FDA approved the first IND request for marijuana use by a paralyzed individual. For years we had heard from paraplegics and quadriplegics who used marijuana to quiet involuntary muscle spasms but few were willing to publicly acknowledge the use. In the rapidly escalating war for medical marijuana Chris Woderiski, a paraplegic from Tampa, Florida, agreed to test our prototype IND for paralysis. In April I joined Chris in Florida to announce his success. He would join the growing list of individuals waiting for supplies from the federal government. As MARS was barreling along we began planning the launch of a second program—PALM—Paralyzed Americans for Legal Medical Marijuana. Chris would be our point man and he was already busy lining up recruits.

For 15 years the FDA had used complexity and paperwork to deflect physician interest in medical marijuana. MARS and PALM radically adjusted the balance by removing the mystery of IND preparation. Physicians treating people with AIDS or paralysis were quick to respond.

March 24, 1991
The Washington Post

An article entitled "U.S. Provides Marijuana for Some AIDS Patients," written by Michael Isikoff, appeared on page A3. The article was unbelievably bland, deftly managing to minimize the plight of patients while constantly relooping to "pro-pot" activists. Isikoff had spoken with Kenny and Barbra ten days before. "Didn't like him much, Robert," said Kenny. "He didn't seem to understand."

Nevertheless the article correctly captured the FDA mantra when it stated "most seriously ill applicants who meet the agency's criteria—a note from their doctor and a signed consent form acknowledging the risks—would likely be favorably considered for legal access."

Associate FDA commissioner for public affairs, Jeffrey A. Nesbit, echoed a long departed Ed Tocus. "I suppose you can say the agency acted compassionately" in supplying the Jenks with legal marijuana.

April 19, 1991
Panama City Beach, Florida

"It's a great relief," Kenny Jenks told the news reporter. "I was worried it wouldn't be resolved before something happened to my wife and me." The Florida Court of Appeals had upheld the defense of "medical necessity" in the treatment of AIDS. In a landmark decision the Appeals Court overturned the conviction of Kenny and Barbra Jenks, declaring them "not guilty." It was the nation's first successful "medical necessity" defense involving marijuana's use in AIDS care.

Barbra received the news in a hospital bed in Pensacola. She was admitted on April 10 with severe bleeding and borderline pneumonia. The news made her very happy.

"I couldn't believe it at first, but it did happen. I feel we made a little bit of history," she said. "If something was to happen to me I didn't want to go feeling like I was a criminal."

April 27, 1991
Washington, D.C.

Eight days later there was another Court of Appeals victory. "DEA Told to Reevaluate Marijuana's Medical Value" headlines *The Washington Post*.

A three-judge panel of the federal appeals court here ordered the Drug Enforcement Administration to reconsider its 1989 decision that marijuana has no medical value, saying the agency acted unreasonably in evaluating the drug's possible effectiveness for cancer victims and other seriously ill patients.

It was a jubilant moment but a careful reading of the 10-page decision gave the Steptoe lawyers some concern. The judges had not quarreled with the DEA's rejection of the facts. It seems the case could hinge, ultimately, on a careful interpretation of the administrator's authority.

This case was not yet over.

Nor was the Jenks case over. During the first part of May the state
of Florida began the process of appealing the Court of Appeals ruling.
It was unbelievable that the state would pursue this matter any further and there was a strong feeling those in charge were reacting to
advice from outside.

May 1, 1991
Washington, D.C.

The Washington Times, the capitol's conservative voice, was anything but conservative in its headline: "Many Cancer Specialists Favor Pot Use."

A survey of more than 1,000 U.S. cancer specialists found that
nearly half had advised patients to use marijuana to control
vomiting associated with chemotherapy.

The results of the Spring 1990 mail survey of members of
the American Society of Clinical Oncology are published in . . .
today's issue of the *Annals of Internal Medicine*.

Of the 1,035 respondents, 44 percent said they had recommended the illegal use of marijuana for the control of vomiting. . . .

The article failed to report that nearly 80% of the oncologists said
marijuana should be legally available by prescription.

It was another salvo in the long spring of 1991. Networks and
newspapers locked onto the story and it became a springboard for
dozens of reports featuring "the local angle." We were generally
pleased with the survey, which had been conducted on behalf of ACT

as part of a master's thesis project at Harvard University. But I was wary of the researchers: Rick Doblin, the student, and his advisor Mark Kleiman, Ph.D. "Drug policy experts," they seemed shallow and opportunistic.

The Harvard report was a featured story on the "Today Show." I was a "part" of the report when old video clips were collected from the Washington affiliate and used in the setup. But the live, on-air interviewees were Dr. Mark Kleiman and Dr. Herbert Kleber, Assistant Director, Office of National Drug Control Policy. Kleber was the assistant drug czar, a man of some authority.

Dr. Kleiman was marginally informative, uncertain under the lights of live TV. Not impressive, but adequate. Herbert Kleber was, from suit to tan, an utterly gray man whose erratic inflections announced the strain running through federal policy. To ease public concerns Kleber boldly defended the Compassionate IND program. He had trouble understanding the problem since anyone could get marijuana who needed it. "Just have your doctor apply to the FDA." "The waiting period," he asserted, "is less than a month."

His comments were decisive. His stern, straightforward reassertion of the promise of care invited patients across America to petition for marijuana. Hundreds of AIDS patients, already armed with MARS packets, took Dr. Kleber at his word. Patients with other ailments called ACT for help. Yes, their doctor would provide "a note." By the end of May the FDA would be inundated with INDs.

In early May, we took MARS on the road. Kenny and Barbra joined us at the 4th Annual AIDS Up-Date Conference in San Francisco. Now well-clad and no longer criminal, they were official MARS spokespersons. Our MARS table, in the entry area of the conference, was immediately swamped by patients and physicians interested in marijuana, AIDS, and "How do I apply?" People really wanted the information. Scores of patients came by just to say "thanks for doing this." Doctors freely admitted patients smoked, one admitting, "I've got five guys smoking now." Nurses always "knew someone" who could use the forms.

It was stunning. Beyond my wildest dreams. I seldom say that. But San Francisco exceeded all expectations. The human reaction to MARS was so warm, thankful, urgent, grateful, intense, and personal.

Kenny was in his element. His notorious "motormouth" was an asset at these events. Like a barker in a carnival crowd, Kenny enticed scores of passing strangers asking, "Wanna see how marijuana looks when it's legal?" He was animated and tireless. Barbra was far less involved. Out of the hospital just a few weeks, we worried if we'd done the right thing in bringing her so far.

She slipped away from the exhibit to wander the inner hall which was filled with tables offering support, services, and medications to the AIDS-afflicted and their caregivers. Lining the walls were panels from The Names Project Quilt, the simple and glorious memorial to those who have been claimed by this 20th century scourge.

Barbra exited the hall looking shaken and tired. I worried she was ill again. "Naw, I'm okay," she said.

"You'll tell me if you want to stop?"

"I don't ever want to stop, Robert." Her reply to my simple inquiry said far more than the status of her energy level. She was on a different plane. I waited, knowing there was more.

"I had a dream, Robert."

"What about?"

"A tree. Just a big, old tree," Barbra replied. "When I was in the hospital."

"Any water nearby?"

"Yeah!" she looked at me, a bit surprised. "A nice little stream."

"What do you think it means, Barbra?"

"Oh. I'm gonna die in the spring, Robert," she was certain and calm.

"Why? What about the tree tells you that?"

"The leaves—they was all fresh 'n new. Like in spring. I'm gonna die in the spring . . . some spring."

Barbra and Kenny's appearance at the AIDS Update Conference generated a massive media release on the West Coast and then reverberated nationally when "CBS Morning News" included the couple as part of their AIDS conference report. As the news flooded out into the country INDs flooded into the FDA.

By June 1991, federal agencies were facing stark decisions. If the FDA kept the government's promise to provide marijuana to people with legitimate medical needs, NIDA had to increase marijuana production. If NIDA increased marijuana production to meet accelerating patient needs, the DEA would lose control over both supply and demand. Once engaged, this cycle of expanding supply and spiraling demand would rip the medical prohibition to shreds.

Bureaucrats were once again meeting in airless rooms to discuss "this medical marijuana thing." But the meetings were no longer public. No special committees were formed to give the sense of "doing something." There was no time for that. These meetings were of the upper echelon and the decision they reached would be a dramatic one.

Fusion or fission?

MARS had reached critical mass.

32 The Collapse of Compassion

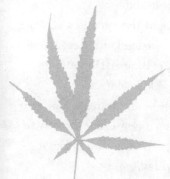

June 14, 1991
Washington, D.C.

"They've stopped sending my marijuana," Corrine's voice was tinged with alarm. "The FDA won't tell my doctor what's going on. Can you help me?"

Corrine Millet, a 58-year old Nebraskan grandmother with glaucoma, had legally smoked the government's marijuana for over a year with excellent results. In early May, however, she went to the pharmacy to pick up her monthly supply. It wasn't there. She had waited for more than a month to call me. Now it was a Friday night in mid-June. There was little I could do on the weekend.

Calls to the FDA on Monday, the 17th, were not returned.

On June 18th I traveled to my pharmacy and discovered Corrine's disruption was not unique. For the second time in three months my pharmacy could not honor Dr. North's prescription. The pharmacist explained that the FDA had placed a "hold" on supplies. He had no further explanation.

My attorney at Steptoe & Johnson, Steve Davidson, immediately phoned the agencies but discovered all the responsible bureaucrats were meeting at the posh Breakers Resort in Palm Beach, Florida.

I was unable to make any sense of this news. Why were federal officials involved in medical marijuana meeting on the beach in Florida? Who were they meeting in such plush and pampered surroundings?

On a hunch I called the hotel and asked for the representative from Unimed. "Which one?" the desk clerk asked.

It was 1981 all over again. MARS had sent the agencies scrambling for synthetic solutions. Only this time, instead of airless rooms in Parklawn, the FDA was at the Breakers, selling AIDS patients to Unimed, the manufacturer of delta-9 THC, a.k.a. Marinol.

Stern messages were flashed to the beach-bound bureaucrats and by early evening my pharmacy was FedExing a new order directly to FDA officials in Palm Beach. Just a glitch, NIDA assured. The marijuana would arrive at the pharmacy by Friday.

June 19, 1991
Panama City Beach, Fla.

"Um, Robert?" It was Kenny's voice and it seemed unsteady. "We went to our pharmacy but they don't have no pot for us."

I explained I was having the same problem. So was Corrine. "How can anyone be this mean?" Kenny wondered.

Barbra took the phone from Kenny. There was defiance in her voice. "They ain't gonna get away with this." Then, a bit frightened, "Are they Robert?"

I knew this was a profound provocation. These multiplying supply disruptions were premeditated, intentional. But to what end? Were the bureaucrats testing the circuits? Corrine had been cut off weeks ago and nothing happened. Did they think they could, one by one, remove the "legal smokers" from the medical marijuana landscape while plotting to release Marinol to appease AIDS patients?

It was time to return fire. It wasn't 1978 or even 1981. Medical marijuana was not an embryonic issue begging to be heard. I lifted the receiver and called "60 Minutes" producer Gail Isen.

The "60 Minutes" medical marijuana segment was "in the can" and waiting for a time slot in the Fall season. Gail knew the story had power and she had grown fond of "the kids" in Florida. She was, as I anticipated, enraged at Kenny and Barbra's supply disruption.

She called the FDA and reached an Assistant Administrator. It must have been a heart-stopping moment for the man. Gail demanded to know why the government was "trying to kill those kids." Excuses were made and blame was focused on NIDA. But the shell game wouldn't work with Isen who responded by giving him the names of specific FDA employees blocking the Jenks' shipment. The Assistant Administrator started to crumble. Then Isen put Morley Safer on the line. It was every bureaucrat's ultimate nightmare.

As darkness fell phone lines between Parklawn and the Breakers went blue. Fingers, no doubt, were pointed. Careers threatened. Amid the chaos one crystal clear order was given: Restore Kenny and Barbra Jenks' access to marijuana.

Immediately!

If I still had any doubt that "something was up" it was dispelled on June 20 with a phone call from Michael Isikoff of *The Washington Post*. It was an unpleasant exchange.

Isikoff was abrupt, abrasive, and appallingly rude. I had dealt with reporters for 15 years, but Isikoff was a puzzle. He was not dumb, but with a major drug story staring him in the face he seemed unable to ask cogent questions.

I listened as Isikoff repeated rumors and searched for an angle. He "demanded" to know what was going on. *The Post*, he says, believed the FDA was planning to close the Compassionate IND system. FDA and DEA were blaming NIDA for lack of supply. But was there another "reason"? Were the pro-pot groups just using this to get legalization?

Isikoff did not grasp the significance of the news he was relating. Fixated on drug war clichés, he was blind to the meaning of this dramatic reversal in policy. For more than 15 years the feds had promised medical marijuana, on a compassionate basis, to anyone with a "legitimate" need. Now, as people have finally been given the means to ask for this promised compassion the government threatened to close the program down. Why? Because there wasn't enough marijuana? The world was awash with marijuana but Isikoff, trapped in a marbleized world, could not comprehend the significance. He spoke of "that couple in Florida"—the Jenks—as if they were abstractions. His tone asked, "what do mere patients have to do with marijuana's medical use?"

Isikoff's call made it clear. The medical marijuana control system was in crisis. Compassion was killing the bureaucrats: murdering their medical prohibition. MARS was pulling interagency arrangements apart.

The FDA approved new INDs while disrupting supplies to existing INDs. Each IND application approved by the FDA eroded the DEA's legal case before the Court of Appeals. NIDA was being drained of supply while being threatened with extinction in the next budget cycle. The control system was fragmenting.

Interagency frictions were so intense that the White House was becoming involved. The bureaucratic plan to kill the Compassionate IND program apparently came as a surprise to the "kinder, gentler" guys in the Bush White House. Herbert Kleber was about to be made a fool, his "Today Show" promise of "legal access in 30 days with a note from your doctor" soon vanquished to the memory hole. It was too late to retreat. What the DEA hoped would become the official government line had already been leaked to *The Post* and they found a willing conduit in the person of Michael Isikoff.

On June 21, I picked up my marijuana supplies at the pharmacy. Hours later, Kenny and Barbra Jenks picked up their supplies in Pensacola. Without the benefit of media or lawyers, Corrine, it seemed, would have to wait.

June 22, 1991
The Washington Post

Isikoff's article appeared on page A14 with the headline, "Health and Human Services to Phase Out Marijuana Program." The subhead—"Officials Fear Sending 'Bad Signal' by Giving Drug to Seriously Ill"— more aptly told the tale.

The U.S. Public Health Service had decided to kill the Compassionate IND program.

A federal program that has provided free marijuana to the seriously ill is being phased out by Health & Human Services officials who have concluded it undercuts official Bush administration policy against the use of illegal drugs, according to HHS officials.

While a small number of patients already receiving marijuana will continue to do so, new applicants will be encouraged to try synthetic forms of delta-9 THC . . . rather than the weed itself, according to a new policy directive due to be signed by James O. Mason, Chief of the Public Health Service.

Mason said yesterday he was concerned about a surge in new applications in recent months, especially from AIDS patients, and the message it would send if HHS were to approve them.

"If it is perceived that the Public Health Service is going around giving marijuana to folks there would be a perception that this stuff can't be so bad. It gives a bad signal."

The article was clear, the directive had not yet been signed. Was this a trial balloon?

The following day *The New York Times* would weigh in with an AP report on the proposed program closing. In an understatement the Sunday *Times* reported, "The government's action seems certain to add fuel to a long standing debate about the restrictive nature of its policy on marijuana as a medical tool."

The *Times* elaborated:

In its announcement on Friday, the Public Health Service said recent publicity that marijuana might curb AIDS patients' loss of appetite had brought a rapid increase in applications to use government supplied marijuana.

The agency said it would not cut off the supply of marijuana to the 34 people who now have government permission to use the drug to cope with the illnesses that include cancer, glaucoma and AIDS.

The government, it seems, was prepared to be compassionate— as long as no one asked.

The government's action did not surprise me although the agency—PHS—was a surprise. In my 15+ year involvement with medical marijuana the Public Health Service had never been overtly involved in the issue other than to provide me with a pharmacy for a few years in the late 1970s. Perhaps Dr. Mason, a Utah native and friend to Senator Orrin Hatch, had been pressed into service by the prohibitionists. Regardless, the PHS chief clearly had the soapbox to stand upon. It remained to be seen whether he had the authority to follow through on his threats.

The gauntlet was cast down and the immediate future was clear. We needed to counterattack in order to clarify the record. The media was confused by a not-yet-signed order to kill compassion. So, while the bureaucrats scrambled for the "right" message, I traveled to the midwest, moving fast and leaving media blisters in my wake. The feds could try and kill compassion if they wished but they would know their victims.

June 26, 1991
Minneapolis, Minnesota

The small conference room was packed with TV crews and print reporters. The halogen lights made AIDS patient Tim Braun claustrophobic and he squinted hard into the bright light. He was uncomfortable with notoriety but mad enough to endure it.

FDA had approved Tim's request for marijuana nearly seven months ago, at about the same time as Kenny and Barbra, but Tim still did not have legal pot. According to the news accounts Tim Braun, because he was FDA-approved, would eventually receive care.

But when? Tim asked at a press conference.

A second AIDS patient, sitting next to Tim, had used MARS to apply for access but his request had not yet been acted upon. He was not one of the FDA's "magic 34." He would be denied care. Is this fair, he asked?

June 27, 1991
Des Moines, Iowa

Another small conference room, another collection of lights and cameras. I sat at the front of the room with George McMahon, a legal smoker approved in late 1989, who suffers from a rare neurologic condition. George had benefited greatly from regular access to controlled quantities of marijuana. His doctor was astonished by George's improvement. His family was delighted. He wanted to publicly tell his story.

Also at the table was Ladd Huffman, wheelchair-bound from multiple sclerosis.

We waited for the nation's first MS patient approved for legal access to marijuana. Barbara Douglass made a dramatic entrance, walking into the room on India rubber legs. Armed with two canes, supported by her husband and another man, it had taken nearly 5 minutes for her to make the 50-foot trek from the elevator to the meeting room. "I wanted you to see how bad MS can get," Barbara told the press.

Barbara Douglass, Republican, well-dressed and well-connected, received FDA approval to legally use marijuana three months ago. Would Ms. Douglass ever receive her FDA-promised supplies? The second MS patient, Ladd Huffman, applied to FDA at the same time as Douglass. But Ladd was still waiting for a response from the FDA. Would these patients receive equal care?

The conference was excellent. The message clear. But the true story on that day occurred twenty minutes after the press conference when I answered a knock at my hotel room door. In walked Barbara Douglass. No canes. No male attendants on her arms. No spasms. "You've smoked?"

"Yes," Barbara said. "You can see what a difference it makes."

You could. Even a nearly blind man could see the difference.

June 28, 1991
Omaha, Nebraska

"Marijuana is such a godsend." The Associated Press reporter scribbled furiously. I watched quietly from across the room.

Corrine Millet, a surgeon's widow, was shy and didn't want to make a fuss. But she was also going blind and was angry at her supply disruption. I arranged for one-on-one interviews. Corrine, clearly worried about losing her vision, was plainspoken and direct. "I can't believe my government would do this to me."

The AP reporter calls Washington for comment. By late afternoon an emergency order was sent from the FDA to NIDA. Corrine's marijuana would arrive within 24 hours.

The total elapsed time of my midwest swing was 60 hours. Local media coverage was heavy and national wires picked up the MS story. Each stop triggered a cascade of inquiries as reporters from Minnesota, Iowa and Nebraska phoned the bureaucrats back in Washington. The questions were the same: Why was the government depriving such fine people access to needed medical care? Didn't the government promise to provide compassionate care to patients in need?

We were defining the battle: grinding down bureaucratic credibility. *The Pilot-Tribune*, Barbara Douglass' hometown paper, succinctly stated it. "Let us continue to wage the war against drugs, but let not the first victim be human compassion."

In one of those quirks of fate, I returned from Nebraska on June 28 and encountered HHS Secretary Louis Sullivan at National airport. We spoke. I told Sullivan, "Killing compassion is not smart policy." Sullivan resorted to the pat answers the FDA gave him. They were not convincing. Secretary Sullivan confirmed he met with PHS midweek, but from his comments it was clear the PHS order to quash the Compassionate IND program had not been signed.

It's difficult to know what the bureaucracies were attempting to accomplish in that fateful month of June 1991. There seemed to be little, if any, coordination among the agencies. Clearly there was growing concern about the influx of INDs and there was, most certainly, a desire to shut things down.

What the agencies did not anticipate was the onslaught of public anger. Hundreds of enraged patients felt betrayed and discriminated against. They let the bureaucrats know it. Many of these patients made it past the switchboard, and tapped deep into the reaches of the bureaucracy. The effect was devastating.

The bureaucrats—operating behind screens of forms and physicians—were insulated from direct human contact. Few of the people administering the medical prohibition had ever encountered actual patients. The sudden flood of incoming anger struck like a riptide. "Why are you killing me?" one AIDS patient demanded of a woman at NIDA. "Why?" By the time he was done she was in tears, sobbing at the craven cruelty of her agency's policy. "I'm sorry," she said. "Very sorry."

This aggressive telephonic battering had a profoundly corrosive effect on institutional morale. There was more to come. While I worked the press in the Midwest, Alice spent the week fielding calls from the National Association of People with AIDS, Cure AIDS Now, and ACT-UP. Mad. Madder. Maddest. These and similar groups were deeply agitated by the PHS announcement. They wanted to vent and federal bureaucrats felt their anger. ACT provided patients with telephone numbers into the FDA, NIDA and the White House.

On June 27, 1991, the nation experienced its first "medical marijuana protest" when representatives of ACT-UP and a drug activist group called the Green Panthers closed Health and Human Services headquarters for an hour by staging a "die-in."

By moving to kill compassion the feds had given the drug reformers and activists a bully pulpit. They wasted little time in clambering on.

• • •

On July 15 the rending sounds of fission give way to the possibility of fusion. MARS has done its job. There was still hope.

I received a call from The White House. Hendrick Harwood, an aide to Herb Kleber, was trying to fathom the problem. He had heard the DEA line, the FDA line, the PHS line, but he knew there was more. Pursuing information Harwood actually began reading testimony from *In the Matter of Marijuana Rescheduling*, the DEA case.

Harwood was impressed by the testimony of patients and asked me to put him in touch with some of the current applicants. He and Kleber were trying to grapple with an influx of information that did not jive with what the drug warriors were saying.

Harwood told me that the FDA had said I (ACT) refused to apply for an NDA—a new drug application, the prelude to marketing a drug. I explained that wasn't exactly correct and relayed, as briefly as possible, the events of December 1990 when the FDA offered me an NDA by threatening my, and others, access to marijuana. Hardly the type of relationship that makes for a speedy and honest resolve of issue, I noted.

What would it take to resolve this issue, Harwood asked?

Someone acting in good faith, I replied. Throughout the entire history of medical marijuana there had never been a federal effort to deal honestly and faithfully with this issue. If Kleber, or someone else at the White House, was willing to work in good faith I was more than willing to discuss some avenues of possible resolution of this conflict, including an NDA.

Harwood was a relative neophyte to the issue but he had already heard enough conflicting information to know that at least part of what I saying was true.

By the end of July a new message was being sent—the PHS decision was on hold. The government became quiet. One or two hapless individuals from PHS were designated to answer media questions. From their responses it was clear the control system was paralyzed. No decisions were being made.

We refrained from aggressive press action, hoping to give Harwood and The White House time to comprehend the situation. The Office of National Drug Control Policy was hoping to limit damage but, in a curious way, they had increased the chance of danger. By engaging the issue they dragged medical marijuana to a new level. Whatever the outcome it would now be seen as Bush Administration policy.

There would be two bright spots in that summer of 1991. On July 20, Barbra's 25th birthday, I delivered the good news that she and Kenny had won the Robert Randall Award for Citizen Achievement from the Drug Policy Foundation.

"An award for us, Robert? You don't have to give us no award." Kenny was confused by the award's name. I explained the award's history and what DPF was. "There'll be a banquet here in Washington in November. We'll fly you up."

The young couple was thrilled. "There's more," I said. "The award comes with a check for $10,000."

Now they were stunned. Kenny was actually speechless. When the news finally sunk in he let go a little hoot and the couple started to laugh and giggle. "Hey Robert," Barbra poignantly joked, "Do you think we can buy me a new body with $10,000?"

The second bit of good news came one month later on August 30, when Iowa MS patient Barbara Douglass received her first supplies of marijuana cigarettes, seven months after her Compassionate IND was approved. Barbara had turned to her Republican friends in Congress—Senator Charles Grassley and Representative Fred Grandy. They had finally shaken her medicine free.

Ladd Huffman, the similarly afflicted but less politically attached Iowan, did not receive his supplies. Barbara was outraged and told the press, "The DEA is playing God," Douglass said with disgust.

"My next job is to get Laddie's okayed. It's too bad that it comes down to who you know."

September 11, 1991
Orange County, California

The editorial in the archly conservative *Orange County Register* must have given the White House pause.

San Francisco voters will have an opportunity in November to tell state and federal authorities that a more compassionate and rational approach is in order regarding the medical use of marijuana."

The editorial referred to Proposition P, a ballot initiative that would mark the first time the American public could vote directly on the issue of medical marijuana.

At any other time the politicians could blithely dismiss the "zanies in San Francisco" but by threatening to kill compassion the feds had created some strange bedfellows. Driving the *Orange County Register* to support a voter initiative for medical marijuana in San Francisco seemed a clear and unequivocal sign that the proposed policy to eliminate Compassionate INDS had badly backfired.

Among the many patients who battered the agencies with incessant calls and relentless attack was an odd but loveable fellow from Cocoa Beach, Florida known as Spacecoast Surfer. The odd moniker was his "cyber-handle," the identity he used while "surfing" the still-relatively young worldwide web. Surfer was one of our first "men from MARS," calling the ACT office on the day the program was announced in February 1991. Surfer desperately wanted to help and he would prove a valuable friend, especially to Kenny and Barbra as he helped guide them through the intricacies of Social Security and Medicaid to secure the maximum benefits possible.

In late September Spacecoast Surfer arrived in Marble City for a meeting of ACT-UP—the AIDS Coalition to Unleash Power. After months of computer and telephone chat he proved to be as wild as his handle. Short, aggressively cute, constantly manipulative, with a buzz cut dyed bright red, Surfer was a hunky, punky homo with attitude.

In exchange for a hotel room and a couple of meals Surfer passed out MARS materials at the ACT-UP meeting. There was great interest.

ACT-UP had planned a march on the White House that finished with angry AIDS activists throwing coffins over the White House fence. As the demonstrators chanted against Bush Administration AIDS policy, Surfer extricated himself from the crowd and walked to the White House Office of National Drug Control Policy. Surfer had often talked with Rick Harwood about medical marijuana and Harwood was happy to make an appointment with the man he knew as Craig Whiteside, Surfer's real name.

There is a strategy in war called "dazzle camouflage." You create a diversion so wild and dazzling that it has the effect of camouflaging an objective. Perhaps unwittingly, Spacecoast Surfer achieved the goal of dazzle camouflage in his White House meeting. Dressed in ripped jeans and leather jacket, Surfer capped the punk look with a graphic "How to Perform Safe Oral Sex" T-shirt. One can only imagine what the Secret Service thought. Harwood's reaction was also a mystery. Surfer would later tell us that several secretaries were grossed out but he noticed they kept peeking over the partition to get another look. While staffers tried to keep their eyes from Surfer's chest, Surfer pelted them with questions. His impression matched my own, "They don't have a clue what to do with us." More ominously he added, "And they don't wanna help."

October 1, 1991

Tampa, Florida

We had been planning the launch of Paralyzed Americans for Legal Medical Marijuana (PALM) for many months but repeatedly delayed it because of the government impasse. Why promise something that may not be there? But, incredibly, the FDA began to approve INDs again in the late summer. It seemed a signal and we moved to capitalize on it.

PALM, like MARS, provided a neat packet of IND forms that could easily be completed by patient and doctor, then filed with FDA. Chris Woderski of Brandon, Florida, had been chosen to head up the PALM effort. His prototype PALM IND, along with that of another Florida patient named Craig Sovine, had been approved by FDA. They were awaiting supplies like so many others.

Nearly a dozen paralyzed vets from surrounding Florida cities attended the press conference to announce PALM. They explained to reporters how marijuana helped control the involuntary muscle spasms that accompany paralysis.

Like MARS, the PALM launch was flawless and powerful. The response from the paralyzed community was enthusiastic and sustained. PALM gave AIDS patients new allies and put new pressure on the government.

October 11, 1991

National Hemophilia Conference

Tampa, Florida

Kenny wanted to bring MARS to the hemophilia community. Thanks to blood companies and their tightly controlled Hemophilia Foundation of America, 90% of the hemophiliacs in the U.S. are HIV-positive. Thousands have already died. It is a monumental scandal that was only just beginning to surface. It made Kenny furious.

Despite the high incidence of infection among conference attendees, MARS was the only AIDS-related exhibit at the National Hemophilia Conference. In this environment of suppressed denial, Kenny and MARS were a draw. Barbra, feeling poorly, took long naps in their hotel room.

On the final day Barbra came rushing in with news. "John Daniel called. The Supreme Court said we won," Barbra repeated John's message.

The Florida Supreme Court had upheld the Appeals Court ruling squashing the State's attempt to reinstate the guilty verdict of Judge Foster. It was now official: in Florida, marijuana is a drug of "medical necessity" in AIDS therapy.

Later that month we traveled to San Francisco to drum up support for Proposition P. Despite the unceasing media coverage of the medical marijuana problem interest in the ballot measure was curiously unfocused.

We took Kenny and Barbra with us and, as usual, they shined. Barbra seemed to be battling a growing list of ailments which, if taken singularly, were not too serious. Collectively, however, they were wearing her down. So were the high doses of medicine she took to counteract the diseases.

At a press conference organized by Proposition P proponents, just a week before the election, we met Jo Daly, San Francisco's first lesbian Police Commissioner. Once called "the wonderful Jo Daly" by columnist Herb Caen, Daly was highly respected and well liked in the City by the Bay. When we met her she was retired, battling cancer and an ardent supporter of medical marijuana. She was a powerful spokesperson and captivated the press with her straightforward, no-nonsense talk.

The compelling comments of Jo, Kenny, and Barbra, together with the presence of nearly a dozen other patients who medically needed marijuana, made for a powerful media presentation.

On November 5, 1991, Proposition P passed with 79% of the vote. The lopsided victory only added to the Bush Administration's confusion over how to handle Compassionate INDs.

33 Bitter Blows

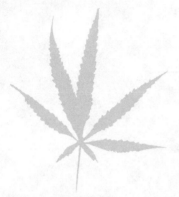

THE OVERWHELMING ACCEPTANCE of Proposition P—79% of the voters—was astonishing, even by San Francisco standards.

It was, in some respects, 1978 all over again. Frustrated by federal intransigence, the people were once again turning to the electoral process—this time expressed through the voter initiative rather than the legislature. There was hope and optimism. The people had spoken and we are, after all, a government of the people.

In the few weeks following the victory of Prop P, the good times continued . . . for a while.

November 6, 1991
Panama City, Florida

Barbra and Kenny stood on the courthouse stairs in the bright autumn sun. The photographers and camera crews encircled the couple. The Jenks had just emerged from the courtroom of Judge Clinton E. Foster, the same judge who, fifteen months earlier, had found the couple guilty of marijuana possession and sentenced them to 500 hours of community service to be spent "loving and caring for one another."

Dressed in the clothes that Rich Dennis had bought them in Chicago and confident in the righteousness of their cause, Barbra and Kenny were a far cry from the scared and confused young couple that Judge Foster had first seen in his courtroom. The proceeding was brief. "When you eat crow," said John Daniel, "you try to make it quick."

"This Court, acting on the decision of the Florida Court of Appeals, rules that in the case of *Florida v. Barbra and Kenneth Jenks* the defendants are found not guilty and are discharged from any further jeopardy in this matter."

Now, standing on the courthouse steps, Barbra and Kenny posed for the news cameras and joked with the reporters, most of whom they had come to know well in the intervening months. Barbra, looking tired, was nonetheless happy.

"I *told* you I wasn't no criminal."

The San Francisco election only intensified intra-agency conflicts over what to do about the compassionate IND program. The firestorm of public criticism accompanying the first announcement of the program closure had lessened but patients and caregivers continued to make their feelings known. "We've had a lot of dying people calling and asking us for help. It's sad." said the chief of staff for the White House Office of National Drug Control Policy (ONDCP).

On November 12 in *The Washington Post* it became publicly apparent that the situation was straining relations in the various agencies. Michael Isikoff's article was starkly frank in portraying a power struggle, citing "a four-month interagency battle between Health and Human Services and the Office of National Drug Control Policy." Isikoff wrote of "alarm among senior officials at the Department of

Health and Human Services" at the prospect of marijuana's medical use by a "new population"—AIDS patients.

James O. Mason, director of the Public Health Service (PHS), was identified as the chief administration official pushing for the program's closure. AIDS patients who medically use marijuana, he said, "might be less likely to practice safe behavior whether it's sharing needles or sexual behavior."

Mason's comment infuriated AIDS and medical marijuana activists. For some who had known Mason since his days as Director of the Center for Disease Control (CDC), the comment reminded them of Mason's difficulties in dealing with AIDS and the homosexual community. In his first days at CDC the Utah native was unable to even utter the word "gay" while meeting with gay delegations.

The article noted that Mason seemed to be winning the debate inside the Administration. ONDCP chief Bob Martinez was reportedly in agreement with the HHS decision to deny all new applications for marijuana, directing patients instead to Marinol. The sticking point was the existing 16 patients receiving marijuana and the applications approved but not yet supplied. The article stated that Mason wanted to cut them off but Martinez's aides disagreed, arguing such a move would be unfair.

"We said it would not be compassionate to cut off people who have gone through this process in good faith," said an ONDCP aide. "We didn't think it would be moral or just."

November 16, 1991
Capital Hill Hyatt Hotel
Washington, D.C.

The banquet room was packed with conference-goers at the Drug Policy Foundation (DPF) annual meeting. It was a glittering affair. Many of the attendees were dressed in formal evening wear while others sported the more expected attire of the activists—blue jeans and T-shirts emblazoned with slogans advocating legalized marijuana and free access to clean needles. Every imaginable style of dress between these extremes could be found in the ornate dining room.

The 1991 recipients of the Robert Randall Award for Citizen Achievement sat at a table in the middle of the room and nervously picked at their food. Barbra and Kenny had arrived two days earlier but generally eschewed the conference for rest and relaxation. They had a room at the hotel but spent most of their time at our home or at ACT's office. Now the big moment was at hand.

"Do you have a speech ready, Barbra?" Alice asked.

"Uh-uh, I don't do speeches. That's motormouth's job," Barbra replied with a poke at Kenny's ribs. "Whatcha gonna say, Kenny?" Barbra teased.

Kenny, uncharacteristically, had no retort. He grinned nervously and took his wife's hand for a moment.

I led them up to the dais and gave a short introduction. The audience applauded warmly as I presented the Jenks with an engraved plaque and an envelope containing the check. Then I stepped aside for Kenny to move to the microphone.

In the audience Alice watched as Kenny's eloquence spilled from him. He always amazed her. He and Barbra could be so chatty, so unfocused and scattered but at moments like these he seemed to draw from a deep well of expression and style that would simply captivate those listening with its simplicity and unwavering focus. Barbra would inevitably underscore his remarks with her own form of comment—short, rougher-edged, and very to the point. Tonight was no exception. As Kenny clutched the plaque and promised it would always be important to him, Barbra snatched the check away, moved to the microphone and said, "He can keep the plaque. I'm happy to receive the check."

The audience was charmed and immediately rose to their feet in laughter, applause, and admiration. We made our way back to the table and sat down. As the applause began to die, Kenny leaned over to Alice. "Did we do okay? What did I say?"

She took his hand and squeezed it warmly. "Fine, Kenny. You did just fine." If she said any more she was sure to cry.

December 1, 1991
Washington, D.C.

Morley Safer introduced the long-awaited "60 Minutes" segment, "Smoking to Live."

"Marijuana is not good for you. It's an axiom. But for some people, marijuana could be the difference between life and death. That's what they and their doctors say. The doctors prescribe it and the patients smoke it to live."

The broadcast came at a perfect time—World AIDS Day.

Barbra and Kenny were at their best, focused and appealing. Safer also interviewed Harvard professor Lester Grinspoon, me, a doctor who tried to give the "government angle," Dr. Ivan Silverberg from San Francisco, and the Jenks' lawyer John Daniel who was remarkably effective when Safer asked him why he took the case *pro bono.* "Because it was the right thing to do," he said. The DEA refused to be interviewed for the segment, thereby underscoring their refusal to play fair.

In Pensacola, Barbra and Kenny watched the segment in Barb's hospital room. The young woman had taken a turn for the worse following their trip to the DPF conference in Washington. When I spoke to them after the broadcast their pride was evident. Barbra termed the show "beautiful."

Across America the story beamed into millions of homes just two days after Thanksgiving. It was the largest single audience yet for the medical marijuana issue.

With the December 1 airing of "Smoking to Live" the medical marijuana question in America went from an "issue" to "a problem." There is a world of difference between the two. The penetration of the "60 Minutes" piece can perhaps best be expressed by comments from a friend's 80+year-old aunt, who watched the show. "I had no idea," she said. "This is terribly wrong. Something should be done about this problem."

December 2, 1991
Frederic, Wisconsin

Among those who watched the story of the Jenks on "60 Minutes" was a Wisconsin cancer patient named Sheila Dinnella. Her IND was one of the requests that had been approved but not yet supplied with marijuana. She had quietly waited for more than a year. Alice and I had encouraged her to "go public," take her story to the people of Wisconsin and, perhaps, the nation. But she always declined. "I didn't want to air my private problems in public," the 36-year-old teacher explained.

After watching the "60 Minutes" piece, Sheila realized she was a pawn in a vicious game. "I resent having to suffer while zealots in Washington block my medical marijuana," she said, "The FDA was hoping I'd die so they could forget about me. It is time for patients to speak out. People are suffering."

So on Monday, December 2, she called and said she was ready to do whatever she must to draw attention to her situation. When asked if that included a press conference in Madison, the state capitol, Sheila said yes. I began to organize another Midwest press swing.

The week of December 9 began with a lengthy video piece at the WUSA-TV station in Washington, D.C. I was interviewed along with two AIDS patients. Dale, a Washington area AIDS patient receiving legal supplies, was nervous about publicity and appeared in silhouette. Another AIDS patient, John Skidmore, was less shy.

John, like Sheila, was among the patients who had been promised supplies but was not receiving them. He felt betrayed by his government and did not mince his words. The report was well done and would capture the attention of Tokyo Broadcast System. Skidmore's story would captivate Japanese audiences in the New Year.

The next day I was in Madison, Wisconsin where I met Sheila and her parents, for the first time. Sheila was a teacher of visually impaired children and lived in a small town near Madison. She was battling ovarian cancer and the cancer was winning. She had been reluctant to try marijuana for the nausea and vomiting, frightened she would jeopardize her job, but the chemo was too excruciating and the marijuana worked too well. "I didn't want to break the law to buy marijuana off the streets. So my doctor and I applied to the FDA for help through the Compassionate IND system," she told a packed press conference.

Her application to legally use marijuana had been approved in December 1990 and she thought her problems were over. "Boy, was I wrong. The bureaucrats who had promised to help me have instead turned my life into a living hell."

For a full year she had waited for the legal joints to arrive. "I'm speaking out now because I'm afraid if I don't speak out, the bureaucrats will just try to sweep me under the rug and forget about me."

Reporters who called PHS after the press conference received the same run around as Sheila and her doctor. In a grand gesture of compassion, James Mason ordered the National Cancer Institute to "get hold of the woman's physician and provide alternative means of relieving symptoms." If he had bothered to consult directly with the physician he would have learned that all means of relief, including the much-touted Marinol, had been tried. But Mason didn't really care about Sheila Dinnella's problems. No one inside the Beltway, it seemed, had time for the medical problems of a middle-aged school teacher in the Midwest. Mason's aide, Raford Kytle, reminded the reporters that the government's chief concern was the large number of AIDS patients who were asking for help and the fear that "marijuana might make the AIDS patients act irresponsibly and spread the virus through unsafe sexual practices." No one, it seemed, ever bothered to ask what that had to do with Sheila Dinnella.

December 11, 1991
Minneapolis, Minnesota

In the small conference room, Tim Braun and Aeren Thomas sat quietly as the press assembled. Gaunt and gray, Braun and Thomas were both afflicted with AIDS. I was telling them of the government's rationale that medical marijuana use by AIDS patients would lead to unsafe sex and spread the disease. The two men gave disgusted laughs. "I'm permitted to take this," said Braun as he lifted the morphine pump that was attached to his body through tubes, "but I legally can't take a couple puffs of marijuana?"

Like Sheila Dinnella, Tim Braun was one of the patients approved for medical marijuana who had never received supplies. His comments were poignant.

"If I buy grass, I can't afford to eat," he told reporters. "If I buy food, I can't eat it."

Braun was living on Social Security and it was barely enough to make ends meet, let alone buy marijuana at $200 an ounce. His weight had dropped to less than 140 pounds and he was battling a lung infection. He was clearly very ill.

The *St. Paul Pioneer Press* called the Public Health Service for a comment and the spokesman, Bill Grigg, squirmed but did not falter. "It's embarrassing to go back on your promise," Grigg said but he went on to insist that marijuana's dangerous side effects justified the government's action.

Looking at Tim Braun that day it was hard to see how the side effects of marijuana could be any more dangerous than the direct effects of AIDS.

From Minneapolis I traveled to Des Moines to draw some attention to Ladd Huffman, the multiple sclerosis patient still waiting for his supplies. Then I flew to Florida to try and bring some pressure on behalf of the two paraplegics Chris Woderski and Craig Sovine, also awaiting their promised care.

On January 31, 1992, *The Los Angeles Times* published the contents of a letter to Public Health Service chief James O. Mason from Ingrid A. C. Kolb, acting deputy director for demand reduction at the White House Office of National Drug Control Policy (ONDCP).

Kolb took Mason and the Department of Health and Human Services (HHS) to task for delaying so long in reaching the decision about whether or not to supply the 30 previously approved patients with medical marijuana. "For HHS to treat this matter as just another bureaucratic decision is unconscionable and, to me, shows an intolerable lack of compassion," Kolb wrote.

In addition to the previously approved patients, Kolb said dozens of patients who would have been eligible for the drug "are suffering from great pain—many are dying."

It was a brutal letter, demonstrating just how deep the split was between the White House and the agencies. At the time we took the letter as a sign that fusion—a melding of patient interests and government policy—was still possible. But it was, in retrospect, a final gasp from the White House. Rick Harwood was on his way out and the other staffers in ONDCP had lost their will to resist. Kolb's letter was the classic CYA—cover your ass. If things went *real* bad when the program closed at least the White House could point to this one moment of humanitarian effort.

Mason would not comment on the letter but his spokesman did say the chief of public health would not be drawn into a public dispute with "an employee" of the drug control office. Clearly Mr. Mason had forgotten that he, too, was an employee.

Significantly the spokesman went on to note the concern of HHS "that harm may result from smoked marijuana for immune-suppressed people." The government had begun to back away from the homophobic notion of medical marijuana inducing unsafe sex but little else had changed.

Ms. Kolb's letter generated a quick blast of news coverage, and we used this as a springboard to call, once again, for Mason's resignation. On February 4, 1992, ten of the twelve legal marijuana recipients sent a letter to the PHS chief demanding that he step down. "You are engaged in a calculated campaign of medical terrorism directed against desperately ill people," we wrote. "Your actions are not merely illegal, they are immoral and have caused much unnecessary human suffering."

Mason again refused to comment. A spokesman said the final decision regarding the Compassionate IND program was with HHS Secretary Louis Sullivan. The Secretary's office had nothing to say. For six more weeks bureaucrats in Washington would drag their feet.

And in Panama City Beach, Florida, Barbra Jenks was dying.

February 28, 1992
Panama City Beach, Florida

Barbra and I sat on the deck of the Jenks' trailer. The air was warm and sweet in the early Florida spring and there was a heavy, earthy smell from the slash pines that graced Barbra and Kenny's yard. Officially Spring was still a month away but in the Sunshine State the first blushes of change had already begun.

It was the first anniversary of MARS. In Washington, Alice issued a press release noting the anniversary but it drew little attention from the press. I had fielded one or two calls that afternoon but it was generally quiet. Kenny had gone off for an evening "with the boys."

The last time I had seen Barbra was in late December. She had been hospitalized for nearly the entire month, battling numerous infections. She had lost a great deal of weight. The hospital had refused to allow her to smoke her legal marijuana, insisting the new drug Zofran would relieve her nausea. Kenny, in agony, had watched as Barbra vomited into a pan even as intravenous Zofran dripped into her arm. Finally he had barricaded the door, stuffed towels around the bottom and lit a joint. Within minutes Barbra's vomiting subsided. The next day he took her home.

When I arrived the following day I found a gravely emaciated and virtually incoherent Barbra. But by the end of my three-day stay in December Barbra was eating, bitching, and making plans.

Now, two months later, her color had returned. She was calm and talkative but no longer mentioned the future. She had despaired of caring for her hair and had most of it cut off. The effect was strangely compelling. There was an odd, almost ethereal, beauty about her. In 1991, Barbra had dreamed she would die in the spring and it seemed to me she might barely make it.

March 3, 1992
Indialantic, Florida

Ron Shaw was lying on his side, looking across a bedside table that was covered with prescription bottles of all sizes containing powerful narcotics like Percodan and morphine. Other bottles contained

Marinol, Valium, anti-spasmodic drugs, and sleeping tablets. None of them eased the post-polio sufferer's pain as well as marijuana. A photographer from *The Orlando Sentinel* furiously clicked away. The result would be a powerful image of yet another American forced to endure hardship because of marijuana's medical prohibition.

Ron was another of the 30 patients approved for medical marijuana supplies who was still waiting for his first legal joint. The 44-year old engineer had designed robotics for NASA, General Motors Corp., and Ford Motor Co. but the cumulative effect of disease and drugs had forced him into disability.

"With marijuana, the spasms subside. The pain is still there but it's in the back of me, not controlling me."

I watched as the photographer went about her business. Another had already left the Shaw's home having collected her images of Ron's handsome family—wife Linda, daughter Sandra, and son Ron Jr. I was impressed with Shaw's family and felt Ron was incredibly lucky to have them. They softened the man's pain-induced anger and made him more appealing.

"My father is no junkie," Ron Jr. told a reporter. "A junkie does it to get high. My father . . . will wait until the pain is unbearable and take a few puffs."

Like many medical marijuana patients, Ron Shaw first used the drug recreationally. In 1983, during the "Just Say No" campaign, Shaw stopped smoking marijuana. Over the next three years his condition had severely deteriorated and pain was wracking his body on a constant basis.

A friend left a marijuana cigarette one night and Shaw felt almost immediate relief after smoking it. Like countless other patients he thought the relief was an illusion but after a few more trials he realized the drug was directly affecting his spasm and pain.

Ron told his doctor, Richard Newman, who agreed to help Shaw. In 1990, Shaw contacted ACT and began the paperwork for a Compassionate IND. In 1991 he became the first black American to be approved for legal, medical access to marijuana. Then the PHS pulled the plug.

Dr. Newman, a former researcher with the National Institutes of Health, told the press that Shaw was a victim of "some so-called moralists [who] say this is a bad precedent."

Once again the bureaucrats in Washington had nothing to say. There would be no comment, they said, until Secretary Sullivan made his decision.

March 9, 1992
HHS Press Room
Washington, D.C.

Five days later, in a routine press conference, reporters learned Sullivan had already made the decision "last week." Bill Grigg, PHS spokesperson, delivered the news in response to a query by the Associated Press. Grigg would not specify exactly when the decision had come down. He would only say James O. Mason had recommended permanent closure of the Compassionate IND program for medical marijuana and Sullivan "did not have any problem with it."

When asked for a copy of the signed order another PHS spokesperson, Raford Kytal, suggested the inquirer file a Freedom of Information request.

Public reaction was fast and furious. In Minneapolis Tim Braun told an AP reporter, "They're giving me a death sentence." Ron Shaw said, "They can lock me up and put me in jail. I will be in pain no matter where I am." Mae Nutt, whose son had worked so tirelessly to pass the Michigan state bill before dying of cancer, said she felt as though "I've been kicked in the stomach." Editorial response was also harsh. *The Chicago Tribune* was typical: "The Public Health

Service's message to these people [who medically need marijuana] is: Drop dead."

Nine days later, on March 18, a second blow was delivered when the DEA responded to the April 1991 request by the U.S. Court of Appeals for clarification of the agency's rejection of Judge Young's 1988 ruling. The Court had found the DEA's rejection unreasonable and ruled the agency used inappropriate criteria. But the agency's March 1992 response was remarkably similar to the first in tone and content. It called medical marijuana a "cruel hoax" and the DEA administrator, Robert Bonner stated, "Beyond doubt, the claims that marijuana is medicine are false, dangerous, and cruel."

The rejection contained some harsh words for advocates of medical marijuana. "A century ago, many Americans relied on stories to pick their medicines, especially from snake oil salesmen," Bonner wrote. "Thanks to scientific advances and the Federal Food Drug and Cosmetic Act, we now rely on rigorous scientific proof to assure safety and effectiveness of new drugs."

ACT quickly issued a press release claiming the DEA and PHS were "acting in concert . . . to force seriously ill people into hiding." It went on, "The federal agencies . . . are seeking to impose a climate of fear in an effort to end the public debate over marijuana's medical use."

These were bold, harsh moves by the federal agencies. It was the final push, a desperate attempt to shut down public debate and silence the opposition. In the same week that Secretary Sullivan quietly signed the order killing the program, representatives from the National Institutes of Health (NIH) contacted each of the remaining physicians who had been granted permission to medically employ marijuana in the treatment of their patients but had not yet received supplies. The physicians were queried about their medical practices.

Had they tried *every* possible medication? Perhaps the patient was addicted to marijuana and just *thought* they needed the drug medically? Was the good doctor aware that marijuana could lead to unsafe sex?

It was a game of medical terrorism and, in some cases, it worked. Ten doctors withdrew their applications but the others held fast. To more rational minds in NIH, this strong stance by attending physicians was no doubt a sign of how critical marijuana could be to the continued health of patients. But rational minds were not listened to in these brutal days.

The bureaucrats were gambling the future of the medical prohibition on a Draconian approach and there was no backing away from it now. They were well aware that media assaults would be harsh and inflict some damage but megawatts alone would not alter the outcome. As far as the bureaucrats were concerned, the debate was over.

March 26, 1992
Panama City Beach, Florida

It was nearly 10:00 p.m. by the time Alice arrived at the small trailer set back in the Florida pines. There were no streetlights and no moon. Picking her way carefully along the unfamiliar ground she walked to the trailer door and knocked. The door opened and there was Kenny, a look of surprise on his face. "Alice! How did you . . . ? Where are the dogs?"

In an instant they were there, not menacing and ferocious but calm and friendly, as if Alice was a frequent guest. The two dogs angled to get close, hoping to edge into the trailer with this newly arrived visitor. As he followed her in and closed the door Kenny wondered aloud, "How did you get past the dogs?"

Alice looked quickly around the tiny space. The hospital bed, with Barbra's frail body, virtually consumed the room. Just inside the door was a large, overstuffed rocking chair. It held a young woman who smiled weakly at Alice.

The door shut behind her and Alice turned to Kenny. They hugged quickly. "Thanks for coming," he said. As they separated he introduced his sister in the chair. She didn't get up. Alice began to offer her hand but then, compulsively, bent down to hug her. Penny clung to her for an instant, like a child who had found a lost parent.

There were some brief, mildly awkward exchanges about plane rides, hotel accommodations, and the unbelievable number of college students that were packed into Panama City Beach, Florida. It was spring break and the migration of drunken, rowdy college students was in full gear. To the uninitiated it was stunning. To PCB it was economic lifeblood. To Alice it was a cruel and ironic counterimage to the shrunken form in the hospital bed.

"Here's Barb," Kenny said needlessly, moving towards the bed in the cramped and cluttered living space. He stroked Barbra's forehead. "Honey, you've got a visitor. Look who's come to see you."

Barbra's eyes opened and looked around. As they found the new visitor's face a look of puzzlement crossed her brow. Alice could see that Barbra was thinking hard. Was this a dream?

"Hey Barb," Alice said as she leaned over the bed and took Barbra's hand. "Barb, it's Alice," she said. Barbra's eyes seemed to focus on Alice's face and then began to open wide as she realized it wasn't a dream. It seemed to Alice that Barbra was absorbing her image more than seeing it. Barbra's eyes moved beyond Alice, looking over her shoulder. "No honey, Bob isn't with me. He's in Washington." Alice took her time speaking the words. As she spoke Barb's eyes moved repeatedly across her face. "I was visiting my Mom in Sarasota. When I heard you were so sick I had to come. I had to come see my traveling buddy."

Alice stroked Barb's forehead as she spoke. Kenny softly cautioned her to avoid the sore that had formed at the hair line. "Shingles," he explained. The frail figure held Alice's hand hard. Alice wondered where all that strength was coming from. Barbra had the sunken form of a concentration camp prisoner. She couldn't have weighed more than 85 pounds. Her lips were parched and dry, her breathing was labored despite the presence of an oxygen cannula.

"Oh friend," Alice whispered, "Look what this has done to you."

In those last 48 hours of Barbra's life Alice would watch a remarkable series of scenes as friends and family arrived and departed. Kenny's mother would insist upon a minister who arrived mid-afternoon on Saturday. He prayed at Barbra's bedside and then asked everyone present to hold hands and say a prayer with him. No one bothered to turn off the stereo or the TV. The elderly minister worked hard to make himself heard above the din, reciting a formal prayer about deliverance and salvation. Alice couldn't help but feel the real message was on the stereo as The Eagles triumphantly sang "I'm Already Gone." She could almost see Barbra's spirit starting to lift from that shattered body.

Barbra Jenks would die on March 28, 1992, just as the sun began to rise on Panama City Beach. She was 25 years old. Kenny was with her in the small hospital bed and he felt her slipping away. He got up and put their favorite song on the stereo, Stevie Nicks singing "Leather and Lace." Then he rejoined her in bed. As the song played and the sun entered the trailer through the small windows, Barbra died, peacefully, in Kenny's arms, in the spring.

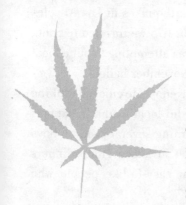

34   MARS on the Mall

THERE WAS LITTLE time to mourn Barbra's death. After nearly a year of protracted feints and jabs, the Public Health Service (PHS) had killed the Compassionate IND program. Anger at the government's action exploded among patients across the country. Many people who had remained silent now came forward to publicly condemn the PHS action. Newspapers across the nation ran local interest stories of patients denied access to care. From Boston to Sacramento editorial writers of every political persuasion crucified the Bush Administration for "killing compassion." *The News Herald* in Panama City captured the pervasive mood: "The decision to ban the use of marijuana . . . is based solely on the political effects of the drug on Bush's ill-advised "war on drugs." The *Star Tribune* of Minneapolis declared the PHS decision "evidence[s] a prejudice against study of this natural drug's medical effectiveness."

The phones at ACT rang constantly as reporters called for comments and patients sought guidance. Radio talk circuits were constantly active; the callers often enraged by the Government's brutal indifference to the welfare of seriously ill citizens. But, barring a miracle, we realized no amount of megawatts and ink would reopen the Compassionate IND program as long as George Bush was president.

A month after Barbra's death we took Kenny to California for some needed rest, relaxation and issue building. We met with many AIDS patients, did some media, encountered earthquakes in Los Angeles and San Francisco. Towards the end of our trip we traveled to Santa Cruz where a local activist, Scott Imler, was attempting to put a local marijuana-as-medicine initiative on the November ballot.

People in Santa Cruz were very kind to Kenny. He enjoyed walking the pier and watching the sea lions. We did local media in support of the upcoming voter initiative. One morning several good ol' boys took Kenny fishing. In the evenings Scott arranged group dinners featuring an abundance of eccentric but easy-to-like people who shared our concerns.

Alice and I were increasingly impressed with Scott Imler, the initiative organizer. Scott was a very tall, very lean man from Missouri, plain spoken and direct, who seemed to have a natural ability to organize chaos. More importantly he had a thoughtful understanding of the issue. Unlike most pot activists he seemed savvy, astute and cautious. An ally?

When we returned from California I asked Kenny if he wanted to stop. "Hell no, Robert. What those bureaucrats did was wrong. People need help and I'm the only AIDS patient in America who gets legal marijuana. That's wrong. I gotta speak out. Besides," he grinned broadly, "If I stop talking Barb would have my hide."

Indeed, despite—or perhaps because of—his faltering health Kenny developed a fervor about "speaking out" and "doing something." We accommodated his desire to remain active and, over the next six months, arranged a series of trips to AIDS conferences around the country where Kenny could speak with other PWAs, promote MARS, and agitate for change.

In the summer of 1992 we learned The Names Project was coming to Washington to display its rapidly expanding AIDS Quilt. The Quilt, which only a few years earlier had been small and comprehendible, now contained over 21,000 panels memorializing Americans who had died from this rampaging plague. When unfolded the Quilt, now the size of twelve football fields, would carpet the Mall from the Washington Monument and the Lincoln Memorial. Twelve football fields of sorrow.

Quilt organizers expected several hundred thousand people would visit their display. They also announced there would be a special area set aside for AIDS-related exhibits. In the past ACT had always communicated with mass audiences via the mass media. Perhaps it was time to ditch the media and meet our audience face to face. After much discussion we decided the Quilt provided MARS with the unique opportunity to directly involve people with AIDS in a protest against Bush administration efforts to kill the Compassionate IND program.

Gauging the gargantuan dimensions of the Quilt display we realized there was no way Alice, I and our part-time helper, Linda Barefoot, could put MARS on the Mall without outside help. It was time to recruit some Men from MARS.

Kenny, despite some incidental infections, was the first to volunteer. We also invited Jim Barnes, the man who had driven to Chicago to be part of our February 1991 MARS launch. Jim, a short, balding man with a bushy beard, lived with his lover, Gil, in near isolation, deep in the cold woods of the U.P. in Michigan. Shy and brooding he had good reason to be angry. FDA had approved his MARS application in February 1991. The bureaucrats even sent him a letter promising to provide him with medical marijuana. But then PHS closed the program and Jim Barnes never received his promised supplies. Accustomed to the wild silences of Lake Superior, Jim immediately accepted our invitation and was obviously excited about coming into the hustle of Washington. D.C.

Kenny and Jim were familiar friends. We also reached out to a newer acquaintance, Ezekiel Ramshur who hailed from Monroe, Louisiana. Ezekiel spoke with the slow, sweet lilt of his region and Alice believed him to be something of a country bumpkin, unfamiliar with big city ways. This image was reinforced when he told her he had never flown before or traveled more than 100 miles from his home. When Ezekiel asked if "a friend could accompany" him to Washington we quickly agreed. The more hands the better.

When Alice picked up Ezekiel and his friend Robert at National Airport she was surprised to find two smartly dressed gay men. Ezekiel was thin, even frail looking with a discreet, pencil-thin braid of hair which hung down the nape of his neck. His lover, Robert, was younger, hyper-blond and far more flamboyant—a Louisiana drag queen fresh from being crowned Miss Monroe. "The city, not the star," he exuberantly explained.

As we assembled our Men from MARS, I realized Alice needed at least one helper who was neither desperately ill nor nearly blind. After some thought I gave Scott Imler a call. By this time Scott had put Prop A on the Santa Cruz ballot and, despite the upcoming election, he jumped at the opportunity to come to Marble City to help us put MARS on the Mall.

Once we lined up the troops we began to consider what we could do. Initially, we planned a petition which visitors could sign. But this seemed static and dull. Besides, people would be forced to stop and stand on line before they could sign. And we would only capture those who took the time to visit our table.

We needed something which would engage AIDS patients in a

more dynamic, less cumbersome enterprise. After much debate we decided to hand out postcards pre-addressed to the Senate Committee on Health chaired by Senator Ted Kennedy. Individuals could sign their cards and leave them with us or take them home and send them on to Congress.

In addition to these postcards of protest we also prepared thousands of MARS brochures and dense packets of information. Finally, we printed large banners for our table and got MARS T-shirts so visitors to the Mall could quickly identify our Men from MARS.

We flew our troops in early and sent them off to Capitol Hill to meet with their respective Senators. Kenny and I visited Senator Kennedy's health aide and were pleased with the reception. "Maybe," the Senator's aide said, "we'll get a new president. Then he could just reopen the Compassionate IND program."

Kenny got excited. More cynical, I thought the man very nice for giving us his time.

October 9, 1992
The Mall
Washington, D.C.

The opening ceremonies of the Quilt display were delayed by a steady, cold rain. MARS also got off to a rocky start when some mean-assed young people stole our large MARS banner to use as an umbrella. They laughed and scattered as Kenny ran after them without success. Alice would arrive to find our Men from MARS wet, cold, and angry.

But the wet day had some redeeming features. The rain forced more people into the exhibit tent and thousands made their way through the mud and maze of tables to our booth. As the crowd increased our Men from MARS began passing out postcards by the handfuls. In exchange they began to receive the gratitude of those who had come to see the Quilt. Their spirits soared. Doctors, nurses, other PWAs (people with AIDS) flocked to our MARS exhibit, anxious to participate in our efforts. Among the clamoring hordes the most touching visitors to our booth were mothers who spoke of buying marijuana off the streets to help a dying son. There were tears of sorrow and solidarity.

By Friday afternoon the sun broke through the gloom and the number of people seeking information began to multiply. Energized by the manic demand we worked late into the evening.

Saturday dawned clear, cool, and bright: a brilliant autumn day. The trees, tinged with changing leaves, created an exquisite backdrop for the multi-colored hues of the Quilt. The crowds were massive. In the exhibit tent our Men from MARS worked non-stop, distributing information, passing out postcards, collecting signatures. The outpouring of support and encouragement was invigorating. Kenny was in his element: laughing, joking, "doing something." Ezekiel, who seemed so frail, blossomed as he and Robert worked tirelessly. All day, from first light to sunset our Men from MARS watched the passing parade of humanity. Jim Barnes, less outgoing, found the flood of people disquieting, but worked hard and was clearly moved by the constant praise he received for his efforts to get legal marijuana to PWAs.

That evening we closed our booth, ate boxed dinners beneath the Washington Monument, then joined 200,000 other people on the Ellipse for a candlelight march past the White House to the Lincoln Memorial. As thousands of marchers filed past the White House they chanted "Bye bye Bush" and "Pack your pearls, Babs," a reference to Barbara Bush's trademark necklace. Watching 200,000 candles flicker down Marble City streets was an awe inspiring sight.

Once we arrived at the Lincoln Memorial people gathered around the Reflecting Pool, their candles turning the water a mellow yellow. Prayers were said. Songs sung and speeches made. The huge crowd was hushed and one could hear the sound of quiet tears spread over the Mall.

Sunday was no less stressful. Hundreds of thousands of people descended on the Mall. The demand for MARS materials was overwhelming. By the time we closed our booth it was clear MARS on the Mall had been a tremendous success. We collected nearly 6,000 postcards on-site and distributed another 10,000 to people who would provide their own delivery. "They was like pigeons on popcorn," Kenny said.

At the end of the day we surveyed our weary volunteers to make certain each was holding up all right. When I took Ezekiel aside and asked if he was okay he replied in his soft, so gentle voice, "Mr. Randall, this has been the best day of my life. I feel great."

Our Men from MARS were very happy, very tired campers.

We had barely recovered from the Quilt exhibit before we were back on the road. To Kenny's delight we returned to California to campaign for Scott Imler's Proposition A initiative. Prop A was the first countywide ballot initiative for medical marijuana. The previous year Prop P had passed in San Francisco. It was a significant victory, but not unexpected in the city of Flower Power and the Summer of Love.

Prop A would test the political strength of medical marijuana in a more conservative, politically diverse environment. The city of Santa Cruz was notoriously liberal and populated with "free spirits" who would be expected to support medical marijuana. But the rest of the county was largely rural and populated by people with strongly conservative inclinations.

Kenny's spirit was indomitable, but AIDS was beginning to get the upper hand. He arrived in Santa Cruz in a great deal of pain.

Despite his legal marijuana, his appetite was failing and vomiting was becoming a serious problem.

On November 2, 1992, Prop A would win decisively, gaining 77.5% of the vote. In the post-election analysis, Scott Imler would note with pride that Prop A carried every district in the county. Medical marijuana, once again, revealed its trans-ideological appeal. Liberal or conservative, Americans believed seriously ill patients should have legal access to needed care.

Immediately following the election, Alice traveled to Florida for two conferences: AIDS Manasota in Bradenton, and Association of Nurses in AIDS Care at Disney World. Kenny, now obviously unwell, joined her in Orlando, continuing his quest to "do something." In a letter to a friend she would note, "He has changed so much since Barb's death. I watch him at these conferences, soaking up positive affirmations, bouncing around the surrealness of his life. These meetings are more therapeutic than any drug he can get but there aren't enough meetings in the world for Kenny and he knows it."

America was about to get a new president. William Jefferson Clinton had squeaked by scandals to win a razor thin victory. It was, many believed, a new day. Certainly there was a change in tone. We were surprised when Clinton tapped a black woman, Dr. Joycelyn Elders, for Surgeon General. In the December 17, 1992 *Arkansas Times* Dr. Elders sent some encouraging signs. "We prescribe morphine for pain and I think doctors should be able to prescribe marijuana as well, if they feel it's medically called for."

Brave words. Reasonable thoughts. Perhaps it was new day.

In December 1992 we began preparing recommendations for the newly elected Bill Clinton, which would evolve into a 50-page booklet titled *Marijuana as Medicine: Initial Steps*. It reviewed the history of the issue and outlined proposed solutions.

As we worked to outline the future it became clear Kenny's health had collapsed. An opportunistic infection of unknown type was ravaging our friend. Kenny took massive overdoses of antibiotics and was given morphine to quell the pain. By Christmas the crisis passed. Kenny would rally, regain lost weight, slowly rebound. But we all knew Kenny had seen his last New Year.

35 False Hope

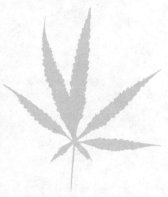

IN THE EARLY part of 1993 we would fly Kenny back to D.C. to hand-deliver the signed postcards from MARS on the Mall to Senator Kennedy. We had hoped to do this before the new year, but Kenny's health was beginning to fail and his strength wouldn't allow a trip.

When we finally arrived at Kennedy's office we learned that thousands of postcards had already reached the Senator independently, fulfilling our hope that people would return home and distribute the cards to others.

Kennedy's aide was encouraging and supportive but he was also wavering. Bill Clinton's election had given the Senator an excuse to "wait and see." "Things are going to change," the aide promised. We'd heard it before.

It would be Kenny's last trip away from his home under the slash pines. He stayed with Alice and me while in Washington. On more than one occasion. Alice would be up during the night comforting Kenny as he coped with terrible pain which brought on waves of nausea and vomiting. Pain seemed to be constantly with him. As

Alice would note, "He was munching morphine like some people eat peanuts."

Kenny was slipping away.

When Alice and I were arrested in 1975 Gerald Ford was president. Now, seventeen years and four presidents later, Bill Clinton was taking the oath. Bill Clinton was our age, our generation. His oblique comments about marijuana use—tried it but didn't inhale— did not cause us any consternation. We really didn't care what Bill Clinton proposed to do for social smokers. We wanted the Compassionate IND program open again and that did not seem like too much to ask.

As we prepared the booklet entitled *Marijuana as Medicine: Initial Steps—Recommendations for the Clinton Administration*, our goal was simple: to provide the incoming Clinton Administration with the history of the medical marijuana problem and suggest three avenues of action: 1) restore compassion, 2) encourage research, and 3) explore options. The 50-page booklet was ready by the end of January, and we began mailings to every incoming member of the Clinton Administration plus all members of Congress. The Compassionate IND program had been officially closed for less than one year and we felt there was a strong possibility of succeeding with our requests. Once again, however, we underestimated the forces at work within the federal marijuana prohibition. The New Year had begun with an announcement that synthetic THC, marketed for nearly a decade as Marinol, would be approved for use by people with AIDS for appetite stimulation and treatment of nausea and vomiting.

The feds had correctly observed that the pressure for medical marijuana was primarily coming from the AIDS community, just as cancer patients had driven the first medical marijuana push in the late 1970s and early '80s. The bureaucrats hoped that by officially approving Marinol for AIDS-related symptoms they could relieve the pressure and quiet the issue once more.

But PWAs were not fooled by the federal gambit. Marinol had been used by AIDS patients for several years, even though the indication was not "officially" recognized in the *Pharmacopoeia*. The synthetic didn't work. The same problems manifested themselves: poor bioavailability, difficulty in determining the proper dose, and the practical problems of keeping down a pill when a patient is vomiting.

The federal shell game also failed because of a radically different patient population. Cancer patients seemed to have an assurance that society and the medical community was doing all that could be done for them. AIDS patients, ostracized and stigmatized by society, had just the opposite impressions. They had grown accustomed to fighting for every treatment available. There was a strong, and sadly, often correct feeling that society could care less about these terminally ill people.

And there was a political savviness that was lacking in cancer patients. This was particularly obvious in ACT-UP, the AIDS Coalition To Unleash Power. ACT-UP was notorious for public demonstrations, particularly at federal agencies such as the FDA. ACT-UP had also begun a service for AIDS patients called "buyers' clubs" where PWAs could purchase needed drugs at reduced prices. In 1992, as the feds moved to shutdown MARS and the Compassionate IND program, some PWA buyer's clubs began to include marijuana as part of their inventory.

This concept of patients helping patients was not new. For years, particularly in the community of paralyzed people, patients had cooperated to obtain quantities of marijuana together. It was more economic and efficient. And in 1979, following the death of her son Keith, Mae Nutt had operated the "Green Cross," a type of "co-op" that provided marijuana to cancer patients throughout Michigan. The Green Cross, and other groups like it, went about their business quietly. They were well-known and often tolerated by law officials.

But in late 1992, when cannabis buyers' clubs first emerged, there was a new feeling, a new stridency. The anger and righteousness that I had counted upon was evident in the news articles, the editorials, and the public's mood. The beast had been unmasked. The decades-old federal lie—"anyone with a legitimate medical need can obtain legal access to marijuana"—was revealed. The memory hole was unearthed.

The feds did not care one single bit about the seriously ill. Their goal was to maintain the total and absolute prohibition regardless of what truth they trampled in the process. In 1977 Peter Bourne had written to me and grandly assured, "The responsible agency staffs and researchers involved . . . all share with me a great feeling of compassion and are pledged to pursue the question."

It was bull then and it still was in 1992. Each successive administration had boldly promised the same unerring devotion to "compassion and pursuit of the truth." Yet the federal government, which controlled medical marijuana utterly, had not a single research project underway that would help answer the questions first posed in the early 1970s. Billions were spent for the war on drugs but not a single cent was allocated for researching marijuana's therapeutic use.

Weary of government people they took matters into their own hands, and the cannabis buyer's clubs were born. The clubs began in San Francisco, which was struggling to implement Prop P, a citywide initiative that recognized marijuana's medical utility but did nothing to provide supplies of the drug to the seriously ill. There was talk of allowing limited cultivation but the talk droned on and no official action was taken. So citizens began to take their own action. Brownie Mary, an elderly woman who volunteered on the AIDS floors at S.F. General Hospital, began bringing marijuana brownies to the wards. There was talk of opening a "marijuana store."

In Washington, D.C., the cannabis buyer's club opened in December 1992. We were under some pressure to endorse these clubs but we resisted for several reasons. We were unwilling to openly encourage illegality and place patients at legal as well as medical risk. Nor did we feel that home cultivation or contraband supplies were the answer to medical access to marijuana. Such solutions were completely inappropriate for the vast majority of those needing medical access. We saw no reason why marijuana should not be available by prescription. The seriously ill needed a regulated, reliable source of medicine. Lastly, we viewed the "clubs" as too loosely structured, allowing many with questionable "ailments" to obtain marijuana. This source of abuse could potentially harm the medical marijuana movement.

ACT was criticized for not embracing the buyer's club concept. We took pains to avoid the conflict but club organizers felt "snubbed." One D.C. activist accused us of "not caring about the sick." After seventeen years of battling to expand the medical use of marijuana it was an odd accusation to hear.

We continued on the path that we had long ago established—attempting to reform the legal barriers that prohibited medical access to marijuana. We placed our fate in the hands of the man from Hope, Arkansas. Across the land there was hope that Bill Clinton would do the right thing.

The year would move on slowly while Clinton settled into the job.

Rumors were flying about his plans for medical marijuana. He appointed Dr. Philip Lee from San Francisco as the head of PHS, James Mason's old job. Activists from San Francisco claimed the Compassionate IND program would soon be reopened by "their good friend." It was promising but not speedy. With each passing month there was a growing sense that our "friends" in the White House didn't much care about medical marijuana. Efforts to meet with administration officials and discuss the issue fell flat.

It was our least publicly active period in four years but there was plenty going on. Press interest in the issue continued to multiply and

I seemed to be constantly engaged in talk radio or press interviews. In March 1993 we captured the unanimous endorsement of the American Medical Student Association. In a strongly worded resolution the association of aspiring doctors called on the new Attorney General, Janet Reno, to abide by the 1988 decision of Judge Young.

"President Clinton . . . should end the medical prohibition against marijuana by creating a rational system of prescriptive medical access to a now-prohibited drug." The group went on to note, "Seriously ill Americans are suffering because of prohibitory federal policies" and asked the Clinton Administration to reopen the Compassionate IND program.

We also spent this time preparing ACT's response to the DEA rejection of marijuana. In the process we enlisted the support of The Physicians Association for AIDS Care (PAAC) and the National Lymphoma Foundation. Both groups filed "friend of the court" briefs on behalf of medical access to marijuana.

As the mechanics of the issue churned on we watched, with heavy hearts, the decline of friends as AIDS continued to take its toll.

In April, returning to D.C. from a visit with her mother, Alice stopped in Panama City Beach to help Kenny contend with a film crew from The Discovery Channel. The cable network was preparing a four part documentary, "In a Time of AIDS" and had first met Kenny on the Washington Mall during the AIDS Quilt display and that wondrous weekend of the Men from MARS. Now, they were conducting more detailed interviews. Kenny was worried about having the strength to make it through the taping and Alice was there to act as a buffer.

The film crew, young and energetic, wanted Kenny to go with them to the beach and walk on the wharf. They had seen this on "60 Minutes" and it was good footage. Kenny, polite by nature, had initially said yes. Alice quietly pulled the producer aside and explained

Kenny was too ill for such exertion. Even the obligatory walk through the front yard was almost more than Kenny could bear. In the small trailer, under the hot spotlights, Alice could see Kenny was having a very hard time concentrating. When the producer asked him to talk about Barbra he became uncharacteristically quiet and asked for a break.

"You okay, Kenny?" Alice was concerned. "I just didn't know what to say, Alice. What can I say about Barb?" Alice looked around the trailer for something of Barbra and found the photographic montage that Kenny's sisters and Barb's friends had prepared for Barbra's funeral. Again she pulled the producer aside. "Get him to talk about the pictures," she advised. With camera and lights off, Kenny and the producer reviewed the montage together. Laughing and telling tales, Kenny found his focus and finished the interview.

Spacecoast Surfer, the impish activist from Florida's East Coast, was also failing. His calls became sporadic, his conversation elliptical. In mid-June, from his hospital bed, Surfer told me he was thinking of "traveling to Bermuda." The next day he had changed his mind. "I think I'll go home," he said. It was our last conversation.

In mid June I traveled to Florida to visit Kenny. While I was away, Alice became alarmed by Surfer's silence. She called the hospital in Indiatlantic. "Whiteside?" the hospital operator said. "There's no Craig Whiteside here."

Perhaps he had gone home but calls to his apartment went unanswered. Alice redialed the hospital and a brusque nurse finally punched up more information on the computer screen. "Craig Whiteside expired."

Alice could not, would not, fathom the word. "Expired?"

"He died," came the cold, abrupt explanation.

Kenny absorbed the news of Surfer's passing with little emotion. He was rail thin, weighing little more than 100 lbs. He was no longer looking to the future. In his cramped trailer we would sit for hours, idly watching TV, reviewing scrapbooks, looking at pictures, chatting about the times in which "we just kept hitting 'em and hitting 'em, didn't we?"

"How are you going to win this, Robert?" Kenny asked. It was a question I heard often in those days. To Kenny I would honestly confide I wasn't quite sure but I was working on plans. "I wish I could help you but . . ." The words trailed off. The sentence did not need to be finished.

Alice would return to Panama City in the last week of June. On July 1 she would say goodbye to Kenny. "I don't think I'll see you again," Kenny said. Alice knew he was right. "Well, Kenny, if we don't meet again in this life be certain you save a place for Bob and me on the other side."

"You know I will. Me and Barb will be waitin' on you. I love you guys."

"And we love you, guy."

Kenny would remain in his trailer, with his dogs and memories. Federal funds, paid under the Ryan White Act, provided Kenny with housekeeping services and Fate sent him a real-life angel named Fatima, a Portuguese immigrant who grew very fond of Kenny and took good care of him.

On July 19 Kenny died in Fatima's arms in his trailer under the slash pines. It was the day before what would have been Barb's 27th birthday. Kenny was 31.

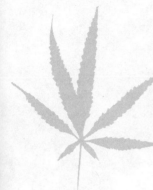

V

Coming of Age

36 Beyond MARS

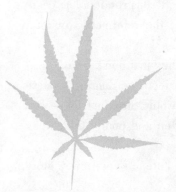

WITH KENNY'S PASSING we were emancipated from a deep meditation on death. Since Steve L.'s call in October 1989 my nights had been a dialogue with now departed spirits. My apprehension of life's fragility was keen; honed as a razor by four years of travel among the young dying.

Our journey along the River Styx had produced tangible benefits. Grand strategies had been played; small lives enlarged. Immersed in mortality we made uncertain plans while bidding farewell to friends rushing to catch the Ferryman's boat.

Now, for the moment, for the first time in four years, my nights were quiet. I was liberated. Alone. Exhausted to the bone. It was a dream time of introspection and reflection.

In the silence that now filled my nights I mused upon the future course. Had we not come far, accomplished much? We could stop here, take up pen and write savagely on the folly of men. Perhaps this is what Fate intends. Perhaps not. Such decisions are made by gods, not men.

Alone along the River Styx I gazed upon the many paths that radiated from this sad place but I could not follow them.

Not yet.

Kenny's death not only left a void in our life, it left a void in the issue. In the weeks following his death a curious question was presented to me over and over again. Some were able to deliver the question with sympathy and tact. Others were incredibly crass. "Who is Kenny's understudy?" they asked. Several AIDS patients phoned to volunteer for the "role."

As if Kenny and Barbra were concocted constructions, as easily fabricated as paper mache stage props, the reformers wondered "Who's the next 'star' of medical marijuana?"

As Barbra would have said, "Robert, they just don't get it!"

Those who saw Kenny and Barbra as icons set against a static backdrop believed endless reproductions would turn the trick—were the trick. But even the best story, too often and poorly told, wears thin and frays.

They do not understand it was time for Fate to weave a new story.

MARS, in final flower, had played its role brilliantly. Medical marijuana was now part of the national dialogue. The battle for hearts and minds had been won.

Our support spanned the political spectrum. In May 1993, the conservative *Orange County Register*, Ronald Reagan's hometown newspaper, polled its readers and reported a whopping 93 % favored making marijuana legally available for medical use. Clearly, our message resonated. The goal now was to translate this preponderance of popular support into useful power. How could this be done?

Alas, such questions were no longer our exclusive concern. MARS had performed as expected, creating vast reservoirs of energy. We had played Tom Sawyer well; making medical marijuana so enticing that everyone wanted to paint our fence. Many were anxious to "get in on the action." There were packs of alpha-pups aching to take a bite. The rush of so many new, discordant voices was jarring. For

years we had been autonomous, able to articulate our message without competing overtones. Now, in the vast vortex of new energies,
medical marijuana was beginning to lose its singular voice.

We watched these new actors with a measure of dread and delight.
While the infusion of new voices was bracing, the danger of mingled
motives was clear. Drug reformers wanted to turn medical marijuana
into a "grow your own" issue. But the desperately ill were not looking
for a unique horticultural experience. They were seeking critically
needed medical care. Drug reformers seemed oblivious to such fine
distinctions.

We reasoned our best strategy was to ignore these newly activated,
somewhat inept actors. By refusing to engage we avoided being drawn
into the petty politics and vicious in-fighting which dominated much
of the drug-reform movement. We had no interest in debating whether
patients should be legally allowed to grow 2 plants or 6 plants. Such
debate trivialized the problem and diverted attention from the Federal Government's intransigent refusal to meet basic human needs.

As drug ideologues prepared for cross-cultural warfare it was time
for us to move Beyond MARS.

Following Kenny's death, several events presented themselves
that allowed us to apply political pressure on the still waffling Clinton
Administration.

California is a mighty political prize capable of swaying the opinions of first term Presidents. We had invested heavily in California
and now we were about to reap our return.

The citizens of San Francisco and Santa Cruz had overwhelmingly
voted to make marijuana medically available. Boards of Supervisors
from liberal Marin to conservative San Luis Obispo endorsed similar
actions. In the Golden State medical marijuana was riding a riptide
of popular support.

In early 1993, shortly after medical marijuana won 77 % of the
vote in Santa Cruz County, Scott Imler received a call. Senate Majority Leader Henry Mello was the most powerful Democrat in the

MARIJUANA RX

nation's largest state and he wanted to help solve the medical marijuana problem.

Scott was quick to realize the potential of such an offer and called for advice. Mello was uncertain about how to proceed and vaguely talked with Scott about legislation that would authorize medical access on a statewide basis. The Senator was aware the implementation of such legislation would likely be blocked by federal authorities but what else could be done?

Scott and I knew this was an opportunity to put pressure on Washington and working together we drafted a resolution which condemned the federal prohibition of medical marijuana. It was exactly what Senator Mello wanted.

Mello's resolution quickly gained broad bipartisan support and, in June, it easily passed in the Senate with a vote of 22–9.

The measure was moving toward a final vote in the Assembly when Scott phoned for help. Hearings in the Assembly had been held in late July. Not surprisingly the Traditional Values Coalition, and a similar group called Committee on Moral Concerns, testified against the Resolution deriding the attempts of "pro-drug groups" to legalize marijuana through "the smoke screen" of medical use. Representatives from NORML did little to dispel this notion when their "supportive" testimony wandered into the area of "the need" for a state law authorizing "personal cultivation." Drug ideologues to the left and right. Suddenly Mello's Resolution was viewed with some alarm. Passage was threatened.

Since there was little hope of taming the pro-pot activists, I took steps to supercede them, offering to testify at hearings and meet with any delegates who might be wavering.

Senator Mello quickly accepted the offer of help. In my conversations with the aging, well-regarded politician, I found an astute and learned champion. It was clear Mello had "done his homework." He had even read *Marijuana as Medicine: Initial Steps* and took the time to praise its moderate, sensible approach. But Senator Mello also had a personal interest. "My two sisters died of cancer," he told me. "If marijuana can help it should be legally available."

Within weeks of Kenny's death I was in California attending the final hearings, meeting with the press and shoring up support. All went well. The hempsters expended tremendous energy to aggravate a few conservatives. The family values representatives managed to aggravate the liberals. The testimony of patients—including myself—kept the message clear, the goal precise.

"The problem is in Washington," I told the committee. "This resolution puts the blame where it belongs."

On August 26, Senate Joint Resolution 8 passed with broad bipartisan support—47–20. The California resolution would be delivered to the White House, the Department of Health and Human Services, the Department of Justice, the President of the Senate, the Speaker of the House and all members of the California Congressional delegation.

Henry Mello was proud of his resolution and determined to do more.

"What can we do, Robert?" the old pol asked.

"Well, sir, the big problem seems to be the DEA. If the Clinton Administration would suspend legal proceedings long enough to objectively review the agency's actions we might be able to take some positive steps toward resolving the problem."

"That seems reasonable. Have you suggested this?"

"Well, Senator Mello, they tend to see my views as biased but if someone outside of Washington, someone with some authority and no ties to this issue were to suggest such an action they might listen."

Senator Mello smiled.

In early September I was hard at work with Senator Mello on a letter to Attorney General Janet Reno.

The letter, dated September 13th, reflected Mello's no-nonsense style. After first "respectfully" requesting a personal review of DEA's effort to block marijuana's legitimate medical use, Mello leveled his sights: "DEA's legal position, that marijuana has 'no accepted medical use in treatment in the United States,' is clearly in error."

Mello's letter was a political broadside. He told Reno:

I am concerned that, unless you act quickly the Clinton Administration may find itself defending this widely discredited Bush Administration policy. Specifically, I am referring to the pending case of *ACT v DEA* . . . which is scheduled for oral argument" on October 1.

Mello sought to assure the Attorney General this was not a "prodrug issue." Referring to his resolution Mello wrote:

Significantly, Senate Joint Resolution 8 secured bipartisan support in both the California Senate and Assembly. During public hearings, several legislators related personal stories of desperately ill friends or loved ones who, because of overzealous DEA policies, were forced to illegally obtain the marijuana they medically required. The California Medical Association and patient-advocacy groups also endorsed Senate Joint Resolution 8.

In light of such support and especially because the filing of the DEA lawsuit predates the arrival of the Clinton Administration, I strongly recommend the Department of Justice immediately reexamine the Drug Enforcement Administration's generally discredited efforts to maintain the medical prohibition. Specifically, I urge you to suspend further legal action in the case of *ACT v DEA* until you and others at the Department of Justice and the Department of Health and Human Services can review Bush Administration actions in this area.

Rather than defending the Bush Administration's failed efforts to enforce the medical prohibition, I am hopeful that the Clinton Administration will be working with credible patients and physicians to find reasonable solutions.

Our experience here in California indicates that the medical community and the American people already know marijuana has important medical properties and strongly believe the natural plant should be legally available for prescriptive medical uses under certain circumstances.

It was a courageous letter that gave us new hope. In addition to Attorney General Reno, the letter was sent to Donna Shalala, Secretary of HHS; Phillip Lee, Assistant Secretary at HHS (and a Californian); Joycelyn Elders, U.S. Surgeon General (who had publicly supported medical marijuana use before her confirmation); Bruce Lindsay, Domestic Affairs Office in the White House; Robert Bonner, Administrator, DEA; and Henry Waxman, Chairman of the U.S. House of Representatives Subcommittee on Health (and a Californian).

Senator Mello's letter tripped through the Clinton Administration then ricocheted around Washington. With Mello's permission ACT released his letter to the national media, sparking new interest.

There was little chance Janet Reno would suspend the DEA case, but Mello's plea could awaken the slumbering Clinton crowd. It belied the bureaucratic claims that medical marijuana was supported only by radical pro-drug advocates. Senator Mello, who played a critical role in Clinton's California victory, was not a pro-drug radical and had never been aligned with drug reform efforts in the past. He was a perfect voice and we were hopeful there was finally someone who could make himself heard above the drug war din.

On the eve of oral arguments before the U.S. Court of Appeals it seemed Senator Mello's letter might have reached its mark when an

HHS spokesperson told a CNN reporter that a "review" of medical marijuana was "in progress."

It was the first public pronouncement on medical marijuana from the nine-month old Clinton Administration.

October 1, 1993
U.S. Court of Appeals
Washington, D.C.

The case of *ACT v DEA* was once again before the U.S. Court of Appeals. Among NORML and the other reform groups there was great optimism.

In the ACT camp things were not quite as cocky. Steve Davidson, our attorney from Steptoe & Johnson, warned the law was against us. He made a forceful argument before the Court that the facts demonstrated DEA's arbitrary handling of the case. But Steve was aware that administrative regulations gave the DEA the right to ignore an administrative law judge's recommendation.

USA Today reported on the Court of Appeals case and carried a sidebar entitled "Cannabis clubs open for medicinal business."

The article reported that clubs were operating in San Francisco, Washington, D.C., New York, and Little Rock, Arkansas. "Other clubs operate underground," the story reports, "but are well-organized."

The San Francisco club was run by Dennis Peron, the author of Proposition P. Peron, a gay pot grower and oft-arrested drug dealer, had moved to the forefront of medpot efforts in California. It had long been Peron's ambition to run a retail pot shop, and his use of sick people to shield his illegal business was bound to attract attention. In exotic San Francisco a gay drug dealer openly peddling pot may be tolerated, even celebrated. But America is not so naïve.

From the prices posted at Peron's Pot Shoppe it was clear that this was no charity undertaking. The article noted marijuana was "free to the poor." Others paid "at cost plus 25%." This translates to $85 per ⅛ of an ounce. Despite Peron's pretense to the role of folk hero we saw him as a drug war profiteer playing a reckless game.

Two days after the Court of Appeals hearing I was on my way to San Diego for the criminal trial of *California v Skipper*. For the first time a California court would entertain a defense of "medical necessity."

I anticipated a quick trip to California but procedural matters extended the case and for two weeks I lived in the lower left-hand corner of America, watching fleet carriers come and go in San Diego Harbor. It would be difficult to find a place more removed from the Capitol or more conservative in inclination than San Diego. A beautiful city.

Sam Skipper was arrested for growing marijuana in his home. I was contacted by his public defender, Juliana Humphries.

Sam, 39, was a gay gardener who had watched 51 friends and lovers die from AIDS. First arrested for marijuana cultivation in 1990, Sam pled guilty because his lover was dying and he didn't want to cope with legal procedures. He was released on probation. Then, in March 1993, vice cops again raided Sam's modest suburban home and found 70 marijuana plants. Facing prison and death, Sam Skipper decided to fight.

After the vice cops collected evidence and left, Sam planted new seeds, then set off to a head shop in Oceanside where he found, and bought, the store's last copy of *Marijuana & AIDS: Pot, Politics & PWAs in America*, which Alice had published in late 1991. "It was such a pretty color," Sam said. The book led Sam to ACT and MARS, just as my article on Steve in *High Times* had led Kenny and Barbra to me.

Sam's story was familiar. He had been HIV-positive for at least 4 years. His 51 friends who faithfully followed doctors' orders and took scores of toxic prescriptive potions were now all stone-cold dead. Sam looked great: healthy, high-spirited, well-nourished with good color. Why?

"Pot's kept me alive," Sam said without a trace of hesitation. Sam used marijuana in a different way than most AIDS patients. He would literally graze his way through his marijuana garden, pinching buds and munching on fresh leaves. He also mixed finely ground pot into peanut butter balls. Of modest height, he was a slightly pudgy 153 lbs.

Sam knew what it was like to slip off the tightrope. On the several occasions when he had no marijuana he lost 2 pounds a day.

Juliana Humphries once saw Sam when he was without marijuana; pale, rail-thin, nauseated, unable to eat. Like Sam, Juliana had watched good friends with AIDS vanish. She was a deeply committed advocate.

Sam's trial revealed the importance of Senator Mello's efforts as well as the overwhelming public support for medical necessity.

In pre-trial motions I testified at length about my medical use of marijuana and that of AIDS patients like Kenny, Barbra, and Steve L. But the judge had only one question: Did I know anything about Senator Mello's medical marijuana resolution? I outlined the Resolution and the recent vote. That was enough for the judge. He concluded since the state legislature, "the voice of the people," had endorsed SJR 8—including marijuana's use in AIDS therapy—Samuel C. Skipper, a citizen of California, must have a legal right to raise a defense of medical need.

As we moved on to the task of empaneling a jury I witnessed an awesome demonstration of how pervasive the acceptance of medical marijuana was in the general populace. Fourteen potential jurors— one after the other—took the stand and bluntly told the prosecutor there was no way they would convict a man with AIDS for the crime of medically employing marijuana. No way!

Sam Skipper's case dominated the San Diego news. A telephone poll conducted by one local TV station found 76% of the good citizens of conservative San Diego believed Sam Skipper had a right to medically use marijuana.

Not surprisingly, the jury acquitted him on all charges.

As the Skipper trial moved forward in San Diego, a medical necessity defense was also under way in England. Within three days of Skipper's verdict a British jury would deliberate for less than 50 minutes and find a doctor "not guilty" by reason of "medical necessity" for providing marijuana to her seriously ill daughter. The nature of the daughter's illness was prohibited from public knowledge by a court order. It was the first successful test of a marijuana-based medical necessity defense in Britain.

Alice worked closely with the doctor, Anne Biezanek, and her attorney. In "Dr. B.," Alice found another kindred soul in our long journey. An indomitable British spirit, Dr. Biezanek was an unstoppable proponent of medical marijuana.

"I became a criminal because my conscience said that it would be wrong of me to obstruct [my daughter's medical use]." Dr. Biezanek explained to the press. "I was following a higher moral law."

Initially Anne Biezanek had been horrified to learn of her youngest child's marijuana use. At 33, Lucy had led a troubled life and modern medicine had done little to contribute to her well being. Setting off on her own to live in Scotland, Lucy, who preferred at the time of her trial to be called Ice Jesus Jones, discovered that cannabis could help stabilize her condition as no other medicine could. Eventually Dr. B. came to see that Lucy was right and, in the course of helping her procure the medication, Dr. B. was "popped" by the local constabulary.

Indeed, in that Fall of 1993, there were many parents who were helping their children procure illegal medication. *The New York*

Times carried a story on 79-year-old Mildred Kaitz who grew marijuana to relieve her son's multiple sclerosis. Unlike Anne Biezanek, however, Mildred Kaitz was found guilty by a judge and sentenced to six months probation.

One chilling line in *The Times* revealed the new direction of the issue. "Groups like the National Organization for the Reform of Marijuana Laws have seized on her case," the paper said, "to argue for allowing the sick to use marijuana."

When Alice contacted Mildred to offer assistance Mildred's only question was: "You don't have anything to do with those NORML people, do you?"

As we entered November 1993 the level of media coverage was off scale. It was "sweeps" month for television, that odd time of year when stations outdo themselves to garner the highest ratings. Medical marijuana was "hot" and it seemed every local, national, and cable network was running a story on the denial of medication to the seriously ill.

From the ridiculous to the sublime the video images seemed nonstop. NBC "Nightly News" weighed in with a piece that was borderline trash. The segment featured Steve Smith, an AIDS patient who had opened the Washington, D.C. Cannabis Buyer's Club. Smith was articulate and compelling but the presence of a bong—a pipe used to smoke marijuana—undercut the message. Then it was on to swinging San Francisco where Papa Peron gathered the pitiful together to party hearty for the cameras. Large groups of people passing joints in a cosmically decorated "cannabis café" hardly conveyed medical need. The NBC story ignored the plight of patients. It was trite, tabloid TV.

CNN weighed in with a story about a Rabbi who delivered pot to dying cancer patients. It was very powerful. In this media-frenzied month talk radio vaulted me around America. A glut of new stories, including several wire overviews, were tumbling out of the media machine.

We were approaching media glaze when The Discovery Channel documentary "In the Time of AIDS" aired. Just seven months before, Alice had helped Kenny through the interviews for this show.

On the first night our old friend Kenny was electronically resurrected and he finally got his opportunity to publicly condemn the blood companies which conspired to murder him and Barbra. It was damn good stuff.

The next night's show contained a jumbled segment on "new therapies" and the marijuana/AIDS connection popped open briefly to file footage of the Jenks trial and Kenny proudly wearing his MARS T-shirt.

The third segment had nothing about Kenny or medical marijuana. The fourth, and last, installment droned out its sad story for almost an hour without any sign of our departed friend.

Then, at the very end of this extensive overview of the global AIDS crisis—after tons of talking heads, endless statistics, and numbing personal stories—then came the show's final images. We were suddenly transported back to MARS on the Mall and there was Kenny at the Quilt, warmly lit in the autumn sun, cheery in his yellow MARS T-shirt and ready smile. He was explaining why he didn't bring a panel for Barbra to the Quilt Display. "It didn't seem right to just have a panel for Barb. My wife and me, we were never separated in life. It didn't seem right to be separated in death."

As his voice-over continued the images faded to Kenny and Barbra in their trailer, happy and full of life, mugging a big kiss for the video eye. The audio shifted to Michael Callan's haunting song, "What We Don't Have Is Time," the song that had moved 200,000 marchers in the candlelight vigil for AIDS at the Quilt Display. And as the video image froze on Kenny and Barbra's kiss, the date of Kenny's death appeared on the screen.

It was sublime. Old friends, gazing back from across the River Styx.

The intense media barrage, the California Resolution, Senator Mello's letter to the Attorney General, Sam Skipper, the death of Kenny Jenks—it was a constant assault on government policies. Once again the bureaucrats were scrambling to get ahead of the public demand for action. But their long-held fallback position—anyone who needs marijuana medically can obtain it through the Compassionate IND program—was gone.

Their second line of defense—we must wait for science to answer these questions—now became the focal point of their endeavor.

Of course the optimum opportunity to scientifically investigate marijuana's medical value—the state-mandated research programs of the late 1970s and 1980s—had all been squashed by the boot heel of drug control agencies. But never mind that. Such efforts had long ago been relegated to the memory hole.

No, it was the '90s now and *this* time there would be a *real* scientific study.

I was supposed to be a part of this latest scientific charade. That was the reason for summoning me to the FDA in December of 1990. The trap was obvious and I wouldn't play. Instead we launched MARS.

But I knew the FDA would look for someone else. They had no choice.

For several years government bureaucrats had promised a marijuana/AIDS study. An FDA designed study called for 50 % of the participants to receive placebo pot to establish "efficacy." Throughout the AIDS community, however, there was no question of marijuana's efficacy. At the 1993 International AIDS Conference in Berlin, Germany, Dr. Donald Kotler of the St. Luke-Roosevelt Medical Center told assembled scientists, "a controlled trial [of marijuana] would be unethical since the efficacy of marijuana is well known."

In December 1993 the San Francisco AIDS Consortium rejected the FDA proposed study, declaring it "unethical." Eventually the ethical problems were resolved and the Consortium approved the study. Researchers, however, were delayed another two years when NIDA refused to provide supplies of marijuana.

This intrusion of ethics scrambled bureaucratic plans. The FDA had hoped to promote a flawed AIDS study as a solution. Instead, its scheme ethically boomeranged, reminding the bureaucrats of their barbarous behavior.

Throughout the country the public was slowly awakening to the grim reality. The federal government really didn't want to know the truth about marijuana. With our fallen comrades, we at MARS had done our job well. We had revealed the corrupt underpinnings of an outmoded prohibition.

Across the nation there seemed to be a societal expectation of change, the first ingredient necessary for change. It was time to meld the collective desire for change into a new foundation. In my mind I began to plot the concept of a medical marijuana fund, fueled by philanthropists and dedicated to completing the research necessary to carry marijuana through the FDA process to the prescription counter. It would take a substantial amount of cash but nothing that a half dozen wealthy individuals couldn't put together with some ease. It would be a group of American financiers who vowed to solve the problem of medical access to marijuana. I pitched the idea to Rich who seemed interested.

But dark forces were at work—both within and without. By year's end Surgeon General Joycelyn Elders was gone. In an overzealous moment at the National Press Club Dr. Elders honestly opined that crime rates would be drastically reduced if drugs were legalized.

Eight days later the Arkansas police arrested her son for his role in a cocaine deal seven months before. A short time afterwards Elders submitted her resignation to Clinton. Suddenly the new administration was, in an eerie way, as drug shy as the Carter camp in the days following Peter Bourne's implosion. Like the proverbial baby tossed out with the bath water, medical marijuana would suffer the sin of association.

And within? Dark forces were working there, too. Things were happening inside my body that I would ignore for months. I entered 1994 expecting it to be the year that all the forces of change would come together.

How can someone so wrong be so right?

37 Going Global

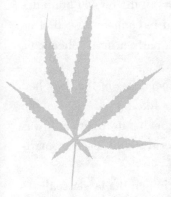

As WE ENTERED 1994 medical marijuana was the star issue of drug reform. New players filled the stage, mimicking scenes that were well-etched in the public's mind, reenacting battles already won. Like an actor who had grown accustomed to a long monologue I was variously distressed, incensed, bemused, confused and stunned numb by the cacophony of so many abruptly babbling voices.

Conspicuously absent were the patients.

And yet there was a more abstract view. For most of the '90s I had been receding, allowing others to move forward in the drama. Now, it seemed, I was the author, sitting in the darkened theater, looking on from the safety of an audience seat. The spotlight revealed raw ambition on the boards: a host of hot hams hoping for center stage. In truth we had enticed these actors to our stage and each player gave our vision new inflexion.

As others jockeyed to be the new star, the new director, and the new writer I found myself looking beyond the footlights of my own drama. The Bard aptly noted that all the world's a stage. It was time to go global.

The seeds of global expansion had already been sown. Marijuana is, afterall, an ancient herb, used by cultures throughout history. Despite the relentless whooshing of the memory hole the drug warriors had not succeeded in obliterating the memory of marijuana's medical use. They could not, for it seems we were born with a memory for marijuana. New research had revealed receptors in the human brain designed specifically for the chemicals found in cannabis. Each of us has tiny neural receptors waiting to find its partner in the chemicals that nature provides in the cannabis plant.

On a less microscopic level, the vast social use of the drug had spawned many serendipitous medical users like myself. None of the illnesses that marijuana could help were specific to America. It was only natural that others throughout the world would discover marijuana's therapeutic utility.

But it was AIDS that focused our attention on the larger scale.

Pandemic AIDS. Threatening to murder millions. In the U.S., HIV-infection had been primarily confined to the gay community, hemophiliacs, and IV drug users. In the rest of the world, however, AIDS was an equal opportunity plague spread by heterosexual encounters. HIV was rampaging through sub-Saharan Africa and rapidly radiating through Latin America, India and Southeast Asia.

Statistical projections were terrifying. AIDS was virtually 100% fatal. There were no cures and few treatments. Available therapies, flawed as they might be, were unavailable to the vast majority of people living beyond the industrial nations. In 1994 there were already double-digit rates of HIV-infection in much of Africa. In Zimbabwe, the U.N. estimated 40% of women of childbearing age might be HIV-positive before the turn of the century. The World Health Organization (WHO) projected global HIV-infection would exceed 20 million, and might crest closer to 100 million by the year 2,000.

Starkly stated, the productive, reproductive young of planet Earth are dying.

The social impact of these stunning statistics cannot be overstated. The deaths of so many millions of people in the prime of life will devastate continents. Developing nation states will be deprived of a healthy labor force. As whole economies dissolve into disease the resources required to alleviate the afflicted will overtax limited healthcare budgets. The sheer cost of caring for millions of orphaned, often ill children is staggering.

Marijuana will not cure AIDS nor global sadness but it can reduce the suffering. In places where transportation, money, electricity and refrigeration are hard to come by a medicinal plant which can be easily cultivated in any clinic's backyard would be of tremendous benefit.

This electrifying thought was manifested in the face of an African woman who visited a MARS exhibit table at the AIDS '92 Meeting of the National Conference of Social Workers. As her puzzled face scanned our exhibit materials Alice could see she was befuddled as to why a marijuana group would attend such a meeting. Alice explained that marijuana stimulates appetite and helps combat the wasting syndrome. Still the confusion clouded her face. "You call it slim," Alice explained, providing the Third World description of wasting.

As if lit from within the Ugandan woman's face began to glow with understanding. "Slim! The cannabis can help people with slim! Ah! We have cannabis in my country. It grows wild . . ." Her speech trailed off but the thought continued.

Britain was the obvious launch point for our global assault: similar language, same culture. In geopolitical terms the United Kingdom is a small country on an isolated island off the edge of Europe. In press terms, however, Britain retains Imperial reach. Some of the biggest media plugs on planet Earth are located in London. If we properly massaged the English media our message would extend into the Commonwealth of Nations giving us information penetration in Australia, India and much of Africa.

As the year began there were promising news reports that seemed to underscore our new international strategy. In early February the British Medical Association (BMA) reported 70% of U.K. physicians supported the legalization of marijuana for medical purposes.

A bit more arcane but nevertheless interesting was a Reuters report about a press conference with the president of Kazakhstan who noted that his country "did not have a pharmaceutical industry" but it did have plenty of opium and marijuana to export to those countries that did.

British media interest had been well primed thanks to the work of Clare Hodges and Dr. Biezanek. Clare, an MS victim, was a polished writer who placed several articles about the medical use of marijuana in English publications. Media interest in Dr. B.'s medical necessity case continued as various legal formalities relative to her criminal case were resolved.

The first big video salvo came on the aptly named television show "The Big Story," a kind of English "60 Minutes" but with longer segments allowing for more intense story development. I had begun working with the producers from the show in late 1993 and the final piece aired in February 1994.

"The Vicar's Desperate Remedy" brought medical marijuana into 5 million HUTs (homes using T.V.) In the U.K., that's a lot of huts. A primarily British-based story with some American angles, it was engaging and cleverly done.

The first segment outlined the situation and introduced several patients, most in wheelchairs, who smoked pot. Then, an inspired producer airlifted three mature British matrons with MS to a canal-side cannabis café in Amsterdam. The women, clearly excited by the unfamiliar surroundings, reviewed the menu, selected several lush buds and were handed a small pipe. After a few puffs they became quite gabby and were variously affected. One loved the strong smell of burning hemp; another was repelled; the third was hungry. How was their MS? No harm done and, looking quite rosy and relaxed, the women admitted they "feel better."

The second segment was "the American story." I was featured smoking legal U.S. government joints along with file footage of the NIDA pot plantation. There was talk of the California ballot initiatives and the focus shifted to Santa Cruz where, with Scott Imler's help, the producers met and interviewed a paraplegic named Scott Hager. As fate would have it, the camera was on when Hager was seized by violent leg spasms that nearly sent him tumbling from his wheelchair. He smoked a small amount of marijuana and, with the video camera still rolling, his violent spasms subsided within a few minutes. It was a Eureka moment, captured on video for millions to see. Hager regained enough muscle control to continue his planned workout in the swimming pool and gracefully slipped from his wheelchair into the cool, blue waters. It was graphic, gripping footage.

In the final segment we returned to England where we met a round, friendly Friar, the middle-aged vicar of a small country church. The vicar suffers from MS, drags a leg, has had little success with conventional therapies. "The Big Story" flew the Friar to Holland for an afternoon in the cannabis cafés. We watched the vicar, unsteady on his feet with cane in hand, awkwardly walking down a Dutch street. He slipped into a corner café, reviewed the variety of marijuana on offer, made a selection, then slowly inhaled his first puff of marijuana smoke. He took a few more puffs, mildly coughed, found it "interesting." Within minutes his stiff frame relaxed; he became animated and chatty. The reporter asked, "How do you feel, vicar?"

"Better," the vicar replied with surprise. "Less shaky." But it is the tape that tells the story. As the vicar left the café the change in his gait was remarkabe. His walk was steady, easy, assured.

A very good piece, "The Big Story" on medical marijuana would rerun in Britain before being exported via syndication to outlets in Australia, New Zealand and other outposts of Empire.

Globalization was under way.

On February 18, 1994, the U.S. Court of Appeals ruled in favor of the DEA, upholding the agency's right to reject the findings of its own administrative law judge. The decision drew some press attention and lobbed the ball straight into President Clinton's court.

The Clinton Administration was in a position to provide the solution but the growing tide of legalizers and reformers made the White House nervous. Clinton could do the right thing and come down on the side of facts and evidence, just as Judge Young had in September 1988. But Clinton had taken a lot of heat for his decision on gays in the military. There was no evidence that doing the right thing had bolstered the President's courage. More than anything Clinton wanted to be reelected and being "soft on drugs" was not a good stance for the incumbent.

We anxiously awaited the President's decision and tried to ignore the growing hiss of the memory hole.

The rejection of Judge Young's decision sent the newly arrived activists into a pique of activity. It is a truism that activists must be active.

Their plan was a mass demonstration of medical marijuana's "power," to take place in Lafayette Park, across the street from the White House, just after the November elections.

ACT was invited to participate in National Medical Marijuana Day by Ethan Nadelman, director of a new drug group called The Lindesmith Center.

Ethan listed an alphabet soup of the nation's drug reform groups and capped it with a list of psycho-active elites who would speak. Absent from the agenda are patients—except me. And maybe I would invite some others to attend and be the masses?

It was hard not to guffaw or gag. Drug reformers who couldn't decide if marijuana should be spelled with an "h" or a "j" were going to coordinate a national rally? And the proposed date—mid-November—defied all logical thought. Cold, dreary weather? Almost certainly. But mostly no one would be there. Congress would be gone. The White House would pay no mind. In October 1992, more than 200,000 candlelight marchers filed past the White House as part of the Quilt Display activities. It was barely acknowledged by the occupant, George Bush. Did Ethan and his merry men actually think they could mount a display that would do any more than capture a few moments of press attention, if that?

With brutalizing honesty I told Ethan, "I think what you're planning is a waste of time."

"Oh, no," Ethan enthused, reading a list of the drug liberation elites who had already signed on. "All of these people are well-intentioned," he insisted.

"Ethan," I responded, "the prohibition is well-intentioned. That doesn't mean it isn't stupid. You'll have to find patients elsewhere."

Our refusal to engage enraged reformers. We were not, it was said, "team players."

Guilty, as charged.

The stampede to exploit patients was on. As the herd headed away we were blissfully alone. Without a legal case to win or a law to be passed or a patient to be saved we were at sea. It had been a fifteen-year marathon, followed by a five-year sprint. It was okay to rest, I told myself. Okay to feel a bit tired.

The activists were rushing towards political activity. Been there, done that. It would not solve the problem.

Nor would research. If the government, as they so often espoused, simply wanted "the science done" then they would have embraced the therapeutic research acts of the late '70s and early '80s. Or they would have welcomed MARS as the way to gather science while indulging compassion.

Federal legislation? Stewart McKinney's efforts had taught us that having support in Congress meant little. One or two individuals could bottleneck meaningful legislation and deny justice.

How to break the back of the medical prohibition?

Money.

Money is the common denominator, understood by all.

For 15 years we operated without substantial financial support. Then we bumped into Rich who, for five years, had generously supported our endeavors. With his financial support we had accomplished a great deal.

Rich's support was a fortune to us but, in the grand scheme of things, it was small change. To resolve the medical marijuana problem would require much more. It would take millions. Moreover, I had come to believe they should be the right kind of millions— millions from millionaires.

Bit by bit the Medical Marijuana Fund was growing in my mind. It was envisioned as a grand philanthropic endeavor, three to four wealthy men joining together to provide the financial support needed to sponsor community-based research projects throughout the U.S.

The money was a critical element but the character of the contributor was even more critical. A consortium of the powerfully wealthy would send a signal to the politicians that it was time to resolve the problem. If there were doctors to do the science and money to support the research how could the feds deny this plan?

I'm not naïve. I figured they might well find a way to deny the plan. That, in fact, was the plan. If the government surprised me and allowed the research cooperatives to go forward that would be swell.

Within two or three years we would have the answers needed to gain federal approval for prescriptive access.

But if, as I suspected, the feds continued to obfuscate and deny the truth, worse yet denied even an avenue to it, then the voices of the weakest of citizens—the seriously ill and afflicted—would be allied with the voices of the strongest. The combination would provide the political will to effect a solution. It was a simple plan, a kind of MARS on steroids. As I began to sketch this idea to Rich he listened carefully and gave me the encouragement I needed.

"Keep working," he said, "keep working."

I did, endlessly going over the same ground. Writing and rewriting proposals that sat in my computer. My focus was myopic and scattered all at the same time. I felt a heaviness of mind and body. My weight had increased in odd ways; I was bloated about the face and belly. There were rashes that wouldn't clear.

Something was happening to me but I was blind to it.

In July the Clinton administration, traumatized by the arrest of Joycelyn Elder's son and emboldened by the Court of Appeals verdict, upheld the Bush administration's decision to void the Compassionate IND program. The decision, not unexpected, intensified activist outrage and editorial scorn.

The radio waves were full of anger but medical marijuana was just one more coal on the fire. The public was weary of do-gooders and government types mandating how they should live their lives. While politicians pandered for approval, people were beginning to realize they did not matter.

My own anger was also increasing. In that summer of '94 it seemed I was constantly annoyed and irritated. Alice urged a vacation and even this simple suggestion angered me.

Alice, visiting old friends in the cool Carolina mountains, tried to explain the changes she saw in me to a friend who had known us for many years. "There's something else happening," this dear friend would say. "This isn't like Robert."

She was right.

In August I flew to California, traveling to Santa Cruz to meet with Scott Imler and attend some political functions. Santa Cruz was one of my target cities for a community-based research project backed by the medical marijuana fund. The August trip was part of laying the groundwork and testing the waters.

I had barely arrived when I received a message from my attorney, Steve Davidson, indicating some problem with my marijuana supply and recommending I return to Washington ASAP. It was a Friday evening and further details were unavailable. I immediately booked a return flight.

The next morning I attended a memorial service for an AIDS patient who had worked hard for Proposition A. I then made apologies to friends and had Scott drive me to San Francisco where there was time to spend a few hours with my old friend, Bobby Evans.

Bobby answered the door slowly, smiled broadly, looked ravaged. He was painfully thin, his face red and puffed from toxic chemicals. End-stage AIDS in all its ugliness.

I sat with Bobby for the remainder of that afternoon, watching the sun walk across the room, talking of old times as he faded in and out of awareness. When the airport limo arrived Bobby unsteadily led me to the door to say good-bye. I realized it was the last time I would see him alive.

I returned to an empty house. Alice was away in Florida, visiting her aging mother and playing golf. On Monday I tackled the supply problem which was resolved with a phone call.

Suddenly it was a quiet time with little to do. On one gentle evening, alone and sad, I fell into a pool of dark humors which inflated, then ignited into an intense rage. Pure anger. Deep, random explosions of emotion. Shouting into the silence of my living room; screaming at nothing and everything.

Alice phoned into the bared teeth of this emotional storm. With fury, I lashed out at her absence. Stunned by the blistering temper of my tone she tried to calm me, to find out what was wrong. Furious, I slammed down the phone, ending her inquisition. Then, like a fever abruptly broken the rage receded.

Exhausted, stunned, I reflected on my utterly uncharacteristic behavior. I had rarely been angry before and seldom raised my voice. Certainly, I have been enraged by some unjust or vile act. But I had never before experienced such a cold, terrible rush of unchecked rage. I could not rationally isolate a particular cause. It seemed as if something deep in the heart of my universe was disturbed. My brain scrambled to logically explain and, in a moment of exhaustion, I concluded that it was just a great fatigue at the folly of the world.

Anger and denial. Classic emotions of the terminally ill.

On the last day of August I received a faxed invitation to speak at the University College of London on October 11. The prospect of international travel was invigorating and quickly pushed to the background the concerns I felt for my recent, unexplained behavior.

We were going to Europe! After a year of pelting Britain with medical marijuana stories, we could now ratchet up the amps through a blitz of London. Clare's fledgling ACT-UK had attracted an upper crust of support, including that of Dr. Patrick Wall, one the country's preeminent pain specialists and the source of my speaking invitation. He had arranged a cozy lecture on "The Therapeutic Uses of Cannabis" that would have an eclectic audience of physicians, BBC producers, pharmaceutical company reps, Fleet Street editors and select patients.

I had been down the international road before and knew the problems I would encounter in attempting to travel with my marijuana. We knew that Holland offered safe haven and settled on an itinerary that would allow some R&R in Amsterdam before crossing the Channel to England. It would also give us a chance to explore the cannabis cafés and speak with officials in Holland about medical marijuana use.

Kevin Zeese alerted us to a conference in Germany and suggested we contact his Dutch friend, Mario Lap, a leading Dutch psychiatrist, who invited us to attend his scheduled seminar at Münster University.

In the morning hours of October 6 Mario Lap collected us from our hotel in downtown Amsterdam for the drive to Münster, Germany. Mario was the picture of a modern European. Witty, well-dressed, well-versed, and well-equipped with technological gadgets. He arrived with two of his psychiatrist buddies which made for a cramped, chatty car ride. Mario assured us it would only take "a short while" but it was a five-hour journey to Münster. In Mario's packed Saab we flew past the remnants of the old Dutch/German border, the customs station savaged by vandals. There were no borders in the new Europe as I imported my U.S. legal marijuana into Germany.

The Münster conference, sponsored by the Dutch and German Health Ministries, brings drug activists and government bureaucrats together. Contrasted with the raging conflict in America, it was heartening to see officials and reformers, treatment specialists and health care professionals endeavoring to work together.

Münster U. looked like any modern American campus. The conference halls were crowded with exhibits. There was much to see and do. It was midnight before we ate dinner in a Chinese restaurant in quaint, bombed out, rebuilt Münster. After five hours of close confinement with three babbling Dutch psychiatrists, and endless hours more of greeting and meeting new people speaking foreign tongues, we were jet lagged into sheer exhaustion.

The next morning the conference seemed more organized. Mario's seminar on marijuana was held in a large lecture hall and drew an overflow crowd of at least 300. The audience, like the conference, was a mix of activists, government officials, physicians and curious students. I was pleased to see that the largest single group appeared to be reporters.

I spoke for nearly an hour, the Germans having no difficulty understanding my English. There were very good questions and obvious interest from the reporters. Following the seminar we did a few interviews. Then, our work done, and having little interest in a drug conference largely conducted in foreign tongues, we hopped a train back to friendly Amsterdam.

It was a lovely weekend at the Amsterdam Hilton and we spent the time touring, wandering museums and the neighborhood streets. It was warm and sunny and we enjoyed a fine dinner at a small Italian-Dutch restaurant. In the civil atmosphere of Amsterdam Alice and I began to relax again with one another. The rage, which exploded in August, had continued to linger beneath the surface but in this relaxed city I found myself opening up for the first time in months. Alice spoke of her concerns about my health. I had developed a nagging cough and was uncharacteristically fatigued.

Over split pea soup and sandwiches Alice talked calmly and rationally about the need to "find out what's wrong." I couldn't disagree. I knew she was right. I promised to see a doctor when we returned to the States.

On Monday we hopped a train for Belgium. We crossed the channel and arrived in London just after dark. Sans pot.

Britain, unlike most of Europe, still maintains border police. I had come to Europe with a Customs Declaration declaring my legal pot. But somewhere in Belgium, while watching the farmland roll by, I decided attending the scheduled lecture in London was more important than playing media games with the British Home Office. Besides, there would be pot in Britain. I consumed what I could of my legal stash and crumpled the rest along the rail bed as the train flew through the Low Countries.

The British also seemed to have no interest in creating a scene. When the Customs agent at the dock asked if I had anything to declare I said "no." He gave me a sharp stare, looked again at his computer screen, then welcomed me into the United Kingdom.

We arrived at our hotel in King's Cross in time to meet our British contact, Clare, for dinner. Clare was an interesting woman, married with two young sons. Well-dressed, stylish and deeply sincere, Clare's focus was, understandably, on the disease which afflicted her, MS. Indeed, to our surprise, and probably because of Clare's efforts, marijuana's use in MS was the focus of most British media attention.

In October 1994 London was beautiful, warm and sunny. We had left our jet lag in Holland and our first day in England we were up early to see the obvious sights. We wandered through Covent Garden and rode double-decker buses. As we walked around Buckingham Palace I found myself exhausted and snapped at Alice momentarily. Just travel fatigue I said to myself, coughing as we entered the cab Alice had hailed.

The University College lecture was scheduled for 5 p.m. The audience was, as promised, diverse, intrigued and attentive. There were no "hard news" reporters present, but nearly half a dozen print editors and television producers were anxious to ask questions. Follow-up interviews were scheduled for the next day. It was a lively, much enjoyed exchange of views.

Dr. Biezanek had traveled from Mersey to hear my speech and after the reporters left we walked a short distance to the Student Union Hall. Clare, Dr. Wall, Dr. Biezanek, Alice and I plus one or two others cheerfully drank pints of beer and discussed our common interest.

The next day was even more interesting when we met Clare in the late afternoon at St. Stephen's entrance to Parliament. We three were ushered through a "Members Only" door, and guided down dark stone corridors to a meeting with Lord Partick Whaddon who greeted us with enthusiasm and invited us into the House of Lords' tearoom. Nice, darkly paneled digs that ooze history. It was a bit late for traditional British high tea, but Lord Whaddon managed to obtain several pots of Chinese green tea and crumpets.

The Lord was an aging peer, highly regarded by his fellow Lords. He was keenly interested in Clare's efforts and marijuana's medical use in spasm control. There was no specific agenda. It was mostly a "get acquainted" meeting to discover if we could work together. We could.

In conversation Lord Whaddon became intrigued by the British Home Office's refusal to allow the importation of my legally prescribed marijuana. He thought it a matter worthy of press attention and promised to make some calls.

Following the meeting we took Clare to catch her train to Leeds. After several days of effort and travel she looked frail as, with mild spasms, she climbed onto the train. She was intelligent, dedicated and anxious to expand marijuana's medical use in Britain. We worried if she had the physical strength to endure such a challenge.

The London Times phoned early in the morning. Lord Whaddon had worked his magic. *The Times* rang off and another publication phoned. The story was taken; photographers were rushed to our hotel for snaps. It was my last scheduled morning in London and it became somewhat frantic. Should I stay another day? No. Eye pressures were rising: it was time for me to go home. As I climbed aboard the airport bus Alice gave me a copy of *The Daily Express*. "Page 4," she says. "See you in a few days."

As the bus rumbled toward Heathrow I read that Richard Branson, founder and chief of Virgin Records and Airlines, one of the world's wealthiest men, declared publicly that he would market marijuana if it were legal. "Of course I would seriously consider marketing it if it was decriminalised . . . I do not view marijuana as dangerous and it is a great pity about the law as it stands at the moment."

A philanthropist for the Medical Marijuana Fund?

• • •

Alice remained in Britain several more days, traveling to Leeds to meet quietly with Clare, then on to Liverpool/Mersey for more talks with Dr. B. and to meet Lucy.

Our European excursion capped our initial globalization efforts. A base was in place, the media was increasingly sensitive to our story, and there were allies at hand. Clare was ready to make a major push. Lord Whaddon would join any reasonable enterprise to resolve the problem, Richard Branson has publicly gone on the record as supportive of change. It is exciting when things work well.

Alice returned from England and I almost immediately flew to Florida to see family, visit with a dying uncle, and vote. She reminded me that I promised to see a doctor about my cough. "When I return from Florida," I said. "Don't worry."

But, in fact, she was right to worry. I was worried. I knew something was wrong but I didn't know what to do about it. I had been denied health insurance because of my glaucoma. The only doctor I knew was Dr. North. Other than my glaucoma I had never been ill, didn't know how to go about entering the medical system.

I lingered in Florida. The November election elevated our once earnest ally, Newt Gingrich, to Speaker of the House. It seemed our government was suddenly in the hands of two not-quite-mature boomers pretending to be adults. It was certain to be an interesting show.

On the 8th I finally returned to Washington and three days later, late in the night, a call came from California. "I'm checking out," my old friend Bobby Evans told me, "Sunday."

His AIDS was too advanced, his life too constricted. Already nearly dead he had decided it was time to leave. The next morning he would call Alice to say goodbye. I had already told her of his call and when she heard his voice she said, "I hear you are planning a trip." It was a graceful entrance to a final farewell. She reported that he seemed happy and relaxed. On Sunday a mutual friend called to report Bobby's death.

• • •

Two days later National Medical Marijuana Day came and went with virtually no media comment. It was a pathetic scene, a friend reported. A handful of antic activists, a few actually afflicted people, the cream of America's psycho-active elite occupying a small square of mud in a corner of the park. Thousands of dollars had been squandered so people only important to themselves could shout their concern for the sick. A pathetic display of cosmic unimportance.

Never mind. With globalization in progress it was time to put the Medical Marijuana Fund in place. We would meet with Rich that weekend to discuss our plans. I actually had several plans for Rich to consider. Everything was on track.

If I could just get rid of this cough. . . .

38 A Passing Shadow

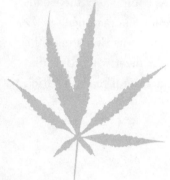

November 15, 1994
Washington, D.C.

"Mr. Randall, the blood test confirms HIV infection. Your pneumonia would suggest you are full blown AIDS but we won't be certain of that until we get the T-cell count in a couple days."

"How long?"

For the second time in my life I am sitting across from a doctor and asking how long. But now it isn't how long will I see . . . now it is how long will I live.

"Well, now that's a bit difficult to say. Let's get the pneumonia controlled and then worry about the next step."

With a 104° temperature there was an impulse to ship me off to the hospital, but when the doctor learned I had no health insurance I was sent home instead, prescriptions in hand.

In the blink of an eye my world was reduced to the size of a waterbed.

The brutality of my diagnosis was buffered by a vagueness in prognosis. Terminal, certainly. But there were tests to run and results to calibrate. Perhaps there would be years of life ahead. Weak in a waterbed, watching the sunlight walk from my room, I pondered what to do when the pneumonia faded.

"We are in this together," Alice said taking my hand. "I will be with you to the end." Fortunately—blessedly—she spoke in metaphors. Her bloodwork, taken the next day, was negative. She was not infected.

"Sorrow comes, not as a single soldier but in legions." The Bard again. That Shakespeare knew the score.

In that sorrowful week in November the news of Alice's good health was the only bright spot. Bobby had been dead less than a week. My diagnosis was less than three days old when my mother called to tell me of my uncle's passing. In a year's time she had lost a sister and two brothers-in-law. As I listened to her weary, sober voice I wondered how we would ever be able to tell her about me.

But there was little time or energy to worry about such things. I was scheduled to meet Rich on Sunday, our annual meeting at which we settle on the next year's goals. Alice went in my place. We had been disinclined to share my sad news with close friends. That would come later. But it would be wrong to deny such information to Rich who told Alice not to worry.

Still uncertain about my future we awaited the results of my T-cell test.

On November 21, 1994, the fiction of my future was foreclosed. The tests returned with an awful audit of my condition. Expecting a much higher number I was spooked to learn I had only 22 T-cells. My immune system was in complete collapse. My defenses, gone. I was on the menu of any microbe that came along. Death was not distant.

Normally, people have 1250 T-cells. As HIV spreads and the immune system declines AIDS usually becomes full-blown and impossible to ignore when the T-cells drop to around 250. Kenny and Barbra, at diagnoses, had 150-200 T-cells. As HIV decimates T-cells the advance of AIDS is marked by night sweats, nausea, vomiting, rapid weight loss, fatigue, mysterious aches, phantom pains, a myriad of major and minor infections and afflictions. A still-mobile man just returned from California, Europe and Florida who was 50 pounds overweight with mild pneumonia and 22 T-cells is something of a novelty. Why such an unusual progression? Clearly, constant access to marijuana had made a difference. But there was little time to expand on this thought. Knowing the debilitating dynamics of AIDS, Alice and I realized I was already deep into dying. There was little time, but much to do.

A bisexually active man in the '70s and '80s, I first thought I might be "at risk" before AIDS had a name. But at what "risk" in a nation with fewer than 500 confirmed cases? By 1985, I was amending my behavior, wondering if I might be ill. By 1988, such fears faded. I was healthy, robust, without the slightest symptom or sign.

As I began working with people with AIDS I carefully checked their many complaints against my own experiences. There was seldom a match. Just enough to cause occasional concern.

Denial and acceptance are curious twins. I accepted denial. Enlightened denial. There is no cure; existing treatments are more toxic than helpful. What good would it do to know? I had friends so damaged by an AIDS diagnosis they could no longer function. Terminality is life-changing. I was delighted with my life. As dozens died around me I felt fine.

Don't worry. Be happy. Still, there is a difference between denial and dumb. After 20 years of diagnosing people's ailments I found slight, subtle signs. Bilateral skin lesions. Increasing fatigue. But contrasted to the ravaging symptoms routinely reported by the actually afflicted it was hard to imagine myself ill. When one is surrounded by dying souls it is easy to be hypochondriacal. Besides, why labor under the limiting yoke of terminality? If I was going to die of AIDS, best it be quick.

The gods now seemed content to grant my unspoken wish.

On the day after Thanksgiving, ten days after my diagnosis, I dressed and crossed the street to our office, a small two-story condo converted into a work space. I labored to climb the stairs and could not get beyond the first level. There was simply no energy.

A German television crew arrived; the first fruits of our Münster madness just over a month ago. The interview went well. After twenty years of medical marijuana interviews there was a certain autopilot quality I could tap into.

After the crew departed I retraced my steps, climbed the stairs to my bedroom and collapsed in exhaustion. The reality of my situation was beginning to set in.

As if to temper the pain, the fates handed us some good news on the final day of the month. The Australian Capital Territory, ironically known as ACT, had just legalized marijuana's medical use in AIDS and cancer therapy.

The flowers of globalization have begun to bloom. I wondered if I would live long enough to enjoy their fruit.

Who to tell? When? Alice, in urgent need of external support, informed her sister and our assistant Linda. Another close friend was told after Alice collapsed in tears when routinely asked, "How's Bob?"

I was in no rush to disclose my pending departure. Terminal news is terrible to convey. When diagnosed with glaucoma I found it hard to tell friends I might go blind. Such a dialogue discomforts both parties and may disquiet the relationship.

Death—one's own death—is not easily interjected into casual conversation. My mother, sister and brother were not told. It was too close to Christmas, and not the kind of news which should arrive by telephone. There would, God willing, be time to tell them in person.

As an alternative to selective silence I could have issued a press release: told everyone at once. But I had no impulse to turn my impending demise into a public declaration. Perhaps when I gained more strength I would play such a card. But not at this point. I was still quite ill and the world was closing down for Christmas.

After a month of many medicines and endless rest I tried to dress every day and make the short trek between home and office. The world beyond my bed seemed an alien, intriguing place. The insights of a visitor. One evening I returned home to find Christmas lights on our small Norfolk pine and across the windows. It was an incandescent delight, even as I realized this would be my last Christmas.

In the quiet of the holiday there was time to consider matters. For years Alice had wanted to return to Florida, to spend time with her aging mother, to play golf in a benign clime, to get us settled "while you can still see." For years I had resisted. From my lovely village in the center of Marble City I could walk my way 'round town. To a near-blind person who cannot drive Florida seemed an asphalt wasteland. I would be isolated. A fair argument at one time, but what does isolation matter to the dead?

By the New Year a plan emerged. It was time to leave Marble City for the land of flowers. I would return home to die.

What of medical marijuana? How easily fate relieved me of obligations. We had already performed our most critical role: knowledge, like a freed genie, cannot easily be recalled. Medical marijuana had melded into mass memory. There were plenty of others to handle the details. Our work was done.

Our plans: we would elusively ease away. Nothing abrupt. ACT would become a phone line. We would set up a small office in Florida.

Or not. It depended. Richard J., ever-kind, accepted this delusional plan and agreed to underwrite "whatever you both want to do." Chicago assured us we were free to use our funds as we desired. A generous gesture from a very good guy.

No need to tell Steve Davidson at Steptoe. My crisis was not legal, but medical. Steptoe & Johnson remained ready to defend my rights. After nearly 17 years many of the once brash young attorneys who, *pro bono*, protected my sight were now becoming powerful men. Notify on demise. Case closed.

Dr. North was an altogether different matter. In February, I phoned him with my sad news. We had also been together for 17 years. A uniquely long and stable association. I still deeply admire his courage in coming to my aid. We shared many laughs together and I tried to maintain some cheer. We both ended in silent tears.

While I wobbled between weakness and worse, Alice moved decisively forward. She had a future to plan. In August '94, while visiting her mother, she viewed a small condo—just blocks from our moms' apartments—that overlooked the intracoastal waterway. As she entered the yard she discovered a Buddha statue sitting amidst the overgrowth. In an instant she felt this was her place. As if to confirm the instinct, six months later she learned the place was still available. She wondered if we should—she should—spend so much. "Buy it," I advised.

Decisions come easily to the dying.

In late March I was much better. I even returned to work of sorts, doing loads of talk radio.

Heartened by my reviving strength Alice, for the first time since November, left me on my lonesome. She was in the final stages of buying her condo on the intracoastal, but had to go to Florida to close the deal. There were papers to sign, contractors, painters, plumbers and electricians to bid, carpets and appliances to buy. On Monday, March 28, I said good-bye, then went to my office to send Rich a fax heralding my astonishing improvement. My last illusion.

On Wednesday I awoke to fire in my gut and pain beyond bearing. Alice phoned and heard my pain. From 1,000 miles away she tried to coordinate my healthcare, even calling a cab to get me to the doctor's office where I was immediately rerouted to Washington Hospital Center Emergency Ward.

Emergency was chaos. Blood was taken, my guts were scanned, an IV was jammed into my arm; saline and—blessed Jesus—morphine. The pain faded.

I awoke in a private room on the oncology ward. Tests revealed a seriously malfunctioning gall bladder and an inflamed pancreas. Surgery was discussed. From the muffled depths of morphine I ask if surgery is dangerous for someone with AIDS. "It certainly adds an element of risk," was the clinical reply.

My urgent condition compelled Alice to tell my mother and sister of my desperate plight. My mother absorbed the horrible news and then, as planned, took Alice shopping for a carpet, an attitude I much admired. Now fully aware of the reasons for our move, my mother and sister rallied to help in whatever ways they could. Alice scrambled to pack five days of work into two.

After a 24-hour period of observation the doctors concluded my gall bladder needed to come out. My urine was the color of cola. Bloodwork was completely skewed. An operation was scheduled for Friday but I refused. Alice had made plans to return late Friday and I want her to be there . . . in case. "Saturday," I said. The surgeons stood above me, haggling over schedules. One stepped forward to accept my request.

"You are very lucky," said the plump Hispanic woman who sat in my room to monitor my care. "He is the best." She spoke gently as I slipped into opium oblivion.

"Is there anything we should know?" My eyes opened. A beautiful black man in a powder blue surgical smock was asking questions. He towered above me, then took a chair close by my bed. His skin was ebony; his face framed by long, snow-white dreadlocks and a well-manicured beard. Very handsome and engaging.

"Is there anything we should know?" he repeated. He was, I assumed, from anesthesiology. "Yes," I murmured. "Phospholine Iodine. I'm on Phospholine Iodine."

For 20 years I have been warned Phospholine and anesthesia can be a lethal combination resulting in respiratory paralysis or cardiac arrest. "I am on Phospholine Iodine."

"Anything else?" he asked.

"Marijuana. I smoke marijuana for glaucoma."

"I see," the beautiful black man smiled broadly as I slipped into sleep. I heard a small chuckle. "Do not worry, Mr. Randall," he said soft as a parent. "Everything is going to be just fine."

Alice arrived early Saturday morning. "Ok, bunky?" she says, brushing the hair from my forehead. "Got any plans?"

I told her of the curious man from anesthesiology as orderlies shifted me onto the gurney for transport to surgery. I stared at the flickering florescent tubes passing overhead, but was unconscious before we reached the operating theatre. Alice spoke briefly with the surgeon. He told her, given my weakened condition, there was a one in three chance I would not survive the surgery. Sobering. Still, absent an operation, there was a 100 % chance I would be dead in days.

These were sad hours for Alice. The surgeon warned it would be a long operation and she returned to the car pragmatically thinking she would go home to "do some work." But as she turned the ignition key her hands began to shake, then her whole body started to tremble. She turned off the key and returned to the waiting area.

For more than five hours she would wait, wander, and worry. It was a beautiful spring day and she found a small inner courtyard outside surgery where nurses and anesthesiologists gathered to grab quick hits of nicotine. One of them was from my operating theatre and said all was going well. Alice asked if the other anesthesiologist was working today, the tall black man with long, white dreadlocks? The technician looked at her curiously. "There's nobody like that here," the young man replied. "I'd remember him," he laughed.

My blue angel. He was right. All went well. The surgeon had never seen a gall bladder such as mine; necrotic and gangrenous, it was shrouded in a sac of milky fluids. He was clearly puzzled by the appearance and, if time had allowed, I might have pursued the matter more thoroughly. For the moment, however, I was happy to be alive and I would spend my recuperative period marveling at the series of events already in motion.

Things were oddly easier now that my family knew. In Florida my mother and sister were supervising the condo renovation, pushing workmen to get the job done before we arrived.

I was released from the hospital on April 5th with orders not to lift anything over three pounds. With movers due in thirteen days this seemed a cruel order, especially for Alice. Friends arrived, literally from around the globe, to help with the endless packing. Our friends from Australia, Craig and Daryl, would do yeoman's duty during their stay with us. There were four floors of possessions; hundreds of files. What to take? What to leave? I watched as other people disassembled my life. Alice's old stage-managing craft would serve her well in this busy time.

Two weeks after my hospital release the moving van arrived. I had been dispatched to a nearby hotel. While I watched talk shows in the safety of my hotel room, Alice monitored the movers. Everything took longer than expected. It was midnight before she returned.

The next day Alice drove me to Washington Hospital Center where

I collected Dr. North's final script: four tins—1,200 marijuana cigarettes.

Since November, I had been squirreling away marijuana. Pneumonia had severely reduced my consumption. Counting my April script I had eight unopened tins—2,400 cigarettes. Another three tins were chock full of loose marijuana; the accumulated leavings of two decades. There was enough government pot to last at least a year. More marijuana than I would need for the journey ahead.

After collecting my cannabis I walked across a courtyard to get my belly staples pulled. The surgeon was pleased by the fine job he had done. "No pain?" He seemed surprised.

A last night in Washington and then we climbed into Alice's car for the short ride to Lorton, Virginia and the auto-train. The day was wonderfully warm: Washington a wonderland of marble buildings and gaudy gardens. I had lived in this Disneyland for adults for half my life. Now, as monuments glided by, I realized it was the last time I would see the Tidal Basin or enjoy the Mall or look at Mr. Lincoln in his great Temple.

I wondered why the passing parade of familiar marble monuments did not make me sad. Perhaps it was the excitement of the journey ahead. My life was unwinding. As the crowding complications of adulthood dropped away I became raw to the deeper rhythms all round.

Homeward bound.

The land of flowers was lush with life, as hallucinogenic as hibiscus. My urban ears were seized by natural sounds. Gulf waters caressing white sand beaches, the baleful cries of exotic birds crowd my nights. Manatees glided beneath the waves out my window. Sitting on Alice's dock, watching silvered slivers of sunlight ripple across Lucky Duck lagoon, I had arrived in Paradise.

Alice's new condo was completely renovated in less than three weeks. New paint, new kitchen, new carpets, an astonishing view. A lovely place in the sun. Our families welcomed us as returning, wounded warriors long gone to a foreign land. There were dinners shared with much laughter.

My surgical wound healed quickly, without pain. Much of me was, I thought, still strong. Daily, Alice and I walked the seawall, holding hands, greeting new neighbors. Nearly fifty, we were nippers newly arrived in a community of octogenarians.

After more than twenty years together Alice and I had our first lawn and garden. There was time spent watering grass and watching flowers grow. Small diversions. I was content. Alice would be happy here.

There was another first. For the first time in twenty years I stopped smoking marijuana. My vital signs were still weak and a few puffs of marijuana caused my already low blood pressure to plunge. The resulting fainting spells were frightening and dangerous. Besides, I was dying; what did blindness matter? In a week or two, when my condition improved, I would begin smoking again.

We had been in our new Florida home for less than a month when my gut exploded with fire once again. It was Memorial Day weekend and we joined the masses of unfortunates at the Sarasota Memorial Emergency Room. After five hours of writhing on a cold aluminum slab I was finally given morphine and shuttled into a private room. The doctors, all strangers to me, diagnosed "acute pancreatitis."

The cause? A pneumonia prevention treatment—inhaled pentamadine—had become toxic. The Florida doctors shook their heads that I was on the drug at all. There were alternatives, inexpensive and less toxic. No one told me. I didn't think to ask.

The treatment for pancreatitis was simple. Morphine for pain, no food and plenty of saline. In a few days, once the pancreas "cooled," things would be fine. That's what the doctors said.

After four days I was allowed to go home. This traumatic event had one great benefit. We were abruptly introduced to the local AIDS clinic, said to be among the nation's best.

In early June I was hunched in pain when I arrived for my first appointment at the AIDS clinic. My weight, a marvel at the time of my diagnosis, was dropping fast. In six months I had lost thirty pounds.

Maureen Murray, a licensed nurse practitioner, ordered blood drawn then gave my belly a few hard pokes which caused me to wince in pain. She vanished, then returned with a container of morphine pills and ordered me to immediately take one. My supposedly transient pancreatitis had returned; perhaps it never left.

Medical care at the clinic was fast and efficient. Over the next several days, as my pain eased, I returned to the clinic for different kinds of help. For the first time since diagnosis I was guided through the complexities of acquiring social services. Florida, we discovered, was among the most advanced states in the country for extended AIDS care. We had unwittingly entered a PWA's (Person with AIDS) Paradise. Fate, it seemed was once again guiding our steps to the best possible place.

But it may have been to no avail. I was on a roller coaster decline. Some days were almost fine. Then pancreatitis flared again.

Throughout the summer of '95 my pancreas smoldered constantly, often erupting in paroxysms of intense pain. There was nausea and vomiting with nearly every meal. I dropped another twenty pounds and began to walk with a shuffle of the aged.

My mind—unhinged from any future—began an archival dump by retrieving and reviewing a maze of memories. How had life been this time around? Not bad. Born in the heartland of a powerful em-

pire, I had never been ill-housed, ill-clothed or ill-fed. I arrived into
Eden, had loving parents and a grand passage from infancy to lit-
eracy. Well-educated, I never pursued a precise ambition, but instead followed as fate led me down an improbable path few others
have traveled.

I had lived the life of a democratic man, successfully defending
my rights against a hostile and brutish state. I had made legal and
medical history, enacted laws, aided the afflicted and altered
global perceptions. Along the way we had encountered an endless
cast of players worked with dying people and rising politicians,
met medical mandarins and toiled with some of the nation's finest
young attorneys.

It seemed upon reflection that the whole of my adult life had
challenged others to make difficult decisions involving ethics and
self-interest.

Good guys. Bad guys. Lots to learn. Law. Medicine. Politics. Media
manipulation. In this life I learned how to cast my voice across continents. Delighted by rhetoric, I practiced ancient arts with powerful
tools. An intensely private man, I played upon a grand stage.

Beyond art and artifice have been the people who had populated
my path. Lynn, Mona, Steve, Kenny and Barbra. Who guided whom?
Great allies in a grand adventure. For every name I knew there have
been thousands of unnamed others who have benefited from our
drama.

Our exploits had been well-compensated. I still had my sight. It
had not been an uninteresting life.

The mind was on rewind. Lots of memories were being remembered for the last time.

What a time!

Alive and young I personally witnessed the most important event
in human history when, on a December morning in 1968, I watched
a Saturn 5 rocket lift three mortals to the Moon. "To see," as Archi-

bald MacLeish would later write, "the Earth as it truly is, small, and blue and beautiful in that eternal silence where it floats."

Alice was with me even then. In the whole of my life I had never been unloved. We had been well mated; constant and tolerant. It had been a better journey shared. A lovely life. But it was time to leave.

In a metaphorical dream I saw myself staring into a mirror framed in lights, looking intently at my reflection as I wiped the grease and paint from my face. As cold cream ripped away the mask of my illusions I was anxious to walk into the cool, dark night beyond the stage door. My play was over.

At the end of July a CAT scan revealed my pancreas—which should have been the size of a small flower—was as big as a child's football. The CAT image also revealed pits and blisters—pseudocysts—covering the swollen surface.

"Grim?" I asked the physician.

"Very grim," he quickly agreed. "Very grim, indeed."

I was abruptly, suddenly very old. Snow white hair above a rapidly receding frame. Reality began to melt; there were gaps here and there. Solid matter seemed little more than an interruption in the flow of photons.

A plane flew high above my bed. I heard the drone and thought, I will never fly anywhere again. No matter. I had seen much in many places.

As death approached there was less fear than fascination. The mystery of tides, a setting sun, a rising moon, a heaven pock-marked by planets and stars mesmerized my apprehensions. The circle of my life was closing as, dying, I wandered into the wonder of unworded beginnings.

August 17, 1995

"You should report to the hospital immediately," Nurse Murray commanded over the phone.

"I want to stay home," I protested. "If it gets worse we'll head for emergency."

"If it gets worse," Nurse Murray bluntly said, "you'll be dead before you get to your car, much less emergency."

I had so wanted to die in my own bed.

Hospitalized again, I was attached to tubes. Morphine through an IV pump with a generous button for extra doses. Lots of saline. Arrangements were made so Alice could wheel me outside several times a day for marijuana breaks. We had told the clinic of our medical marijuana exploits and there was the usual fascination. I omitted the fact that I was no longer using the substance. Our trips outside were a chance to savor sunlight and smoke sweet nicotine. Sitting in my wheelchair, IV bottles swaying above my head, surrounded by a sunny circle of luminous plantings, Alice and I were saying goodbye.

Efforts to "cool" my pancreas failed. The slightest bite of food, the clearest of broths, even the smallest sips of water provoked gut-wrenching vomiting. Like a caterpillar in a chrysalis I was dissolving from the inside out.

My family visited constantly. My brother flew in from Alaska. Death was imminent. "We are," the nurses assured, "going to do everything possible to keep you comfortable."

I was between here and there. Talkative, cheery, alert but ready to leave. My bags were packed for the great beyond. No fear now. I felt homeward bound.

After a week of no food and only ice to munch there was a terrible night when a vein blew and the IV technician could no longer find an alternative site. As Alice stood outside my door, a second technician was called. For an hour they slapped my arms and legs, probing, poking, searching for a place to put the needle.

They finally succeeded and left. Alice came in to comfort me. As she left I realized my bed was immediately above the place where I was born. It was a last memory. The circle closed. I was done.

Death seemed certain. At some time in the night a pseudocyst erupted and Robert Carl Randall, 48, suffered a massive hemorrhagic rupture of the pancreas. A rush of blood and toxins flooded into my gut. There was an instant, searing pain as my soul was released into the care of the Ferryman who arrived to take me from myself.

It was over.

39 What Seems Certain

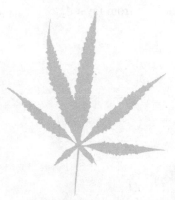

ADRIFT IN MYTH; on dark waters there was peace. Overhead a bright light beckoned.

The River Styx?

No. I was afloat in a boat on the intracoastal. A full moon overhead turned limpid seas to silvered mercury. Three years past dead it was good to be alive.

What seemed certain, changed. Death seemed certain, but I did not die. You remember, I'm tan as a red man and fat as a Buddha of Happiness. Alive in the land of flowers; living in a condo on the intracoastal.

In a slick theatrical trick fate flew me out of death's grasp. Magic. Or so it seemed. A deus ex machina mystery which warrants explaining. Death scene/Take 2.

August-November 1995
Sarasota, Florida

Weary of being slapped silly by IV technicians searching for a puncture point, I consented to the insertion of a Hickman dual-line catheter. Simple surgery. A small incision was made over the left breast. A thin plastic tube was threaded through the chest wall where it was anchored inside a major vein near the heart. Externally, five inches of white vinyl hose hung from my body.

A new umbilical cord. The procedure was not intended to save my life, merely to make my demise more manageable. Through one port a small pump delivered a steady stream of morphine. I was not "locked out"; there were no restrictions on amount. The second Hickman port was used to infuse TPN (total parenteral nutrition) which would keep me hydrated and nourished while we waited for my pancreas to explode. I was sent home. No one expected me to live two weeks.

Pat Kelly—a home care nurse—joined my primary treatment team of O'Leary and Nurse Murray. Pat's arrival seemed a fulfillment of attorney John Karr's droll, long ago observation to Judge Washington that "Perhaps Mr. Randall has a penchant for Irish women."

I adored my Hickman. After months of pincushion injections the hose hanging from my chest provided physicians with easy access to my interior. Drug delivery was less painful, more direct, and the Hickman could also be used to draw blood for tests. No more needles and blown veins.

In addition the Hickman provided a perverse sense of security. For months I had puzzled over my choices, should I decide to commit suicide. The Hickman afforded an elegant answer. The dual ports, if left uncapped, quickly drain blood from the body. Death was suddenly as near as a short walk to the dock, a super jolt of morphine and the easy release of my blood into the bay. No clean-up required. The plot gave me great peace of mind.

But no suicide was attempted. Instead, I confounded my physicians, infusing my daily 3-liter bag of TPN without adverse effects. My digestive system was intentionally shut down. I was not allowed to eat or drink anything. Only ice shavings and an occasional banana popsicle passed my lips. Embryonic existence.

After three months my long fast came to a delicious turkey-dinner-with-all-the-trimmings end on Thanksgiving Day 1995. There was much to celebrate. TPN had maintained my weight at 130 pounds and allowed my pancreas to "cool." CAT scans were clear. By Christmas I was weaned from TPN. A week later I toasted the New Year with sips of champagne.

Much improved, I was still dying. The hose hanging from my chest remained in place. Physicians—utterly certain of my prognosis—feared pancreatitis might return. I continued to receive morphine. No logic in putting a dying man through the stress of withdrawal. I was down to 6 T-cells, death close at hand. We were well-acquainted.

Spring-Fall, 1996
Sarasota, Florida

Year upon year AIDS had ruthlessly murdered my friends. Upon diagnosis the only expectation was certain death. But, what seemed certain, changed. Suddenly, as I was halfway through the doorway to doom, a new class of exotic and marvelous medicines rushed from the labs: Protease inhibitors.

I had never taken any antiviral drugs. All the better. In late April 1996 I began AZT, then protease was added. There was much anxiety inside me as these magic medicines began to work. "What," I wondered for the first time in a year, "does the future hold?"

In June, efforts to add a third antiviral drug provoked a brutal bout of pancreatitis. Morphine murdered my pain, but all antiviral treatments were suspended. Then, slowly, I resumed taking AZT and protease which I tolerated well.

As blood pressure and temps returned to near-normal I was, for the first time in a year, visited by tricolored haloes in the night. My glaucoma was flaring. Time to start smoking marijuana.

The first joint produced an unsettling effect: I felt normal. Having been numbed by terminality, feeling normal felt very odd indeed. Despite some onset apprehension I managed to adjust, relax and enjoy euphoria. It felt very queer.

There were other side effects. As eye pressures declined, my appetite roared. I become an eating machine. Craving calories of any kind I thought nothing of downing multiple double malt shakes between meals. I remembered my stock line: "To the unintentionally anorexic the munchies can be a lifesaver."

The mix of marijuana and effective antiviral drugs produced dramatic results. My weight soared. By August, I was a hefty 180 pounds and had 44 T-cells: precisely twice as many as when diagnosed. I was dying in reverse. Coming alive. Incredible. And very disquieting. I tried to articulate my alarm.

"Disappointed?" an insightful nurse asked.

Disappointed. Precisely right. My bags were packed. I had my Trip-Tik to oblivion. Death was my destination; I was ready to leave life behind. Beyond a certain point dying is easy; automatic. No decisions required. But living—living is hard work. I was apprehensive about reengaging all the chaos and clutter which comes with the territory.

Throughout 1996 I slowly recovered from my addiction to death. Strength returned as T-cells multiplied like rabbits. Yet I remained uncertain. How much could I trust this new world into which I was, however reluctantly, being reborn?

November 12, 1996
Los Angeles, California

I was sitting in a studio at CBS Television City in Los Angeles. Tom Snyder was interviewing me on the 20th anniversary of my first legal toke. Wasn't this where we came in?

There was a news hook: California and Arizona voters had just enacted ballot initiatives favoring medical marijuana. It was an easy interview. Snyder, eyes twinkling, played with the angles before deftly introducing AIDS into our conversation. It was the first time I had publicly addressed my diagnosis. All went well.

It was good to be alive.

40 Growing Pains

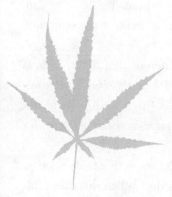

BEING REBORN PROVIDES an interesting vantage from which to monitor the aftermath of one's life. Medical marijuana, much changed, survived my demise but remains unresolved.

Once a morality play of intimate dimensions, medical marijuana has become a didactic drama driven by drug war motifs. The principal players are no longer the sick and afflicted, but a chattering collection of prohibitionists and reformers.

As AIDS snatched us from the stage in November 1994 an ACLU poll revealed no public support for drug reform . . . except, of course, for medical marijuana. The poll found 84% of the American people believed marijuana should be legally available by prescription.

An astonishing figure—84%! In a polyglot nation obsessed by ideological divisions and deep cultural conflicts, 8 out of 10 Americans believe doctors and patients, not bureaucrats and policemen, should decide when marijuana is medically appropriate.

Such vast public appeal is a tribute to those who have peopled our stage—Lynn Pierson, Jim and Mildred Ripple, Anne Guttentag, Mona Taft, Steve L., Kenny and Barbra—actors of incredible integrity and awesome powers of persuasion. But these noble players have moved on. A new cast of characters now crowd the boards.

In April 1995, a group of wealthy men, drug policy analysts and political consultants met in Santa Barbara. All agreed medical marijuana was the only drug reform "opportunity" available. The problem: no one had "a plan."

Fickle Fate. The meeting was MARS come to fruition. The moneymen arrived right on schedule, looking for a plan. We have a plan. But I am dying and we are in no position to make a presentation. The vacuum in our wake was quickly filled.

While plutocrats and policy pimps pondered what to do, Dennis Peron and the happy Hempsters pushed blindly ahead. Peron's speakeasy for the sick—a.k.a. the Cannabis Buyer's Club—was doing a brisk business, pleased to serve all patrons without regard for illness. Peron was looking to expand.

In early 1996, Peron, Scott Imler and other activists decided to put medical marijuana on the California ballot. When this effort faltered Ethan Nadelman, backed by billionaire currency speculator George Soros, moved in, hired professional political consultants and abducted Peron's initiative. With the aid of paid signature collectors Proposition 215 was placed on the California ballot.

Polls revealed overwhelming support for the measure. But infighting soon erupted between the East Coast pros and the West Coast activists. It quickly spilled over into the press. This public firefight between unappealing factions rightfully frightened the electorate. California voters were not amused.

Despite lavish funding, Proposition 215 received only 56% of the vote. In neighboring Arizona, where reformist angst was less intense, Proposition 200, a broader drug reform initiative featuring a medical marijuana plank, won 65% of the vote.

"Great victories!" said drug reformers who had seldom won anything before. It was, of course, victory. Winning beats losing. But the cost in dollars and damage done to the public sense of medical marijuana was immense. In Arizona, for example, the conservative state legislature, offended by the influx of "outside money," overturned Prop 200 in favor of federal controls.

Peron, instinctive, impulsive, occasionally inspired, immediately sought to exploit Proposition 215. "After all," he told the press, "all marijuana use is medical." So much for meeting patient needs. To retain public attention Peron then outlined a provocative plan to franchise his Buyer's Club concept statewide.

Operating under the cloak of Prop 215 Peron's Buyer's Club did a roaring business providing patients and non-patients with marijuana. This reckless behavior, and Peron's rash disregard for consequences, undermined public confidence. Eventually, even the home-town press tired of his endless antics. In a May 1998 editorial the *San Francisco Chronicle* wrote, "We all support the premise of the club, but it was never run properly—or legally. That never seemed to matter much to Peron—at least until the state and federal authorities began closing in. But it certainly mattered to other pot clubs around the Bay Area that began feeling the heat because Peron saw himself as a martyr unaffected by the law."

By mid-1998 the jig was up. Peron's so-called Buyer's Clubs was closed by the courts. Many imitation efforts around California also collapsed. Criminal charges were brought. Trials are pending. Not a promising plot.

The reform pros who deplore Peron's antics are hardly more heroic. Sensing a steady stream of revenue the consultants recommended more political action, i.e. more state initiatives. What a surprise. But since winning California and Arizona the up-scale politicos have spent masses of money to achieve rapidly diminishing returns. While the generosity of their patrons is obvious, the outcomes they finance are less than impressive.

In 1997, the reform pros tried to export their defective, legislatively-rejected Arizona initiative to Washington state where polls indicated strong public support for medical marijuana. Instead of sticking to basics the reform pros stretched public tolerance by trying to use medical marijuana as a ploy to lure voters into also legalizing LSD and heroin. The good people of Washington, offended by pushy pro-drug politicos fat on out-of-state cash, rejected the inane initiative by a resounding 60–40%.

Defeated, but far from humbled, win or lose the pros made a profit. Only seriously ill patients were injured by their reformist zeal.

Voter initiatives could be useful tools for change. A simple statement proclaiming "the people of (fill in the state) find marijuana has medical value and call on the federal government to end legal prohibitions against its lawful, prescriptive use" would suffice. Such initiatives would send a powerful message to Washington and undermine marijuana's Schedule I status as a drug "with no accepted medical use in treatment in the United States."

But the political pros, absorbed in polls and aphasic with focus group awareness, are incapable of articulating the obvious. Instead, they craft coy and convoluted plans of "medical relief" which simply ignore patient needs. The resulting efforts are a case study in cringing liberalism. For example, a proposed, but thankfully abandoned ballot initiative in Maine would have allowed seriously ill patients to legally grow 1.25 ounces of marijuana.

What an idiot idea! First, it is medically meaningless. I smoke two ounces of marijuana per week. Being allowed to legally grow 1.25 ounces hardly seems helpful. Second, as anyone who has grown tomatoes knows, nature is fickle. How can a person plan to grow precisely 1.25 ounces of anything? A bumper crop and, dying or not, you're busted?

Finally, why should seriously ill Americans have to grow anything? Is it not enough they are seriously ill? Do drug reformers expect cancer patients to endlessly worry over who will water their marijuana plants while they endure chemotherapy? Should paralyzed people in wheelchairs be made to tend medical victory gardens?

This is not medicine. Or even rational drug reform. Indeed, such ill-conceived schemes are, as many hard-line drug warriors warn, just a ruse for drug legalization. As one hardliner told the *Las Vegas Review-Journal* (June 14, 1998) " 'That's really the point behind this: To legitimize marijuana; and full legalization would be the next goal.' Legalization groups, he contends, don't really care about sick people but rather use them as props in the propaganda war against drug prohibition. 'It's just a scam to legalize dope—that's all it is.' " Obligingly, drug reformers accept this cynical assessment of their efforts. An unnamed but "leading marijuana strategist" told *The New York Times* in July 1997, "From the beginning our thesis has been that the medical marijuana issue will get people to start questioning the larger war on drugs."

Patients as stage props! The American people do not like such clever ploys. There is no public appetite for drug reform or much affection for drug reformers. Given the above quotes it is easy to see why. Put simply, the American people are not interested in cultural conflict. As far as medical marijuana is concerned all they want is a sane solution which provides seriously ill people with medically supervised access to marijuana.

While drug reformers squander great opportunities for trivial political gains, other less ideological people, sensitive to patient needs, continue to expand the debate. Our old friend, Scott Imler, now operates the Los Angeles Cannabis Resource Center. A patient-based treatment cooperative, the LACRC works closely with physicians to provide several hundred seriously ill Angelenos with medically authorized supplies of marijuana. While not technically legal the LACRC's responsible attempts to meet basic human needs have won public praise and the effort enjoys broad community support. In addition to responsibly aiding patients Scott continues to work with

local politicians and state officials to define workable long-term solutions.

Overseas our efforts are also bearing fruit. In Britain ACT-UK
continues to press for expanded research and patient access to care.
Polls in England suggest overwhelming public support for these efforts, and many British physicians are demanding change. As a result
of these efforts in mid-1998, Her Majesty's government authorized
the private sector cultivation of marijuana for medical research and
future patient use. Though it is too early to know the outcome of
these undertakings, the British action threatens to end the U.S. Government's monopoly control over legal supplies of marijuana. Similar
efforts are evolving in Holland, and there is increasing German interest.

All these things taken together suggest medical marijuana is coming of age; experiencing growing pains. The influx of so many new
voices, the convergence of so much money and so many mixed motives was bound to cause concerns. While it would be easy to dismiss
many of these characters as blundering, inept, often self-serving
louts, they are all "well-intentioned" individuals. However inartful
or exploitative some may seem they are not the villain of this piece.
That role is reserved for a Government which refuses to simply acknowledge it has made a dreadful mistake.

41 A Consistent Message

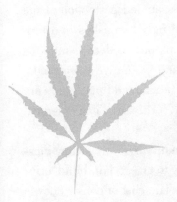

THE STATE, IN pursuit of Orwellian absolutes, demands "zero tolerance." Medical marijuana and the plight of patients are to be ignored in favor of "sending a consistent message."

We are treading a dangerous, but well-worn path. Centuries ago an august bureaucratic body—the Roman Catholic Church—confronted a similar dilemma. Galileo, a curious and enterprising man, looked through his telescope and carefully charted the contours— the mountains, craters and seas—of the Moon. The Church was appalled by his drawing. Heaven is perfection, the Cardinals said, filled with flawless crystal spheres. The moon could not be pock-marked by craters. Galileo must be wrong. "Look for yourselves," Galileo protested. The Church fathers reflected on the offer, refused the opportunity and promptly condemned the telescope as an instrument of the devil. Galileo was put on trial as a heretic and placed under house arrest. The knowledge he unlocked was censored. Case closed.

Of course, we all know how this story turns out. Odd, how such a small, seemingly obvious observation could threaten such a huge and complex system of Belief. Odder still is the inability of such a complex system to incorporate unwelcome information. History indicates the most trivial of facts can implode the most powerful dogma.

We are not immune from such madness. Our own century is blood stained by the search for State-sponsored certainty. In the name of "a consistent message" eugenic Nazis condemned millions to cremation and Scientific Socialists sent millions more to Siberian gulags.

Our Government's "consistent message" about marijuana is a bald-faced lie, as erroneous as the once-assumed perfection of the heavens. Medical marijuana has revealed ugly blemishes in a prohibition packed in lies. Like aging bishops our modern mandarins dismiss the facts with caustic comments and pejorative propaganda. The nation's drug czar says doctors who recommend marijuana are engaged in "Cheech and Chong medicine." The DEA calls medical marijuana "a cruel hoax."

Unable to admit fallibility, anxious to maintain a "consistent message," federal drug bureaucrats are willing to arrest, jail, blind, cripple and even kill seriously ill Americans. The cost of consistency is paid in human suffering. The bureaucrats can live with that.

The drug war is fought by crusaders who seek to maintain the moral order. Order is orthodoxy. America's law enforcement elite live in a black and white world. Marijuana is an "evil weed." Admitting that marijuana has redeeming medical value would violate this order. Besides, the drug war is profitable to many. The police require much equipment and big budgets to bust down doors of hapless citizens and confiscate private property. Prison construction booms. There are great career opportunities in corrections, addictions and rehabilitation. While everyone knows marijuana has medical value there is no profit in such knowledge.

Those who find the cult of coercion too absolute worship at the far more subtle and sophisticated cult of synthesis. FDA and the pharmaceutical complex are dedicated to the proposition that nothing untouched by the hand of man can possibly be a medicine. While brutish DEA bullies enforce the law, the brainier bureaucrats at FDA and NIH are devoted to developing artificial medicines.

In FDA's orthodoxy drugs are invented, owned, patented, produced in factories and sold at monopoly inflated prices by large corporations seeking gross profits. A God-given herb owned by no one, which grows easily and has multiple medical applications threatens the entire science of synthesis. Who, other than patients, would profit? Marijuana, rationally prescribed, could diminish the demand for Valium, damage the profit profile of Prozac and erode the need for hyper-expensive anti-vomiting drugs. Such thinking could, FDA flacks warn, undermine "modern medicine" and even adversely affect the stock market.

One brief example. Zofran, a synthetic anti-vomiting drug, costs $600 per dose and is usually given by IV, so patients are generally hospitalized at $1,500 a day. By comparison, marijuana controls vomiting better than Zofran but only costs 50 cents per day. Zofran requires hospitalization. Marijuana can be used by patients at home. Zofran can cause intense anxiety. Marijuana is a mild euphoriant. Unlike Zofran, marijuana also enhances the appetite.

On a human level patients, not bureaucrats, should decide their course of care. Some may want hospitalization and infused synthetic drugs. Others might prefer to stay home, smoke marijuana and enjoy a meal with loved ones.

On the societal level, however, there are vast implications. As mentioned above, Zofran is expensive; marijuana costs next to nothing. Multiply these costs by 10,000 treatment episodes per week. It adds up. Way up. The difference is staggering. Billions for synthetics vs. several thousand dollars worth of weed. Little wonder the medical mandarins in our pharmaceutical elites have not rushed marijuana to market.

The American people know these things are true. They know the drug war is a corrupt, corrosive failure. They know their government is dysfunctional, increasingly anti-democratic and, in all too many cases, run by self-aggrandizing liars and crooks.

We are told America is a democracy. But the medical marijuana problem belies this assumption. In the late 1970s and early 1980s two-thirds of the States legislatively mandated that marijuana had medical value and should be available for patient use. The unelected drug warriors in Washington blocked these popular state efforts.

In 1996 when the people of California and Arizona voted in favor of medical marijuana unelected bureaucrats in Washington told the electorate to "drop dead." The Attorney General then threatened to arrest any doctor who dared to even mention marijuana's medical use with a patient.

Authoritarians pursuing a policy of "zero tolerance" are imposing their will over that of the electorate. The drug warriors would, if they could, flush medical marijuana down Orwell's memory hole. To hell with facts, reason and simple compassion.

To disguise their evil fraud the drug warriors couple their "consistent message" mantra to their "save the children" chant. The odd notion that little Sally Ann, aged 10, will become a drug addict because a 55-year-old woman with breast cancer is allowed to legally smoke marijuana under medical supervision is absurd!

No doubt the good cardinals of Galileo's time were deeply concerned about the damaging effect his drawings might have on young minds.

You think the Galileo analogy is a stretch? In order to assure "a consistent message," the drug warriors want science stopped. In an astonishing act of arrogance some in the House of Representatives— many former medical marijuana supporters—have actually proposed a congressionally mandated ban on any and all research into the prohibited plant's potential benefits. In effect, Washington is trying to take away the telescope.

If ignorance is bliss, drug warriors are in hog heaven. Is it any wonder the American people distrust their government?

Seriously ill Americans are caught in the crossfire as drug warriors on both sides of the cultural divide try to turn the sick into ideological cannon fodder. In a sane society the possibility that an easily grown plant could ease human suffering would be cause for celebration. But we do not live in a sane society. Instead, we live in a society distorted by drug war demons and unresolved cultural conflicts. Our national policy of "zero intelligence" is enforced by a drug control elite which increasingly views seriously ill citizens as "the enemy." To maintain this deluded behavior our government even pretends that our high tech civilization, which routinely alters genes and sends rockets into space, is scientifically unable to fathom whether marijuana has medical value.

Marijuana has medical value. That is a simple, historically recognized and easily verifiable fact. A person with AIDS who smokes marijuana and stops throwing up does not need a white-coated bureaucrat from the FDA to recognize the medical benefit. But marijuana will never be medically available to the seriously ill so long as the debate is dominated by irrational men who, for the sake of a "consistent message," evade the truth and sacrifice the sick.

Afloat in a boat on the intracoastal this entire situation seems a bit silly and ever so sad. Reclining into reclusion we are far removed from the madness. What role, if any, we have to play in this still unfolding drama is difficult to say. Fate has treated us well. It has given us interesting lives and, in the process, I have evaded criminality, blindness and death. There is an impulse to rejoin the battle. But my year of marijuana abstinence damaged my eyesight and my AIDS recovery is less than certain. Perhaps we have done all Fate intended. Perhaps not. Such decisions are made by gods, not men.

Afloat in a boat on the intracoastal we know it is good to be alive.

We are together and grateful to have enjoyed a measure of time to recollect the adventure of our lives; to tell you the stories of brave men and women who, despite their own desperate plight, labored under the illusion that they could create a more sane and compassionate world.

In our quest for justice we have wandered through the last quarter of the first century of the Radio Age. We have survived to tell you the history of medical marijuana in America. What will it take to resolve this problem? That is simple. Rational men with courage, compassion and just a bit of common sense. Unfortunately, such men are in short supply.

Two decades ago a big, burly Samoan approached me in a Honolulu bar and took away my marijuana because "it was bad." Terrified of the consequences, legal and medical, I told the ex-wrestling champ I smoked marijuana to save my sight. Slowly, the Samoan let go of his anger. "I am sorry," he said as he gently returned my medicine, then embraced me in a crushing bear hug I still recall.

"I am sorry," he repeated, "I did not understand."

Is there anyone in the American government who has the simple courage to do the same as my Samoan friend?

We shall see.

Index